The **A** to **Z** of Children's Health

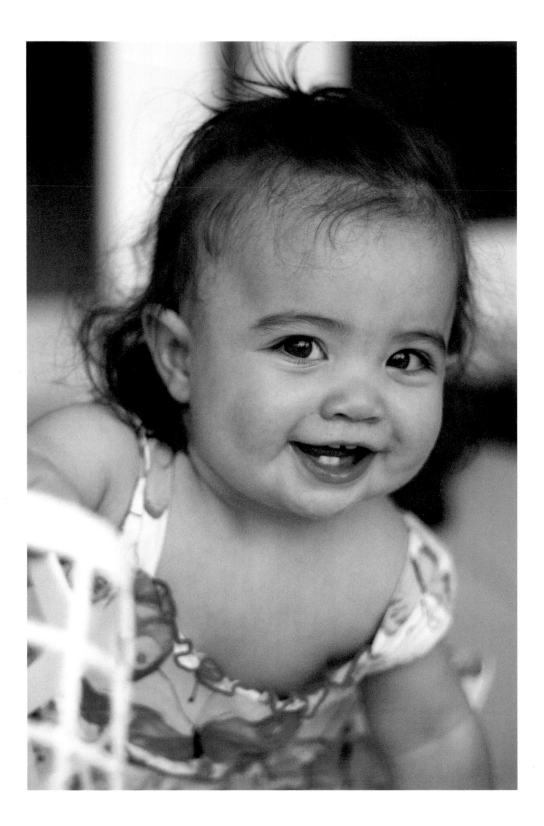

The **A** to **Z** of Children's Health

A parent's guide from birth to 10 years

Dr. Jeremy Friedman, MB.ChB, FRCPC, FAAP,
Dr. Natasha Saunders, MD, MSc, FRCPC,
with **Dr. Norman Saunders,** MD, FRCPC

The Hospital for Sick Children

Robert
ROSE

For a complete list of photo credits, see page 433.
For complete cataloguing information, see page 434.

Disclaimer

This book is a general guide only and should never be a substitute for the skill, knowledge, and experience of a qualified medical professional dealing with the facts, circumstances, and symptoms of a particular case.

The nutritional, medical, and health information presented in this book is based on the research, training, and professional experience of the authors, and is true and complete to the best of their knowledge. However, this book is intended only as an informative guide for those wishing to know more about health, nutrition, and medicine; it is not intended to replace or countermand the advice given by the reader's personal physician. Because each person and situation is unique, the author and the publisher urge the reader to check with a qualified health-care professional before using any procedure where there is a question as to its appropriateness. A physician should be consulted before beginning any exercise program. The author and the publisher are not responsible for any adverse effects or consequences resulting from the use of the information in this book. It is the responsibility of the reader to consult a physician or other qualified health-care professional regarding his or her personal care.

Design and Production: Kevin Cockburn/PageWave Graphics Inc.
Editor: Bob Hilderley, Senior Editor, Health
Copyeditor: Sheila Wawanash
Proofreader: Sue Sumeraj
Indexer: Gillian Watts
Illustrations: Kveta/Three in a Box

Cover image: © iStockphoto.com/Photolyric

We acknowledge the financial support of the Government of Canada through the Book Publishing Industry Development Program (BPIDP) for our publishing activities.

Published by Robert Rose Inc.
120 Eglinton Avenue East, Suite 800, Toronto, Ontario, Canada M4P 1E2
Tel: (416) 322-6552 Fax: (416) 322-6936
www.robertrose.ca

Printed and bound in Canada.

1 2 3 4 5 6 7 8 9 TCP 21 20 19 18 17 16 15 14 13

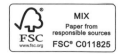

To my parents, Norman and Lynn Saunders,
whose unconditional love, wisdom, and passion
for living each day to its fullest continue to guide me.

To my husband, Justin Fluit, for being the best and
most supportive partner anyone could ever wish for.

And to my children, Nathan and Hailey Fluit,
for reminding me daily how much I love being a mother.

— NRS

To Norman Saunders, a great colleague, friend and inspiration.

To my A to Z: Shelley, Sam and Dani

— JNF

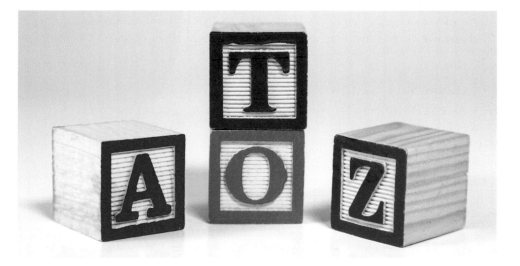

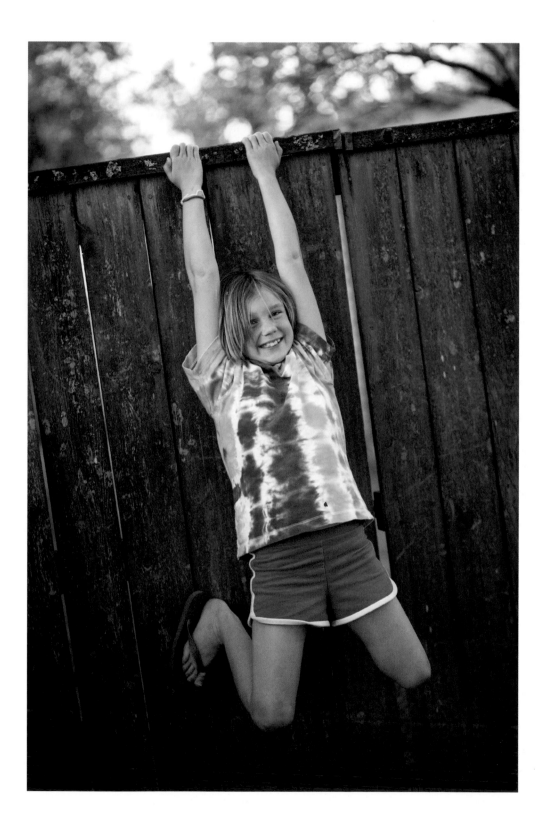

Contributing Authors

Sherri Adams, NP-Paediatrics, MSN, CPNP
Division of Paediatric Medicine
The Hospital for Sick Children
Adjunct Lecturer
Faculty of Nursing
University of Toronto

Carolyn Beck, MD, MSc, FRCPC
Division of Paediatric Medicine
The Hospital for Sick Children
Assistant Professor
Faculty of Medicine
University of Toronto

Stacey Bernstein, MD, FRCPC
Division of Paediatric Medicine
The Hospital for Sick Children
Associate Professor
Faculty of Medicine
University of Toronto

Zia Bismilla, MD, MEd, FRCPC
Division of Paediatric Medicine
The Hospital for Sick Children
Assistant Professor
Faculty of Medicine
University of Toronto

Mark Feldman, MD, FRCPC
Division of Paediatric Medicine
The Hospital for Sick Children
Associate Professor
Faculty of Medicine
University of Toronto

Jeremy Friedman, MB.ChB, FRCPC, FAAP
Associate Paediatrician-in-Chief, Department of
Paediatrics
Head, Division of Paediatric Medicine
The Hospital for Sick Children
Professor
Faculty of Medicine
University of Toronto

Beth Gamulka, MDCM, FRCPC
Division of Paediatric Medicine
The Hospital for Sick Children
Assistant Professor
Faculty of Medicine
University of Toronto

Sheila Jacobson, MBBCh, FRCPC
Division of Paediatric Medicine
The Hospital for Sick Children
Assistant Professor
Faculty of Medicine
University of Toronto

Irene Lara-Corrales, MSc, MD
Section of Dermatology
Division of Paediatric Medicine
The Hospital for Sick Children
Assistant Professor
Faculty of Medicine
University of Toronto

Elena Pope, MD, FRCPC
Head, Section of Dermatology
Division of Paediatric Medicine
The Hospital for Sick Children
Associate Professor
Faculty of Medicine
University of Toronto

Daniel Roth, MD, PhD, FRCPC
Division of Paediatric Medicine
The Hospital for Sick Children
Assistant Professor
Faculty of Medicine
University of Toronto

Natasha Saunders, MSc, MD, FRCPC
Divisions of Paediatric and Emergency Medicine
The Hospital for Sick Children
Academic General Paediatrics Fellow
Faculty of Medicine
University of Toronto

Norman Saunders, MD, FRCPC
Division of Paediatric Medicine
The Hospital for Sick Children
Associate Professor
Faculty of Medicine
University of Toronto

Michael Weinstein, MD, FRCPC
Division of Paediatric Medicine
The Hospital for Sick Children
Associate Professor
Faculty of Medicine
University of Toronto

Contents

This table of contents includes symptom chapters with cross-references to associated conditions to make it as convenient as possible to find the information you need to care for your child. The symptom chapters are listed in bold type.

Introduction

There has been an enormous increase in the amount of information at our fingertips since the growth of the Internet and, more recently, social media. The majority of parents in North America now have access to medical and parenting advice at the click of a mouse or with the touch of a fingertip. So why publish a book of medical advice for parents on how to deal with all of their children's symptoms from A to Z and everything in between?

In some ways, the need is greater now than a generation or two ago, when Dr. Spock was one of our only options. The reason is that much of what you read on the web and information shared through social media is sincere in its intent but generally strongly held personal opinion and conviction. Convincing yes, but not always in context, accurate, or even true. Certainly, in most cases, not based on the latest scientific evidence or consensus among children's health-care providers.

Our book meets this need for evidence-based information and advice published in an accessible format. We will guide you through your questions about your child's health, advise you when you should be seeking help, and give you practical tips and strategies that will help you to avoid having to spend countless hours in your provider's waiting room or, even worse, in an emergency care center.

This book is written by a dozen of the top pediatricians at the Hospital for Sick Children (a.k.a. SickKids), recognized internationally as one of the best children's hospitals in the world. SickKids is not only renowned for the outstanding clinical care provided to its young patients and their families, but this hospital is a leader in educating patients, families, and the next generation of pediatric health-care providers, as well as a powerhouse of research, providing the evidence behind the latest and best treatments and care for children worldwide.

We have tried to present the information you will need in an easy-to-find, easy-to-read, consistent format to walk you through what we see as the most common problems that we encounter on a daily basis in our offices, clinics, and emergency rooms. In addition, most of us are parents of young children ourselves and have tried to bring that perspective to our writing as well; not to mention using many of our own children to demonstrate the common pediatric day-to-day issues!

You will find the answers to your questions – What is this? What causes it? and How should I treat it? — as well as a clear list of "red flags" that signify varying levels of urgency for which to seek medical attention. In our DYK (Did You Know?) and Doc Talk sections, we give you a few useful and interesting facts and take-home messages. For the more complicated complaints, you will find algorithms and tables to guide you through your approach to getting to the bottom of what is causing the problem or how to treat it. Our FAQs (frequently asked questions) address some of the questions that parents ask us on a regular basis. We have cross-referenced the various diseases so that you can easily read more about a problem if you feel the need. We realize that no one source can provide all you need to know, so we have highlighted some of the general resources online in North America that we feel represent excellent, reliable, and trustworthy information.

How does this book work? To start, we focus on symptoms and their prevention and treatment rather than systems and conditions. Parents will recognize a symptom, such as a cough, before they pursue an understanding of the related condition, such as pneumonia, or learn that this condition is part of the respiratory system. Still, we provide an extensive table of contents that lists symptoms cross-referenced with conditions. This book can be sampled at quiet times out of curiosity, studied in depth as you look for answers to help a sick child, or consulted in an emergency like a first aid guide. You will likely find other ways to access and apply the information in the *A to Z of Children's Health*.

Finally, we'd like to recognize the huge influence that Norman Saunders had on the writing of this book. Norman passed away a few years ago from cancer after a courageous battle, while still in the prime of his career and life. He had represented the gold standard of what we all aspired to as general pediatricians. Some of the content of this book was actually written by him prior to his passing, and some other parts reflect his teaching and philosophy of care. This book is dedicated to his memory.

— Jeremy Friedman and Natasha Saunders

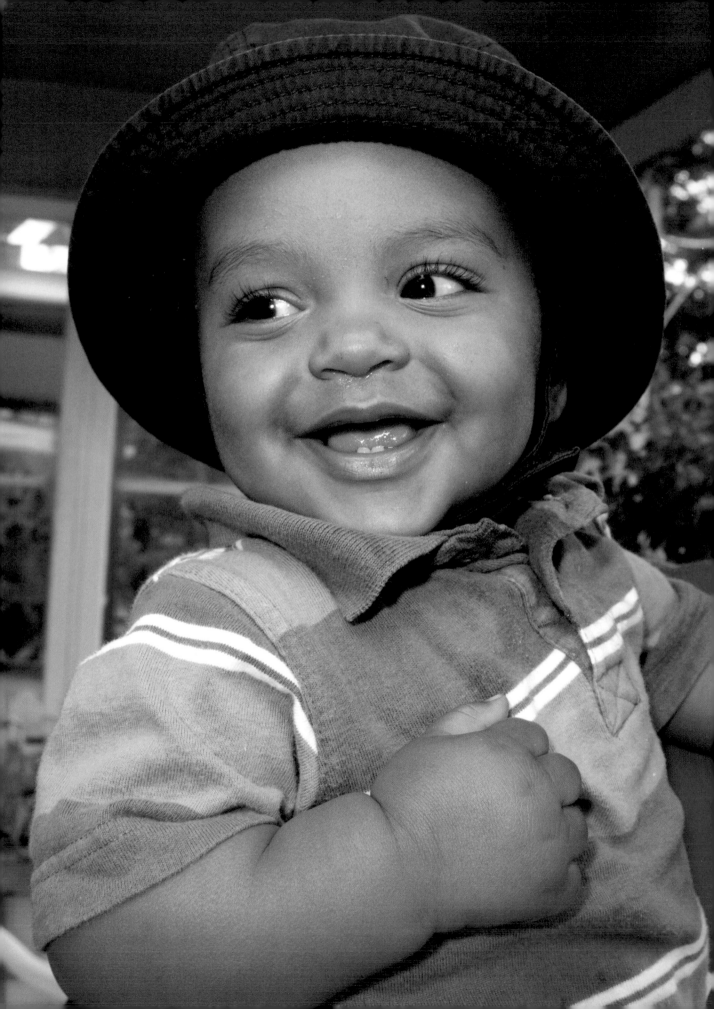

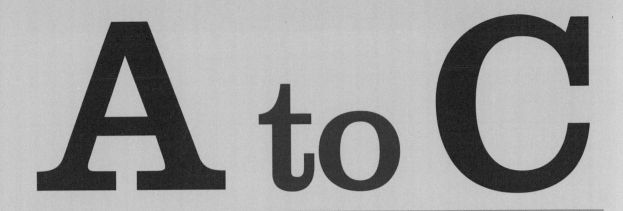

A to C

Abdominal Pain (Acute)

What Can I Do?

▶ If the stomach pain appears suddenly and lasts for a few hours, comfort your child by giving her a gentle massage and reassuring her that the pain should pass.

▶ Try giving her acetaminophen or ibuprofen for the ache.

▶ Determine if your child has any red flag symptoms that require immediate medical attention. These symptoms continue to get worse and worse until treated!

▶ Ensure she is drinking enough fluids to prevent dehydration.

▶ If the pain has been there for weeks or months, consult the next chapter, on Abdominal Pain (Chronic or Recurrent).

RELATED CONDITIONS

- Appendicitis
- Colitis
- Constipation
- Gastrorenteritis
- Henoch-Schonlein purpura
- Intussuception
- Kidney and bladder infection
- Midgut volvulus
- Pneumonia
- Strangulated hernia
- Strep throat
- Testicular torsion

❶ What Is Acute Abdominal Pain?

Most parents will be faced with the challenge of deciding what to do with their child who has a stomach ache. Actually, the term "stomach ache" is not always correct because the pain could be coming from anywhere in the abdomen, from the bottom of the rib cage down to the groin, including the stomach, intestines, kidneys, bladder, liver, and other organs. It could even be referred pain from pneumonia at the base of the lung, causing irritation of the diaphragm and giving the impression that the pain is coming from the abdomen.

Acute or Chronic

Determining the kind of pain your child is experiencing is a first step in relieving the pain. When medical professionals talk about acute pain, it refers to pain that has been present for a short period of time, usually hours or days. Chronic abdominal pain has been present for weeks or months and has a very different set of causes. See Abdominal Pain (Chronic or Recurrent).

When should we contact our doctor or local hospital?

The difficulty with acute abdominal pain is deciding if your child might have a serious problem — such as appendicitis requiring immediate medical attention — or something harmless that may not require any treatment at all. The latter will be the more common experience. You can start by recognizing red flag symptoms that you can report to your doctor.

> ## ⏩ Acute Abdominal Pain Red Flags
>
> Seek medical care immediately if your child shows any of these signs or symptoms:
>
> - Sharp and steady pain that moves from the belly button to the lower right groin area and gets progressively worse. Suspect appendicitis.
> - Sudden periods of cramping and inconsolable crying while your child seems happy and comfortable otherwise. Suspect intussusception.
> - Bloody stools that look a bit like red currant jelly. Suspect intussusception.
> - Painful swelling in the groin or scrotal area. Suspect a strangulated hernia or torsion of the testicle.
> - Vomit that is a dark green (bilious) color. Suspect volvulus or other causes of bowel obstruction.

Duration of Pain

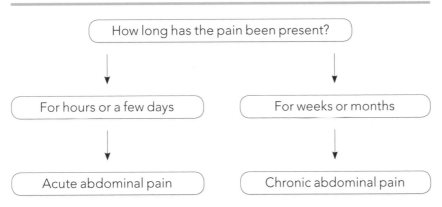

How long has the pain been present?

For hours or a few days → Acute abdominal pain

For weeks or months → Chronic abdominal pain

❷ What Causes Acute Abdominal Pain?

There are a few causes that may require surgical treatment and generally need immediate attention. Even though these causes are quite rare, it is the possibility of these conditions that tends to provoke concern in parents when their child has acute abdominal pain.

Appendicitis

Appendicitis is the most common surgical problem associated with abdominal pain in children. It is very uncommon in the first few years of life, and it almost always begins with vague, hard-to-localize pain around the navel (belly button) accompanied by nausea. In a matter of hours, it moves from there down to the lower right side of

Did You Know?

Eating Pain
Often, a child will complain of a stomach ache after eating too much, eating too quickly, or eating something that didn't "agree" with him. These pains settle down rapidly within a few hours.

Midgut Volvulus

This is a very rare but important cause of pain requiring surgery. Volvulus is the fancy term for twisting of the small intestines on their own stalk. These children will have severe pain and will vomit a dark green bile-containing liquid, as will most children with a blockage of their intestines.

the abdomen. The pain becomes sharp and steady, continuing to get worse over time. Any movement — coughing, jumping, or pressing down over the affected area — tends to be very painful. Children will often have a low-grade fever, poor appetite, nausea, and vomiting.

Intussusception

This relatively rare condition occurs when a piece of intestine telescopes into the next part of the bowel and then becomes stuck. This condition is most common between the ages of 6 months and 3 years. One clue to this condition is the episodic nature of the pain. Your child's behavior will alternate between being relatively comfortable, even playful, with having periods of inconsolability due to spasms of severe, crampy pain. As the condition worsens, you may see bloody stools that can be described as looking like "red currant jelly."

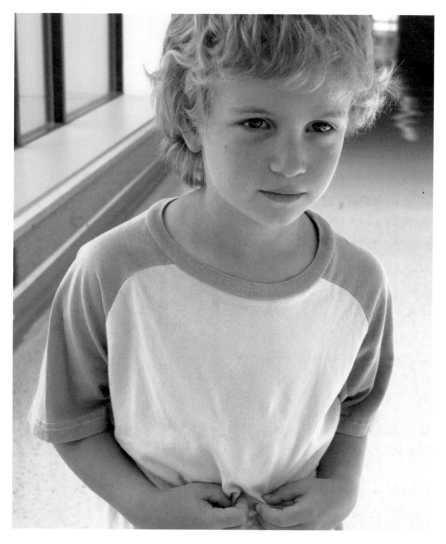

More Common, Less Serious Causes of Abdominal Pain

There are a number of less serious and very much more common reasons to explain why children complain of acute abdominal pain.

Symptoms	Possible Condition	Treatment
Very hard stools ("rabbit pellets") that are difficult or painful to pass	Constipation	Increased fluids, fiber in diet, and if that doesn't work, occasionally a mild laxative is needed (see page 124 for details).
Vomiting with watery diarrhea and/or low-grade fever	Viral gastroenteritis	Acetaminophen or ibuprofen if uncomfortable. Ensure adequate liquids to prevent dehydration (see page 150 for details).
Cramping (where the pain comes and goes) and/or fevers with blood in the stools	Colitis (bacterial or inflammatory)	See your doctor for a thorough examination and possible stool culture.
Pain following the consumption of possibly contaminated/spoiled food	Food poisoning	See your doctor for a thorough examination and possible stool culture.
Lower back pain and/or fever. Vomiting with a change in the color or smell of the urine or an increase in frequency of peeing, or burning with peeing	Kidney or bladder infection	See your doctor for a thorough examination and possible urine culture. If infected, an antibiotic is required.
A sore throat or swollen glands in the neck and/or fever	Strep throat	See your doctor for a thorough examination and possible throat culture. If positive for strep, an antibiotic is required.
Cough, breathlessness, or breathing distress with fever	Pneumonia	See your doctor for a thorough examination and possible chest X-ray. If a bacterial pneumonia is suspected, an antibiotic is required.
A rash made up of little spots or even "bruising" that doesn't blanch when you push on it — especially over the legs and buttocks	Henoch-Schonlein purpura	See your doctor for a thorough examination and discussion regarding what further tests may be required.

Strangulated Hernia or Testicular Torsion

Hernias in the groin occur when part of the intestine protrudes through a hole in the inner layers of the abdominal wall. Usually the intestines move in and out through the hole quite freely, but if they become stuck, then your child may have pain, vomiting, and possibly a swollen, red lump in the groin or scrotum. A swollen and painful scrotum should also raise concern of testicular torsion, particularly in the newborn period or during early puberty (see page 328). The cord leading to the testicle gets twisted, cutting off the blood supply — which means it needs to be dealt with ASAP!

Constipation

This is a very common condition and can cause quite severe abdominal cramps. A child with constipation will generally have a history of infrequent, very hard stools that can also be painful to pass. There may be some blood on the toilet paper after wiping or in the toilet bowl. See Constipation (page 124).

Did You Know?

Sore Throat and Earache

Sometimes children with a strep throat or otitis media, commonly known as middle ear infection, complain of stomach pain in addition to their sore throat or earache. See Earache and Ear Infections (page 169).

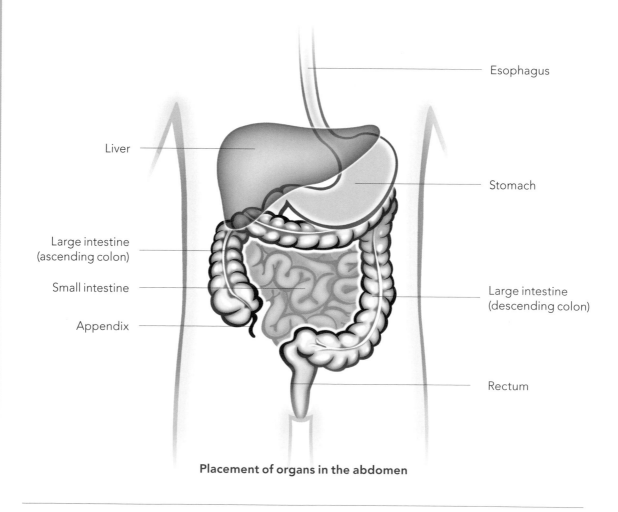

Liver
Large intestine (ascending colon)
Small intestine
Appendix
Esophagus
Stomach
Large intestine (descending colon)
Rectum

Placement of organs in the abdomen

Viral Gastroenteritis

Many different types of infections can also cause acute abdominal pain. Pain that is associated with vomiting of stomach contents and is often followed the next day by watery, foul-smelling diarrhea is usually due to viral gastroenteritis (stomach flu). These children will generally not feel well, have a low-grade fever (often, although not always, below 101.3°F/38.5°C), and a poor appetite. Because it is quite contagious, a friend or family member might have similar symptoms. See Viral Gastroenteritis (page 209).

Bacterial Bowel Infections

These infections cause inflammation of the large intestine, called colitis, which can cause cramping associated with high fevers and bloody stools in a sick-looking child. This is more common in returning travelers (often from "developing" countries) or those exposed to potentially contaminated food (food poisoning) or water.

Kidney and Bladder Infections

These infections should also be considered as the source of abdominal pain. Kidney infections can be accompanied by fever, vomiting, and lower back pain; bladder infections can cause pain on urination, increased frequency of urination, and new onset bed-wetting at night. See Urinary Problems (page 404).

HSP

Henoch-Schonlein purpura (HSP) is an uncommon condition that occasionally occurs in children, caused by inflammation of the blood vessels. Most parents have not heard about this before, but it is an important cause of severe acute abdominal pain. Inflammation produces a characteristic rash and, often, crampy abdominal pain, frequently with bloody stools. The rash is usually most prominent on the legs and buttocks, and it resembles bruising (purpura).

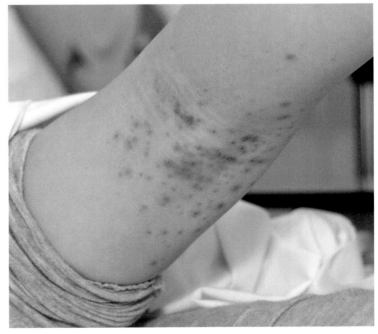

Henoch-Schonlein purpura

❸ How Is Acute Abdominal Pain Treated?

If your child shows any of the red flag symptoms, fairly urgent medical attention is required. A feature of all of these surgical causes of abdominal pain (meaning that they will usually require a surgical procedure to fix) is that they generally continue to get worse until appropriately treated. So get some help!

FAQs

After eating out at a fast-food restaurant last evening, my son began to feel nauseous and vomited during the night. Does he have food poisoning?

Food poisoning is an intestinal infection that can look quite similar to a viral stomach flu (gastroenteritis). In food poisoning, the problem is usually due to toxins that are ingested in food that is contaminated or spoiled due to poor sanitation or inappropriate preparation practices. Your child may present with profuse vomiting, abdominal cramps, and diarrhea within hours of ingesting the food. A big clue to diagnosing this condition is often that others who ingested the same food will also tend to have symptoms, even if not as severe.

What are "staph" germs? We've heard they are especially bad.

One of the more common contaminating germs causing food poisoning is staphylococcus. This can cause rapid onset of nausea, severe vomiting, dizziness, and abdominal cramping. These bacteria produce a toxin in foods, especially in pies, salads (for example, potato, macaroni, egg, and tuna salads), and dairy products. Contaminated salads at picnics are a common cause if the food is not chilled properly.

Doc Talk

Fortunately, most abdominal pain in the majority of children is not an emergency and does not require immediate medical attention or an operation! These pains will likely settle down after a few hours; some reassurance and distraction can help. If your child would prefer not to eat, do not force him; just ensure that he is drinking enough fluids to prevent dehydration. See Dehydration (page 150). If your child's pain seems different or more severe than usual, it is always safest to discuss this with your physician.

Abdominal Pain (Chronic or Recurrent)

What Can I Do?

▶ Acknowledge the presence of your child's chronic pain. Although the cause may be hard to find, the pain is real.

▶ Reassure him that this pain will improve with time and encourage him to carry on with normal school and social activities to the best of his ability.

▶ If your child shows any red flag symptoms, seek urgent medical advice.

▶ If this is your child's first episode and has lasted for several hours or days, refer to page 18 for an approach to Abdominal Pain (Acute).

❶ What Is Chronic Abdominal Pain?

In most children, tummy or abdominal pain is acute (sharp and severe pain) and settles within minutes, hours, or days. Unfortunately, sometimes it doesn't. In these cases, it may stick around for weeks or months (chronic abdominal pain), it may wax and wane, or it may go away but frequently come back (recurrent abdominal pain). As a parent, you likely want to know what is causing the problem, whether you should be concerned and see your child's doctor, and, of course, how best to help your child. We will try to navigate you through this sometimes frustrating and difficult course with some tips and strategies.

RELATED CONDITIONS

- Celiac disease
- Dyspepsia
- Inflammatory bowel disease (Crohn's disease and ulcerative colitis)
- Irritable bowel syndrome
- Lactose intolerance
- Recurrent functional abdominal pain (RAP)

When should we contact our doctor or local hospital?

About 15% of school-aged children, more often girls, suffer from chronic abdominal pain. Only a very small percentage of the abdominal pains are found to be caused by a specific and recognizable problem, such as inflammatory bowel disease, celiac disease, or lactose intolerance. In other cases, the symptoms may be suggestive of less specific causes, such as irritable bowel syndrome, dyspepsia, or constipation. It is important to realize that not every illness is caused by a known disease that can be proven by medical testing. Many individuals have symptoms for which no illness can be identified. This is often the case in recurrent abdominal pain. If you see any of the red flags listed on page 26, seek urgent medical attention. Even if none of these are present, if the pain is interfering with your child's daily life, you should discuss this with your doctor.

A B C D E F G H I J K L M N O P Q R S T U V W X Y Z

➤➤ Chronic Abdominal Pain Red Flags

Seek urgent care if your child presents with these signs and symptoms:

- Pain that consistently wakes your child from sleep
- Pain that affects one particular part (not the entire abdomen)
- Weight loss
- Poor growth or delayed onset of puberty
- Recurrent vomiting
- Unexplained fevers
- Joint pains
- Blood in the stool
- Family history of inflammatory bowel disease (IBD)

Symptoms, Causes, and Treatment Options for Chronic Abdominal Pain

Possible Cause	Symptoms	Why do they get these symptoms?	Possible Treatment Options
Irritable bowel syndrome (IBS)	• Stools are either loose and frequent (more than 3 times daily) or else infrequent (fewer than 3 times weekly); pain may be relieved by a bowel movement (BM) • After BM, child may feel that she still needs to go	• Theories abound, but the exact cause of the problem has not been established	• If loose stools, cut back on excess sugars (for example juices) as well as the sweetener sorbitol (found for example in sugar-free gum) • If constipated, then try to increase dietary fiber or consider trying a mild laxative
Constipation	• Infrequent, hard stools • Large stools that may plug the toilet • Stools that are difficult or painful to pass	• See Constipation (page 124)	• Increase natural or supplemental fiber in the diet • May require laxatives • See Constipation (page 124)

Possible Cause	Symptoms	Why do they get these symptoms?	Possible Treatment Options
Gastro-esophageal reflux disease (GERD)	• Pain under the ribs, centrally or on the left side • Heartburn • Sour taste at back of mouth • Pain associated with eating • Nausea, vomiting, bloating	• GERD produces heartburn when the stomach's acid contents regurgitate back up the esophagus • Can be indistinguishable from a peptic ulcer, which is very rare in children unless there is a strong history of ulcers in the family	• Avoid spicy, fatty foods • Eat smaller, more frequent meals • Trial of antacids or acid-blocking medication may help • May require assessment by a gastrointestinal (GI) specialist
Recurrent abdominal pain (RAP)	• Most often occurs in girls 5 to 10 years of age • Most often occurs in those with high-achieving, intense personalities • Nonspecific location of pain (usually belly button or all over) • Not related to meals or time of day • Child is growing well and appears generally healthy • May also have headaches or family member with headaches	• Your child complains of moderate to severe recurrent tummy pain, but despite a thorough review of symptoms, a physical examination, plus any tests felt to be necessary, no diagnosis can be found • Although the exact cause of this pain is not clear, the child is experiencing real pain	• Reassurance that the pain will settle down over time • Maintain normal school and social routines whenever possible
Celiac disease	• Poor appetite • Poor weight gain and growth • Vomiting • Greasy, loose stools • Pallor • Irritability	• The small intestines are unable to tolerate gluten, which is a protein found in barley, wheat, rye, and possibly oats — hence, celiac disease's other name: gluten-sensitive enteropathy • Symptoms can take months or years to show up; they can develop at any time — from late infancy to adulthood	• If screening blood tests are positive, proceed to endoscopy (scope) • If bowel biopsy confirms diagnosis, a strict gluten-free diet is required

Possible Cause	Symptoms	Why do they get these symptoms?	Possible Treatment Options
Inflammatory bowel disease (IBD) Ulcerative colitis	• Bloody, slimy stools • Poor appetite • Joint pain or swelling • Eye pain or redness • Weight loss • Multiple flare-ups, with settling down (remission) • Fever • Poor growth	• Involves inflammation of the colon • Commonly runs in families • Exact cause is unknown • Can present at any age but more commonly in preteens and teens	• Diagnosed by combination of barium studies (X-rays) and endoscopy • Will require various medications and occasionally surgery
Inflammatory bowel disease (IBD) Crohn's disease	• Poor appetite • Weight loss • Poor growth • Diarrhea, may be bloody • Nausea, vomiting • Fatigue • Abscesses or ulcers near the anus • Mouth ulcers • Fever • Painful or swollen joints • Eye pain or redness • Delayed puberty	• Similar to ulcerative colitis, but Crohn's disease can involve any part of the gastrointestinal tract, from mouth to anus	• Diagnosed by combination of barium studies (X-rays) and endoscopy • May require dietary changes, various medications, and occasionally surgery
Lactose intolerance	• Loose stools • Gas, cramps • Bloating • Flatulence • Symptoms 30 minutes to 2 hours after eating foods with a lot of lactose (dairy products)	• Child has difficulty digesting milk products because of low lactase activity; it is not a milk allergy • Lactase is an enzyme found in the small intestine that digests lactose, the sugar found in milk and milk products • Lactose intolerance can be inherited (primary) or acquired (secondary) • Primary lactose intolerance is more common in people of Asian and African ancestry • Secondary lactose intolerance may occur after gastrointestinal infections, such as the stomach flu; this is usually temporary	• Avoid lactose-containing products • For primary lactose intolerance, lactase replacement therapies (for example, chewable pills)

❷ What Causes Chronic Abdominal Pain?

There are many causes of chronic abdominal pain. You will want to become familiar with them, but in most cases, you should have your doctor examine your child if symptoms persist. These are invariably tough conditions to diagnose and treatment is often not straightforward.

Irritable Bowel Syndrome (IBS)

There are different criteria that have been used to define IBS, but the key features are common to most definitions. IBS is associated with recurrent or persistent abdominal discomfort that is relieved by a bowel movement. Typically, there is a sense your child's tummy is swollen, and her stools are occasionally accompanied by the passage of mucus. The stools are either loose and frequent (more than 3 times daily) or else they are infrequent (fewer than 3 times weekly). After the bowel movements, the child may also feel that evacuation was not complete.

How Is Irritable Bowel Syndrome Treated?

If constipation is a feature, a high-fiber diet is often helpful. Laxatives can also improve symptoms. See Constipation (page 124). If soft and frequent stools are present, eliminating excess sugar, such as fructose and lactose, may help. You should also avoid using the sweetener sorbitol. Various medications have been tried for IBS, particularly in adults, but their role in childhood IBS is less studied. You should have a careful conversation with your child's doctor before deciding whether to use them.

Dyspepsia

Dyspepsia refers to a recurrent or persistent pain or discomfort that is most noticeable above the belly button. It can be caused by an ulcer, which is relatively rare in children, by gastro-esophageal reflux disease (GERD), which produces heartburn when the stomach's contents regurgitate back up the esophagus, or by a disease that involves the upper bowel, such as Crohn's disease (IBD). Finally, it can be functional, with no known cause.

Pain may be your child's major symptom, or your child may have nausea or vomiting, bloating, and a sense of having had enough to eat early in the meal. Heartburn and the refluxing of food suggest GERD, but ulcer disease and functional dyspepsia are often indistinguishable.

Did You Know?

Imperfect Treatment
The treatment for IBS is imperfect, which can be frustrating. A medical examination can provide an explanation of the problem, give reassurance, and rule out serious disease.

Did You Know?

Referral
Sometimes, your child will be referred to a pediatric gastroenterologist, who is an expert in bowel disease. Occasionally, examining the esophagus, stomach, and duodenum with a scope will be necessary to rule out an ulcer or another serious condition.

How Is Dyspepsia Treated?

Your child needs a careful medical examination — but even that may not be enough. Symptoms can often be reduced by avoiding aggravating foods, often spicy or fatty ones. Often, your child's physician will prescribe a trial of medication that reduces stomach acidity. Medications known to upset the stomach, such as ibuprofen, should also be eliminated. Smaller, more frequent meals may relieve the sense of bloating and early satiety.

Recurrent Functional Abdominal Pain (RAP)

The majority of school-age children with recurrent or persistent abdominal pain will have RAP. The patient is more often female than male, with symptoms beginning between 5 and 10 years old. RAP is a symptom-based diagnosis rather than a pathological one. It has distinctive features, although the exact cause or causes have yet to be found.

Classically, the pain is located around the belly button and is quite variable in its intensity. Although it can be severe enough to disrupt activity, often it is present as a low-grade discomfort. Meals, exercise, and the time of day don't appear to influence the pain. There may be other symptoms, such as headache and limb pain. In spite of all the complaining, the child appears physically healthy. Many of the children are described as intense, conscientious, or "highly strung." There is also a tendency for other family members to suffer from functional painful symptoms, such as tension headaches.

Treatment

It is important to realize that in RAP, although there is no distinct disease diagnosis present, there is still a lot of pain. Obtaining a typical history and finding nothing physically wrong during the exam are usually sufficient to establish the diagnosis. The reassurance that nothing serious is causing the pain is often enough to reduce the severity of the problem, with no additional therapy. Laboratory testing has little value in identifying unsuspected disease. Except when an actual disease is suspected, tests are probably unnecessary. Medication is of little proven value in treating RAP. Constipation and lactose intolerance, if they coexist, can be treated appropriately.

Celiac Disease

Celiac disease is a condition where the small intestines are unable to tolerate gluten, which is a protein found in barley, wheat, rye, and possibly oats. The technical name is gluten-sensitive enteropathy.

Did You Know?

Normal Lifestyle

Once the diagnosis of RAP has been made, the goal of therapy is to attain as normal a lifestyle as possible. Your child needs to attend school regularly. Obvious stressors should be eliminated or, at least, reduced. Reassurance and lifestyle adjustments seem to help. Within a few weeks of diagnosis, 30% to 50% of children will notice that their pain has disappeared or significantly decreased, enough so that it no longer disrupts activities.

Exposure to gluten in the diet (which usually starts with the introduction of infant cereals) and a trigger, such as a viral infection, are also necessary to start the ball rolling. When these features are present, your child's immune system makes antibodies that attack the small bowel and damage its lining. The injured intestine has a diminished capacity to digest food.

Sign and Symptoms of Celiac Disease

Symptoms can take months or years to show up; they can develop at any time from late infancy to adulthood. It is rarely seen in young babies because it takes time for the symptoms to develop after gluten is introduced into the diet. If a few of the symptoms are present, it may be best to do the screening blood test. Some children may have very few, nonspecific, or vague symptoms, and it can take a long time before your child's doctor makes the diagnosis. Here is a list of the common signs and symptoms of celiac disease:

- Poor appetite
- Crankiness
- Poor weight gain and growth
- Vomiting
- Greasy, loose stools (some children may have constipation)
- Pallor
- Mouth sores
- Delayed tooth eruption
- Delayed puberty

Diagnosis of Celiac Disease

Some of the antibodies that are particularly associated with celiac disease can be measured in your child's blood through a screening test, but the presence of these antibodies by themselves is not diagnostic. The best test is an upper endoscopy with biopsies. During this procedure, conducted while your child is under anesthetic, the doctor will examine the small bowel through a small flexible camera placed in the mouth and passed through the bowel to the small intestines. Small tissue samples (biopsies) are taken for analysis under the microscope to check for specific signs of injury.

Treatment of Celiac Disease

The main treatment for celiac disease is a lifelong strict avoidance of gluten in the diet. Gluten is found in foods like bread, pasta, and cookies. A dietitian will help you and your family learn about this special diet, teach you to read food labels, and learn about

Did You Know?

Prevalence of Celiac Disease
Your child may have inherited a predisposition to this disease. Close family members are also at risk of developing celiac disease. About 10% of first-degree relatives have damage to the intestines without symptoms, and about 2% to 5% have celiac disease with symptoms.

hidden sources of gluten in foods (for example, in additives and preservatives). Only if your child has been diagnosed by blood tests and biopsies should she be committed to this restrictive diet. The special diet can be challenging for parents and children. There are organizations, support groups, and cookbooks to help with the challenges.

The best confirmation that your child has the disease is when her symptoms clinically improve (usually over a few months) and when damage to her bowel is reversed while she is on the diet. A repeat biopsy is not routinely necessary. People with celiac disease can develop other autoimmune conditions, such as diabetes mellitus and hypothyroidism. They are also at higher risk for bowel cancer, although it seems that the risk is less if they follow a gluten-free diet.

Inflammatory Bowel Disease (IBD)

Inflammatory bowel disease is a term used to describe chronic conditions that involve inflammation of the gastrointestinal tract. Crohn's disease and ulcerative colitis are two distinct yet similar conditions that fall into this category. The intestine's immune system cannot adequately control inflammation, causing the inflammation to wax and wane throughout life. Although both ulcerative colitis and Crohn's disease can be diagnosed in children as young as 4 or 5 years of age, it is most often seen in preteens, teens, and young adults.

Ulcerative Colitis

The inflammation of ulcerative colitis is limited to the colon (large bowel) and involves only the inner layer of the bowel wall. Some individuals can suffer from inflammation involving the entire colon, and others might have only rectal inflammation. Generally, the rectum and the lowest parts of the colon are the most affected. There is tremendous variability with respect to severity and response to medication. Individuals with ulcerative colitis may also experience inflammation in the eyes, joints, and skin.

Signs and Symptoms of Ulcerative Colitis
- Bloody, mucusy stools; stools are often loose and a lot of blood can be lost
- Symptoms can begin and progress quickly
- Abdominal pain, poor appetite, joint pain or swelling, eye inflammation, and weight loss are also common; fever, vomiting, and skin lesions are less frequent
- Multiple flare-ups and remissions
- Nighttime stooling, stooling urgently

Crohn's Disease

Crohn's disease can involve any part of the gastrointestinal tract — from a child's mouth to anus — not just the colon. This inflammation typically involves all the layers of the intestinal wall (not just the inner layer, as in ulcerative colitis) and is usually patchy in distribution, with healthy areas of intestine interspersed with inflamed areas. Involvement of the small bowel can prevent normal absorption of nutrients, leading to nutritional deficiencies and growth problems. There is also an increased incidence of lactose intolerance in individuals with Crohn's disease. Your child with Crohn's disease can also have inflamed skin, eyes, and joints, which may precede any obvious involvement of the gastrointestinal tract. The degree of symptoms can vary from individual to individual, and flare-ups and remissions are often experienced.

Signs and Symptoms of Crohn's Disease
- History of chronic abdominal pain, poor appetite, weight loss or poor growth, and diarrhea
- Blood in the stool, nausea and vomiting, fatigue, abscesses or ulcers near the anus, mouth ulcers, fever, painful or swollen joints, eye inflammation, and rare skin rashes that are specifically associated with IBD
- Delayed puberty in preteens and teens
- If colon involvement is significant, your child can have an urgent feeling prior to bowel movements (that she must have a bowel movement immediately or she'll have an accident), or pain with bowel movements
- Thickening of the intestinal wall might narrow the inside of the intestine to the point that the bowel becomes obstructed

Diagnosis of Inflammatory Bowel Disease

Two types of tests are very helpful in evaluating the gastrointestinal tract for signs of inflammation: barium X-rays and endoscopy.

Did You Know?

No Clear Cause
IBD has no clear cause. Like other inflammatory diseases, IBD can run in families. It is believed to occur in individuals with a predisposition to the condition and who experience some type of environmental trigger that leads to intestinal inflammation.

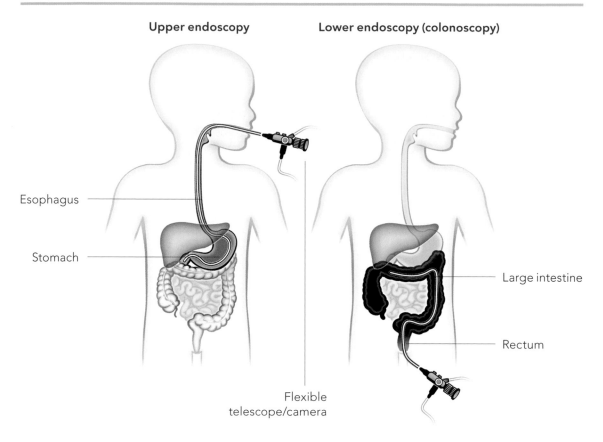

Upper endoscopy **Lower endoscopy (colonoscopy)**

Esophagus

Stomach

Large intestine

Rectum

Flexible
telescope/camera

Barium X-rays use barium to outline the lining of the intestines. Your child will be given a barium enema that will pass through the rectum and colon and she will swallow a barium drink that is followed through the esophagus, stomach, and small bowel in what is called an upper GI series.

Upper and lower endoscopy are more invasive tests and require your child to be sedated or under general anesthetic, and they require a special preparation for the bowel. Upper endoscopy involves the insertion of a long flexible telescope into the esophagus, stomach, and duodenum (first part of the small bowel). Your child's doctor or a specialist can see the lining of the tract and take biopsies (small samples of tissue). Detailed information about the inflammation is provided by examination of the biopsies under a microscope. Similarly, through lower endoscopy, the rectum and colon can be examined. Because chronic infections can mimic some of the symptoms of IBD, stool samples can differentiate the two: in IBD, there is no evidence of bacterial or parasitic infection.

How Is Inflammatory Bowel Disease Treated?

Whether your child has ulcerative colitis or Crohn's disease, the experience of having a chronic illness can be quite overwhelming. You can find support through your pediatrician, gastroenterologist, and the local chapter of the Crohn's and Colitis Foundation.

Ulcerative Colitis

Various medications are used to decrease the inflammation in ulcerative colitis. For those who respond poorly to medications, a surgical operation to remove the inflamed bowel may be necessary.

Crohn's Disease

No treatment at this time can provide a permanent cure. Your child's treatment is aimed at controlling symptoms, improving nutrition, and promoting normal growth and puberty. Your child's doctor will choose therapies based on the severity and location of gut inflammation. The therapies will likely combine nutrition, medications, and, occasionally, surgery.

Lactose Intolerance

Lactose intolerance can be either primary, which means it develops without obvious cause, or secondary, which means that it results from some disease. Lactose intolerance is the term used to describe difficulty digesting milk products because of low lactase activity. It is not a milk allergy.

FAQ

What is lactose intolerance?

Lactase is an enzyme found in the small intestine that enables the human body to digest lactose, the sugar found in milk and milk products. The amount of lactase in the small intestine is highest in infancy, when milk is the main food, and then it begins to fall at about 3 years of age. In some individuals, lactase activity can drop to a level that may prevent proper digestion of large quantities of lactose-rich foods.

Primary Lactose Intolerance

Primary lactose intolerance happens when the level of lactase production gradually declines to a degree that prevents the digestion of all the lactose consumed. It is more common in certain ethnic groups, particularly people of Asian and African ancestry, and, as such, can run in families. However, children and adults from any background can develop lactose intolerance. It can develop at any age in childhood, adolescence, or adulthood, but it rarely develops in infancy.

Secondary Lactose Intolerance

Secondary lactose intolerance is a condition arising from gastrointestinal infections, such as a stomach flu (viral gastroenteritis) or inflammatory bowel disease, which lead to a decrease in the lactase activity level of the lining of the small intestine. In the case of gastrointestinal infection, the intolerance is a temporary condition and gets better after the lining of the small bowel heals.

Symptoms of Lactose Intolerance

In primary lactose intolerance, symptoms vary from one child to another. Lactose that cannot be digested travels through the intestines and causes more water to be expelled in stools, thereby making them loose. Bacteria in the intestine can digest the lactose, producing gas, which can cause cramps, bloating, and flatulence. Most children develop symptoms 30 minutes to 2 hours after consuming foods with a lot of lactose, such as milk. However, because lactose is found in many different foods, it is sometimes difficult to correlate symptoms with the ingestion of lactose. Some children have enough lactase to digest some lactose-containing foods, like cheese or yogurt, but they have more symptoms after consuming high-lactose products, particularly a glass of milk.

Elimination Diet

If secondary lactose intolerance occurs after an infection, temporarily removing milk products from your child's diet and slowly reintroducing them after the diarrhea settles may help. Doctors might suggest following a soy formula or lactose-free formula for a brief period if your baby is still dependent on milk as a major source of

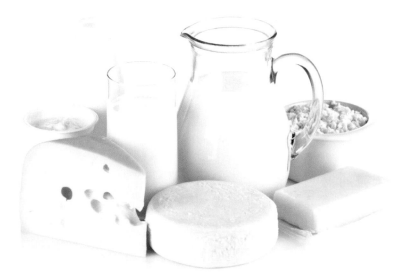

nutrition. After the fever and vomiting settle and the initial diarrhea improves, cramps and looser stools may recur when she drinks milk or consumes milk products. This settles after a few days or weeks as the cells that line the gastrointestinal tract regenerate.

Hydrogen Test

Diagnosis of lactose intolerance is best made using a breath hydrogen test, which is a noninvasive test that involves measuring the amount of hydrogen that is breathed out of the lungs. If the hydrogen, released by the gut bacteria after exposure to the undigested lactose, in your child's breath rises after she eats or drinks lactose, this suggests lactose intolerance.

Lactose Intolerance Treatment

Primary and secondary lactose intolerance related to inflammatory bowel disease require long-term changes in your child's diet. The goal of treatment is to restore your child's ability to enjoy her food and to live without symptoms.

- Step 1: Involve your family and caregivers in learning how to read ingredients on food labels and to identify milk products in foods.
- Step 2: Let everyone become acquainted with the types of lactose-free products and lactase replacements that are available. Lactose-free milk, nondairy cheese, and lactose-free ice cream are available in most grocery stores.
- Step 3: Use chewable lactase replacements, which are available without a prescription and are usually found in the drugstore aisle with other digestive medications. Your child should chew these lactase pills before eating or drinking regular milk products, to aid her digestion and prevent symptoms.
- Step 4: Once symptoms are controlled and your child is happier, slowly reintroduce small amounts of lactose to identify which foods and what volumes of lactose she can digest without suffering any symptoms. Yogurt, cottage cheese, and hard aged cheeses may be easier to digest. It is important that her nutritional need for calcium is met. In some cases, she might have to take calcium supplements.

Doc Talk It is important to realize that not every illness is caused by a known disease, one that can be proven by medical testing. Many individuals have symptoms for which no illness can be identified. Such is sometimes the case in recurrent abdominal pain. It is really frustrating! If any new symptoms develop, it will be important to review these with your child's doctor.

Allergic Rhinitis (Hay Fever)

What Can I Do?

▶ Avoid the offending allergen or trigger if possible.

▶ Use indoor air conditioning and reduce humidity in the home.

▶ Enclose mattresses and pillows in a hypoallergenic mattress slip and pillow slips, and wash bed sheets and blankets in hot water once a week.

▶ Discuss with your doctor the use of antihistamine medication and/or inhaled steroid nasal spray.

❶ What Is Allergic Rhinitis (Hay Fever)?

Allergic rhinitis, more commonly called hay fever, means inflammation of the nasal passages caused by allergies. This condition most often occurs each year in a seasonal pattern, when pollens, from grass, trees, or ragweed, are in abundance. It is called perennial allergic rhinitis when it occurs year-round. Children with hay fever frequently have a history of other allergic problems, such as asthma and eczema. Often, many family members have allergic rhinitis, suggesting a genetic component to this condition.

Did You Know?

Prevalence
Symptoms usually develop after two seasons of exposure to the allergen; for this reason, it is more common to see symptoms of allergic rhinitis after the age of 2. Allergic rhinitis affects 5% to 15% of children.

Signs and Symptoms

- Nasal congestion (stuffy nose)
- Runny nose
- Cough due to postnasal drip
- Sneezing
- Itchy nose and eyes
- "Allergic shiners" (dark, puffy lower eyelids)
- "Allergic salute" (children rub their dripping nose upward with an open hand)
- Persistent mouth breathing (can lead to dental problems)

When should we contact our doctor?

If you suspect that environmental allergens are causing hay fever in your child but are not sure exactly what the triggers are, see your doctor to arrange for possible allergy testing.

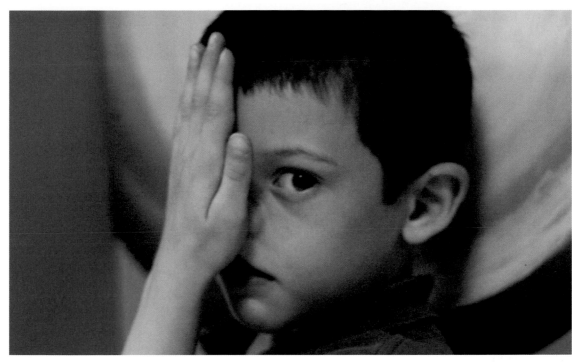

Allergic salute

❷ What Causes Allergic Rhinitis?

The main triggers for allergic rhinitis are airborne particles from the natural environment.

Pollen

Many flowering plants rely on the wind to disperse their pollen, and some of these pollens can cause allergies. Tree pollens are the first of the allergy season, often appearing before the leaves unfold. Grass pollens are the next to appear. In late summer, the final pollens to appear are those from weeds, such as ragweed.

Fungi

Several fungi (molds), both outdoor and indoor, can cause allergic rhinitis. Outdoors, fungi grow on dead plant material. Activities that disrupt such material, such as cutting grass or raking leaves, can be associated with the release of fungi into the air. Indoors, fungi grow in humid environments, including poorly cleaned humidifiers.

Pets and Rodents

Animals can shed allergic particles into the environment that can become airborne and cause allergic rhinitis. The source of these

Did You Know?

Airborne
Dust mites are tiny transparent bugs that are related to ticks. They feed on skin scales shed by humans and require a humid environment. In homes, dust mites live in beds, carpets, and upholstered furniture. Cockroaches and other insects can also produce airborne particles that can cause allergic rhinitis.

A B C D E F G H I J K L M N O P Q R S T U V W X Y Z

allergens varies by animal. For example, the allergic particles from cats come from their skin, and the allergen from rats is from their urine.

❸ How Is Allergic Rhinitis Treated?

If it is clear that the allergic rhinitis symptoms are caused by a specific allergen, such as ragweed, further tests might not be required. Simple avoidance of the trigger will help reduce symptoms. If a clear seasonal cause cannot be identified, or if the symptoms are year-long, your child might be referred to an allergist, who could undertake specific allergy testing to identify the triggers.

Antihistamine Medications

Antihistamines are the most frequently recommended medications for allergic rhinitis. Newer antihistamines that don't cause sleepiness should be the first option. If your child has significant nasal congestion, prescription nasal steroids applied directly to the inside lining of the nasal passages might be recommended for occasional use.

Oral Treatment Options for Allergic Rhinitis

Treatment	Examples	Advantages	Disadvantages
Nonsedating antihistamines	Loratadine (Claritin), cetirizine hydrochloride (Zyrtec, Reactine)	• Nonsedating • Lasts up to 24 hours • No prescription required	• Cost
Sedating antihistamines	Diphenhydramine (Benadryl), hydroxyzine (Atarax)	• Readily available • Inexpensive • Rapid onset of action	• Sedating • Requires 3 to 4 times daily dosing
Leukotriene receptor antagonists	Montelukast (Singulair)	• Nonsedating • Also helps with asthma symptoms	• Requires prescription

Doc Talk The use of over-the-counter oral or topical decongestants in children is not recommended by pediatricians, despite their availability on the shelves of drugstores. Their use in children has not been shown to be beneficial and may, in fact, cause harm by producing unwanted side effects.

Allergies and Food Intolerances

What Can I Do?

▶ If your child has symptoms of anaphylaxis, this is a medical emergency! Inject your child with an epinephrine self-injection pen (such as an EpiPen) if you have one and call 911 immediately.

▶ Try to identify the most likely trigger. The best treatment is avoiding the allergen.

▶ If your child is found to have a true allergy, ensure that all caregivers are aware and get a medical alert bracelet for her to wear and an epinephrine self-injecting pen to carry — it could be lifesaving.

❶ What Are Allergies?

Allergies occur when the body's immune system reacts to specific proteins in the environment that we ingest, touch, or inhale, identifying them as foreign. These proteins are normally not harmful to most people, but a select group of individuals may have an allergic reaction to this "invading protein" or allergen.

There is a wide spectrum of reactions, ranging from a mild allergic reaction with a little bit of itching to a full-blown severe allergic reaction with throat and mouth swelling, a drop in blood pressure, and loss of consciousness, known as anaphylaxis. Anaphylaxis refers to a severe and life-threatening reaction to an allergen.

RELATED CONDITIONS

- Anaphylaxis
- Conjunctivitis
- Hives
- Itching

Common Allergens

Food allergens	*Environmental allergens*	*Other allergens*
Peanuts	Molds	Bee stings
Tree nuts	Dust mites	Insect stings/bites
Shellfish	Pollen	Medicines
Eggs	Pet dander	Chemicals
Cow's milk	Cockroaches	

When should we contact our doctor or local hospital?

During an anaphylactic reaction, a child may experience swelling of the face, lips, and throat. This swelling can block the airway, making it difficult, and sometimes impossible, to breathe. Some children may experience difficulty breathing from spasm of the bronchial tubes in the lungs. This may sound like wheezing, a musical whistling noise heard when trying to exhale.

➤➤ Anaphylaxis Red Flags

Anaphylaxis is a medical emergency! If you suspect your child is having an anaphylactic reaction, call 911 and use an epinephrine self-injection pen, if available.

Allergy Symptoms

Food (and Insect) Allergies

Symptoms typically occur within minutes of eating (or being stung) and include:

- *Hives:* Blotchy, raised, red, itchy rash, which appears and disappears in random places all over the body
- *Swelling:* Often occurs around the mouth and face
- *Breathing:* Difficult, labored, or noisy breathing
- *Vomiting:* Can occur shortly after ingestion of the allergenic food (but vomiting in isolation is not likely caused by an allergy)
- *Low blood pressure:* Dizziness, light-headed, fainting, loss of consciousness

Environmental Allergies

Symptoms can occur at any time with exposure to environmental allergens:

- *Itching:* May occur anywhere, with or without the presence of a rash
- *Conjunctivitis:* Red, burning, itchy, or teary eyes
- *Breathing:* Wheezing, coughing, and chest tightness, usually slower in onset than with a food allergy
- *Cold-like symptoms:* Congestion, runny nose, itchy throat

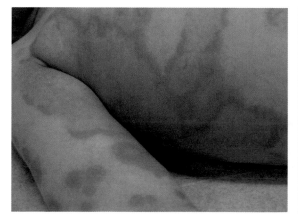

Hives

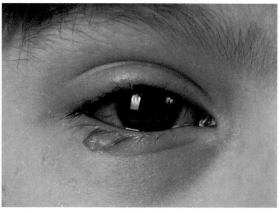

Conjunctivitis

❷ What Causes Allergies?

Allergens trigger an immune reaction in the body. The reaction to allergens will vary between individuals. Most commonly, the eyes, nose, throat, lungs, and skin are affected. Reactions to foods and insects tend to differ from reactions to environmental allergens.

Allergic Immune Cascade

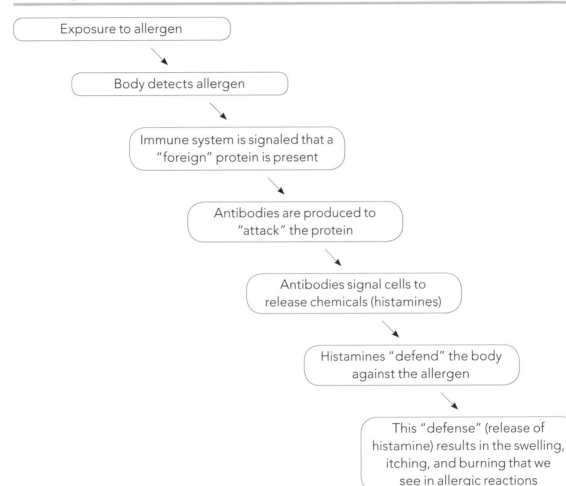

Exposure to allergen

Body detects allergen

Immune system is signaled that a "foreign" protein is present

Antibodies are produced to "attack" the protein

Antibodies signal cells to release chemicals (histamines)

Histamines "defend" the body against the allergen

This "defense" (release of histamine) results in the swelling, itching, and burning that we see in allergic reactions

Drug Allergies

Some children will experience unwanted side effects during or after treatment with a drug. Most drug reactions are a side effect of the drug itself, and only a few are a result of an allergic reaction. This is very important to remember so that not all reactions to drugs get labeled as allergies.

Not a drug allergy if:

- Your child has symptoms of another illness, such as a rash, while taking a drug, and these symptoms are attributed to the drug — in error.
- Your child received two drugs that interacted with one another.
- Your child experienced an unwanted known side effect of a medication.
- Your child received too much of a drug, resulting in a drug overdose.

❸ How Are Allergies Treated?

How To: Prevent an Allergic Reaction

If your child has a food allergy:

- Avoid all foods your child is allergic to.
- Read all food labels to check ingredients.
- Ask about ingredients in foods being served to your child.
- Teach her to read food labels (when your child is old enough) to avoid the foods she is allergic to.
- Teach her to ask about ingredients served in foods.
- Instruct all caregivers about your child's allergy and the need for certain dietary restrictions.

If your child has an environmental allergy:

- Wash linens in hot water to reduce dust mites.
- Vacuum and dust your home often to reduce dust mites.
- Use hypoallergenic linens, pillows, and mattresses.
- Seal pillows and mattresses to reduce dust mites.
- Eliminate pets from the home. If this is not possible, bathe your pet and vacuum floors frequently. Keep the pet out of your child's bedroom.
- Close windows during pollen season and use an air conditioner with a high-quality filter or air purifier.
- Remove carpets from your child's bedroom to reduce dust.

How To: Manage Allergic Reactions

If your child has mild allergic symptoms, you can:

- Administer antihistamines — for example, diphenhydramine (Benadryl); these can make your child sleepy.

- Administer non-drowsy antihistamines — for example, loratadine (Claritin) or cetirizine (Reactine or Zyrtec).
- Apply cold compresses for rashes.

If your child has severe allergic reactions:

- If you have a self-injection pen, use it immediately.
- Call 911.
- If you have given your child his epinephrine, and he is feeling better, he still needs to be transported to the nearest hospital for assessment.

How To: Use an Epinephrine Self-Injection Pen

1. If there is a history of anaphylaxis, don't wait for signs of a severe reaction before injecting epinephrine.
2. Unscrew the cap from the container and remove the pen.
3. Grasp the pen in a fist.
4. Take off the safety cap from the back of the pen.
5. Push the rounded tip hard into the outer muscle of the thigh, aiming it perpendicular to the thigh.
6. The pen can inject through clothing if necessary.
7. Hold the pen in place while slowly counting to 10.
8. Gently massage the area.
9. Call 911 or rush to the nearest hospital.

The child may need more than one injection. If there is no improvement or there are ongoing symptoms after the first injection, give a second one, if available.

Immunotherapy

Some children who have severe allergic reactions to stinging insects may be offered desensitization injections (allergy shots, or immunotherapy). These injections — given in response to the specific stinging insect — have a very high rate of success (over 95%) in preventing a future anaphylactic reaction. Talk to your child's doctor about this if your child has had a life-threatening reaction.

> **Did You Know?**
>
> **Seasonal and Perennial**
> Allergy shots can also be offered to children with seasonal or perennial allergies who still have symptoms in spite of taking medication on a daily basis. In these children, avoidance of the allergen may be virtually impossible. Injections are given every 1 to 2 weeks over several months to years.

> **Doc Talk**
>
> Can you prevent a child from developing an allergy? Probably not. The results from many studies are contradictory, creating a confusing picture for both parents and physicians. The most consistent evidence suggests that breastfeeding may help to protect against the development of allergies.

How to Use an Epinephrine Self-Injection Pen

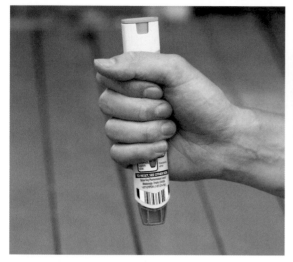

Step 1: Hold the epinephrine self-injection pen in your fist.

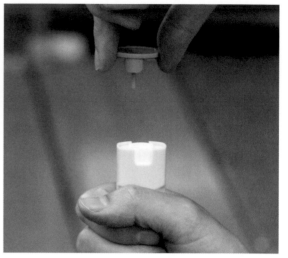

Step 2: Remove the safety cap from the back of the pen.

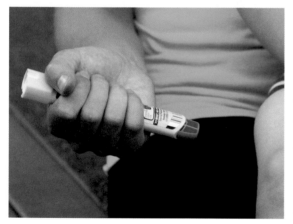

Step 3: Aim perpendicular to the thigh.

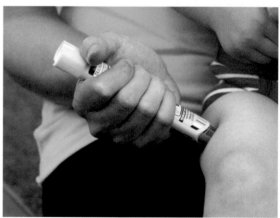

Step 4: Push the tip hard into the thigh muscle and hold in place while slowly counting to 10.

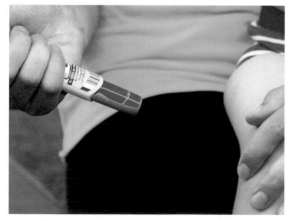

Step 5: Remove the pen.

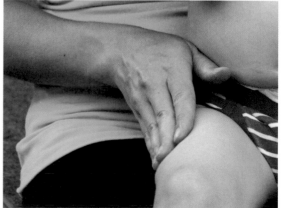

Step 6: Gently massage the area.

❹ What Is a Food Intolerance?

Food allergies are not, in most cases, a true immune response but rather an intolerance to a specific food or ingredient. Food intolerance can cause a variety of symptoms, such as abdominal cramps, changes in behavior, and diarrhea in children. Some children are lactose intolerant, meaning that they are unable to digest milk products because a digestive enzyme is not available in their digestive system. See Lactose Intolerance (page 35). Some children develop a rash after eating fruits or drinking fruit juices, but these have not been proven to be caused by allergies.

❺ How Are Food Allergies and Intolerances Treated?

The best way to avoid a reaction to a food is to avoid it altogether. For example, in an infant with a cow's milk allergy, breastfeeding mothers might try a dairy-free diet to prevent cow's milk protein allergy. Formula-fed babies might be switched to a hypoallergenic formula. With peanut allergies, a child should avoid any peanut product, including all tree nuts (because they may have been cross-contaminated with peanut protein during processing and packaging).

Allergic Shiners (Dark Circles Under the Eye)

Just because your child has dark circles under his eyes does not mean he is sleeping poorly. In children, dark circles under the eyes suggests the possibility of nasal congestion from allergies. With nasal congestion, blood doesn't flow as easily through the veins draining from the eyes to the nose. This results in a darker appearance under the eyes, called allergic shiners.

Allergies are the most common identified cause of dark circles. Other causes of nasal congestion, such as chronic sinus infections or enlarged adenoids and tonsils, may contribute to this condition. Often, dark circles under the eyes runs in families.

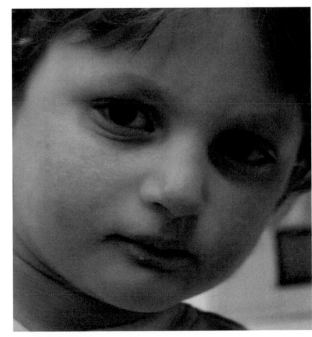

Allergic shiners

Drug Reactions

The most common drug reaction is a skin rash. Many different types of rashes can occur, and they are often difficult to distinguish from rashes seen in many common viral illnesses. Do not give any more of the offending medication. If the reaction is mild, such as with a rash, call your doctor for further directions. He may advise that it is okay to continue the medication if the symptoms of the reaction can be managed, or he may suggest an alternative form of treatment for the initial underlying problem.

FAQs

Will my child outgrow her allergy?

The most common food allergies in infants are allergies to cow's milk and eggs. Cow's milk allergy is seen in about 2% to 5% of infants, usually in the first month of life. Many children will outgrow allergies to cow's milk and eggs. In fact, 80% to 90% of those allergic in infancy will tolerate these foods by 3 years of age. Allergies to other foods, such as peanuts, tree nuts, and shellfish, tend to persist throughout life, with only a small percentage of children outgrowing them.

If I am allergic to something, does this mean my child will be allergic to it too?

We know that genetics plays a role in the development of an allergy. A family history of allergies puts a child at increased risk for developing allergies too, but it does not necessarily mean that a child will become allergic.

Doc Talk

Some children are atopic — that is, the child is predisposed to developing heightened immune responses to common allergens. The classic triad of symptoms includes eczema (atopic dermatitis), hay fever (allergic rhinitis), and allergic asthma. These children also have a tendency toward food allergies. Atopy has a strong hereditary component, tending to run in families. More recent evidence in the literature suggests that pregnant and lactating mothers do not need to avoid any particular foods for the prevention of allergies in their child. Additionally, there is no current convincing evidence that delaying the introduction of solid foods (including nut products, fish, and eggs) beyond 4 to 6 months of life plays any role in preventing the development of atopy or allergies in the majority of children.

Ankle Injuries

What Can I Do?

▶ If the pain is severe, not improving with time, or your child is unable to put any weight on the affected side, seek urgent medical attention to rule out a broken bone.

▶ If the pain is manageable and your child can still walk, elevate the leg and apply ice to reduce swelling.

▶ Administer ibuprofen, which is helpful in reducing pain and swelling.

❶ What Is an Ankle Injury?

Ankle injuries are very common during sports. Most kids have, at one time or another, rolled their ankle playing soccer, football, or basketball, or while running on uneven surfaces. The child will usually complain of pain and swelling around the ankle area.

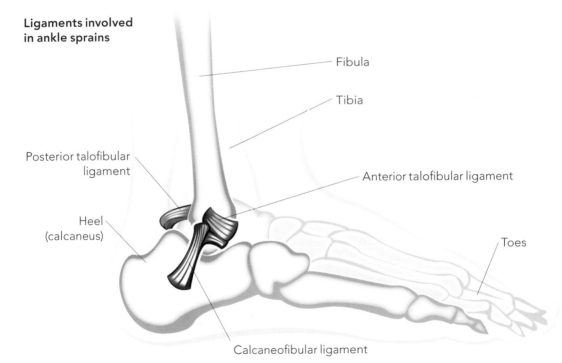

Ligaments involved in ankle sprains

- Fibula
- Tibia
- Posterior talofibular ligament
- Anterior talofibular ligament
- Heel (calcaneus)
- Toes
- Calcaneofibular ligament

Common Signs and Symptoms of Ankle Sprain
- Limp
- Pain on the outside of the ankle
- Pain with moving the ankle
- Swelling and bruising on outside of the ankle

When should we contact our doctor or local hospital?

Other symptoms might indicate a fracture of the ankle or a more severe injury. If any of these features are present, see your doctor as soon as possible:

- Severe pain
- Inability to walk or put any weight on the ankle
- Pain when pressing over the bones of the ankle
- No improvement seen by 48 hours after the injury

Did You Know?

Patience
Returning to sports too early can cause a more long-standing injury, so patience is important. If there is no pain with hopping, running in an easy zigzag, or light jumping, healing is probably sufficient to return to sports.

❷ How Is an Ankle Injury Treated?

If the pain is not severe, if your child can walk with no more than a mild pain or limp, and if there is no pain or large swelling over the bones, you can manage your child at home.

- Rest the ankle.
- Elevate the leg to reduce swelling.
- Apply ice packs to the sore area for 20 minutes at a time, every 3 to 4 hours while your child is awake, for the first 24 hours.
- Administer ibuprofen to reduce pain and swelling.

Although it will not completely heal right away, the ankle should start to feel better during the next 48 hours and your child can do light stretching exercises. It can take several weeks for the ankle to feel back to normal, even after a minor sprain. Complete healing of the ligaments can even take a few months.

Doc Talk   Injuries to ligaments and bones are extremely common in children. Your child might have had an obvious injury, such as a fall, but sometimes no obvious event is recalled that might explain the pain. Toddlers may even develop a small fracture of one of the bones in the leg after jumping. Sprains and fractures may cause pain, swelling, limping, or bruising. Some children will simply refuse to use their leg or will resist movement without complaining of pain. Ligaments are like elastic bands that are attached to bones and that help control movement of joints. Like elastics, they can be stretched or torn — this is what happens in a sprain. A small stretch causes a mild sprain; a severe sprain might tear the ligament.

Anxiety, Fears, and Phobias

What Can I Do?

▶ If you have concerns that your child's anxiety is significantly interfering with her social life, learning, or happiness, speak with your doctor or a child psychologist.

▶ Help your child to cope with everyday social interactions by anticipation, preparation, and role playing.

▶ Understand that most children have some anxieties and fears. This is a normal part of child development. Support, patience, and encouragement are usually all that is needed.

❶ What Is Anxiety?

All children get anxious from time to time and all kids experience fear. It is natural for infants as young as 7 months to appear apprehensive when encountering strangers. It is also normal for toddlers to display some reluctance at being left alone in their rooms at bedtime. During such times, we worry about how our children are feeling and we may wonder if their anxiety is excessive or abnormal. How do we know? Anxiety disorders are common; approximately 5% to 10% of children will suffer from them at some time. Anxiety becomes a "disorder" when it interferes with normal functioning and social development.

When should we contact our doctor or local hospital?

When anxiety interferes with normal functioning and social development, the term "anxiety disorder" is applied. For example, it is normal for a child not to want to try something new initially (a team sport or day camp, for example). If, however, this apprehension cannot be overcome, and despite reassurance and encouragement, your child steadfastly avoids the activity because of anxiety, this would be considered "functionally impairing anxiety."

Types of Anxiety

Anxiety may be generalized (feeling anxious most of the time about a wide variety of things) or it can be more specific:

- Separation anxiety disorder
- Social phobia

A B C D E F G H I J K L M N O P Q R S T U V W X Y Z

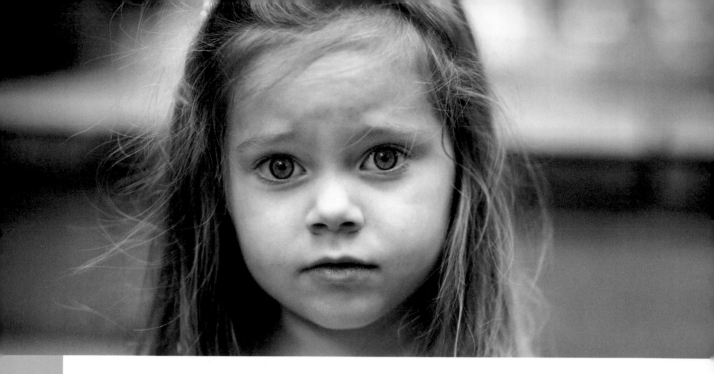

- Generalized anxiety disorder
- Obsessive-compulsive disorder
- Phobias
- Post-traumatic stress disorder
- Panic attacks

Did You Know?

Development
Among those children with significant anxiety disorders, as many as 30% may later develop another mental health issue, often a different form of anxiety.

Occasionally, usually manageable, generalized anxiety erupts abruptly, producing a panic attack characterized by sweating, a racing pulse, shortness of breath, and panicky fear. One form of anxiety disorder — obsessive-compulsive disorder (OCD) — is defined by how an individual tries to deal with stress. A person with OCD uses rigid and repetitive, but restrictive, routines to cope.

❷ What Causes Anxiety and Phobias?

- Some forms of anxiety appear to be the result of a particularly stressful event, such as the death of a parent or witnessing an accident, manifesting as acute stress disorders and post-traumatic stress disorders.
- Some kids are just anxious by nature (born with it).
- Anxiety disorders may run in a family.

❸ How Is Anxiety Treated?

There are several treatments commonly used for anxiety disorders.

Commonly Used Treatments for Anxiety Disorders

Modality	Cognitive behavioral therapy (CBT). Ask your doctor for a referral to a CBT counselor or therapist.
What this means	Child is taught strategies to recognize and better understand the thoughts that result in anxiety. The therapist will help the child develop improved reactions to the triggers of anxiety.
Most often used for	Generalized anxiety disorder, post-traumatic stress disorder, obsessive-compulsive disorder
Comments	One of the most successful forms of counseling
Modality	**Relaxation techniques or breathing exercises**
What this means	Child is taught techniques for progressively relaxing muscle groups or controlling his breathing. When "fight or flight" response sets in, breathing usually speeds up. These techniques can work to purposefully slow breathing and halt the anxiety from escalating.
Most often used for	Panic attacks, phobias
Comments	Once techniques have been learned, they are an inexpensive, simple way for a child to control his anxiety.
Modality	**Systematic desensitization**
What this means	Gradually confronting a phobia or anxiety-provoking stimulus in manageable but increasing amounts.
Most often used for	Phobias
Comments	Can be combined with other modalities, such as relaxation techniques.
Modality	**Medications**
What this means	SSRIs (selective serotonin-reuptake inhibitors) are taken daily to help with anxiety symptoms.
Most often used for	Most forms of anxiety that are sub-optimally controlled with counseling alone.
Comments	Should always be used in conjunction with counseling.

Doc Talk

Anxiety in children tends to settle down after a month or two. If your child seems generally happy and is progressing well, and if the occasional anxiety can be satisfactorily managed with a little extra support, reassurance, and encouragement, no further assessment or treatment is needed. Many seemingly anxious behaviors, such as nightmares or separation anxiety, are simply a normal stage of child development.

Arm Injuries (Fractures, Pulled Elbow)

What Can I Do?

▶ Do not swing your child around by the hands or yank him by the arms.

▶ If there is significant pain, swelling, or deformity, or your child is unwilling to use his arm, seek urgent medical attention to see if an X-ray is required.

▶ If the area is swollen, apply some ice, elevate the arm, and encourage your child to rest.

▶ Use ibuprofen to alleviate any pain.

❶ What Is an Arm Injury?

It is not unusual for your young child to trip and land on an outstretched arm or injure himself in another way while exploring his world. Thankfully, on most occasions, he'll pick himself up, dust himself off, and recover before your heart rate has returned to normal. On other occasions, there may be a small graze or bruise over the affected area. But what do you do in the less common scenario when a part of his arm or hand is really swollen or looks crooked, or when he is just not willing to use the arm at all? Read on to see if you need to have him assessed to rule out a broken bone or a pulled elbow.

Case Study

Ben's Arm Fracture

Ben is a healthy, very active 4-year-old. He was upstairs playing tag with his older sister, Danielle. In an effort to get away from Danielle, Ben ran down the stairs, tripped, and fell onto his outstretched arm. He cried immediately, but — being a brave little boy — he "toughed it out" for the afternoon. By dinnertime, Ben's arm was a bit swollen, just above his wrist, and he didn't want to use his hand to eat his meal. Ben's mother took him to the local urgent-care center, where he had an X-ray. The diagnosis was a simple buckle fracture.

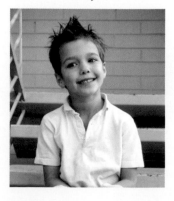

Ben had suffered a small break to the forearm bone (the radius). The bone "buckled" with the force of impact when he tripped down the stairs. Ben needed to wear an immobilizing splint for 3 to 4 weeks to allow the bone to heal completely. The doctor reminded Ben and Danielle that although he liked that they were active and playing together, playing tag on the stairs was probably not the best idea!

❷ What Is a Fracture (Broken Bone)?

A fracture is a partial or complete break in the bone. Some fractures result in complete separation of the bone into two pieces, whereas others buckle and bend but do not break completely.

Greenstick and Buckle Fractures

Because children's bones are softer, they often buckle or bend rather than break completely. These fractures are called buckle fractures if the bone buckles from the force, and greenstick fractures if there is a partial break in the bone (similar to the partial break that occurs when you try to bend a young tree branch). Buckle and greenstick fractures may cause less swelling or deformity than other fractures and they may be harder to recognize as fractures. Sometimes the only signs in a child might be pain and a refusal to use the affected limb.

Did You Know?

Bone Ends
Although children's bones heal faster than adult bones do, special attention may be required for fractures involving the ends of bones, which may disrupt the growth center and interfere with normal bone growth.

When should we contact our doctor or local hospital?

If there is significant pain and swelling over the affected area, if your child is unwilling to use his arm, or if you can actually see some deformity to the bone, then you should seek urgent medical attention to see if an X-ray is required to rule out a bone fracture.

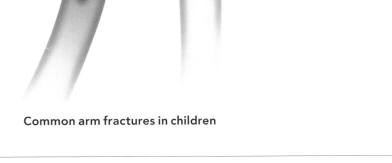

Greenstick fracture

Buckle fracture

Common arm fractures in children

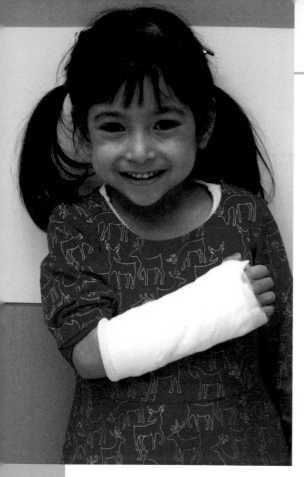

Signs of a Fracture

- Pain
- Swelling
- Deformity
- Difficulty using — or a refusal to use — the affected limb
- Significant warmth, bruising, and redness of the affected area

❸ How Is an Arm Fracture Treated?

If any of these fracture signs or symptoms are present, your child should be seen by a doctor. Most fractures will be diagnosed with a regular X-ray. Treatment of a fracture involves pain relief to make your child comfortable, and the arm's immobilization in a cast or splint. Surgery may sometimes be necessary to ensure the bones continue to grow properly if they are not straight enough or the fracture involves the bone's growth center.

❹ What Is a Pulled Elbow?

Pulled elbow (sometimes called a nursemaid's elbow) is a very common injury in children between 1 and 5 years of age. It occurs when a bone in the forearm, called the radius, slips through the ligament surrounding it, caused by a sudden pull or twist on the arm or wrist. This can happen when swinging a child around by the hands or even by a very minor awkward twist while pulling on the outstretched hand. Children may cry and complain of pain or simply stop using the arm. They will often hold it close to their side. There is no visible swelling or deformity to see.

When should we contact our doctor or local hospital?

If after a "swinging" game or twisting movement of the arm as described above, your toddler refuses to use his arm, then you will need to seek medical attention to confirm the diagnosis of pulled elbow and have it manipulated back into place.

Case Study

Andy's Pulled Elbow

Andy is a 2-year-old boy. One day he was at the park with his father. It was time to go home, but Andy insisted on staying at the park. He pulled his father's arm to get him to join him at the swings. Andy's father pulled back, telling Andy that playtime was over. Andy cried out immediately, and held his arm limply by his side. He refused to move it. His father brought Andy to the doctor for assessment.

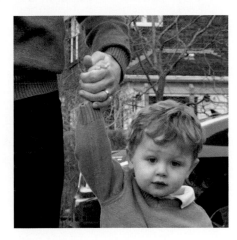

Andy was diagnosed with pulled elbow. Andy's doctor explained that the forearm bone had slipped out of place when he was pulled away from the swings. He did a quick maneuver to put the bone back in place and Andy felt better immediately. He began using his arm normally and no further treatment was needed.

Don't pull or swing your toddler around by the hands!

❺ How Is Pulled Elbow Treated?

It can usually be treated quickly and effectively by a health-care provider by manipulating the arm. No X-ray is needed, and children usually return to normal within minutes. The treatment for this is quick. Your child will be smiling and back to normal in minutes! Some children are susceptible to pulled elbows. Prevention is the best treatment!

Doc Talk Why a bone breaks is sometimes mysterious. Children are more likely than adults to suffer a fracture because their bones are softer and their ligaments are relatively stronger. The same force that causes a fracture in a child is likely to cause a sprain in an adult. Children's bones also differ from adult bones in that they continue to grow in length through growth centers found at the ends of the long bones. Sometimes there is nothing to see in terms of injury or swelling, but the child refuses to move her arm. To be safe, get medical attention.

Attention Deficit Hyperactivity Disorder (ADHD)

What Can I Do?

▶ If your child has ADHD, work with teachers and doctors to identify any coexisting disorders in order to put together the most effective management plan.

▶ Know that treatment can help prevent the cycle of negative interactions between a child with ADHD and his peers, his parents, and his teachers.

▶ Understanding ADHD can help you to be patient with your child — don't give up.

❶ What Is Attention Deficit Hyperactivity Disorder?

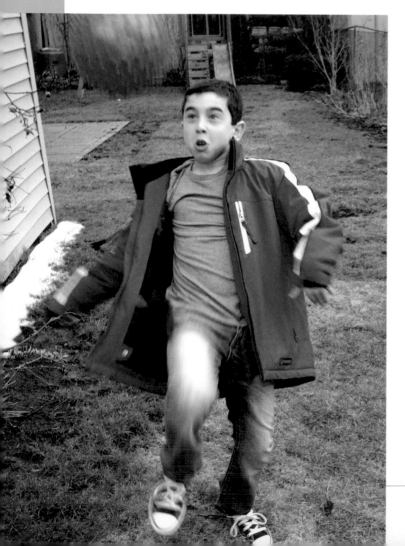

ADHD is a developmental disorder that occurs to varying degrees of severity in 5% to 10% of school-aged children. Children with ADHD tend to be impulsive, distractible, inattentive, and, in many cases, fidgety. These behaviors usually interfere with learning and create difficulties in interpersonal relationships at home, in school, and with peers.

Types of ADHD

- *Inattentive:* Children who are easily distracted
- *Hyperactive-Impulsive:* Children who are hyperactive and/or impulsive
- *Combined type:* Children who have features of both inattention and hyperactivity/impulsivity

Symptoms of ADHD

Inattentive symptoms	• Careless mistakes, poor attention to detail • Trouble keeping attention on task • Does not listen well when spoken to • Does not follow instructions, has difficulty finishing schoolwork and chores	• Avoids tasks requiring a lot of mental effort (homework) • Often loses things (toys, homework, pencils) • Easily distracted • Forgetful in daily activities
Hyperactivity symptoms	• Fidgets with hands, squirms in seat • Gets up from seat when supposed to be seated • Runs about and climbs when not appropriate	• Difficulty playing quietly • "On the go" or "Driven by a motor" • Talks excessively
Impulsivity symptoms	• Blurts out answers • Trouble waiting one's turn	• Interrupts others (in conversations or games)

When should we contact our doctor or local hospital?

ADHD is not a medical emergency. If your child has symptoms of ADHD, arrange meetings with your child's doctor, teachers, and caregivers to assess your child's behavior.

Social Consequences

In the classroom, if the underlying problem is not well understood, children with ADHD — with their hyperactivity and impulsivity — are often viewed as difficult children who are wilfully disobedient. At home, problems following through with instructions, forgetfulness, and impulsivity can result in conflict with parents and siblings. Children with ADHD talk before they think, resulting in fights with peers or difficulty maintaining friendships.

❷ What Causes ADHD?

The exact cause of ADHD is unknown, but several factors have been identified.

• Heredity plays a role, as ADHD is more common in families that have another child or a parent with ADHD.
• Children with ADHD may have differences in the balance of chemicals in the brain called neurotransmitters.

Did You Know?

Stimulation
Children with ADHD often seem engaged in a chosen activity at home, such as watching TV or playing a video game. They are able to maintain focus well because these types of activities are actually very stimulating with lights, sounds, and pictures.

Though commonly present in ADHD, hyperactivity, impulsivity, and inattention can occur for other reasons. It is essential that the health-care professional who makes the diagnosis of ADHD evaluate your child carefully for other possible causes of his difficulties.

- Learning disabilities
- Anxiety
- Hearing problems
- Vision problems
- Home stressors, parental conflict
- Depression
- Oppositional defiant disorder
- Conduct disorder

Diagnosis

The diagnosis of ADHD is made by a physician or psychologist, based on the assessment of information provided by parents and school personnel describing the child's functioning at home, in social situations and at school.

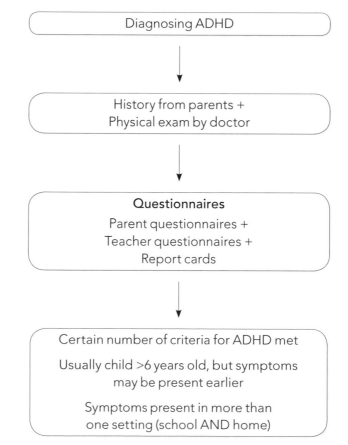

Diagnosing ADHD

↓

History from parents +
Physical exam by doctor

↓

Questionnaires
Parent questionnaires +
Teacher questionnaires +
Report cards

↓

Certain number of criteria for ADHD met

Usually child >6 years old, but symptoms may be present earlier

Symptoms present in more than one setting (school AND home)

❸ How Is ADHD Treated?

ADHD is a long-term problem for which there is no quick solution. A coordinated management plan with good communication among parents, teachers, physicians, and mental health professionals is essential. Treatment can include both behavior management and medication. The goals of treatment should be specific for each child and family, and clearly established before initiating a management plan. Patience, perseverance, close monitoring of the management plan, and frequent reassessment are important.

Goals of Treatment

- Improvement in school performance
- Decreased disruptive behaviors
- Increased independence
- Improvement in relationships with family members, teachers, and peers
- Improved self-esteem
- Improved accident and injury prevention

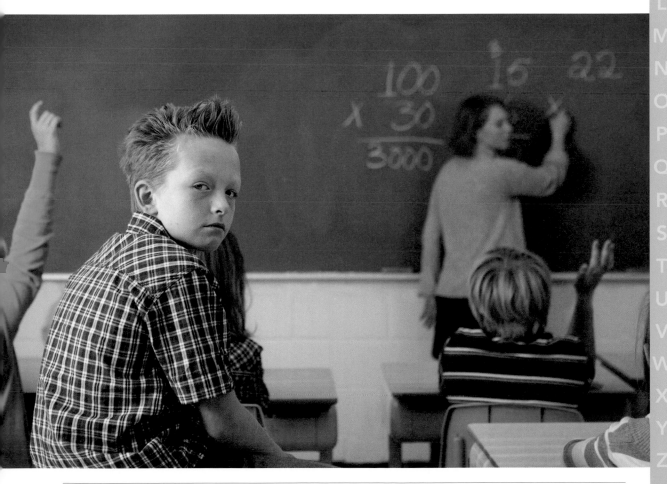

Medications

The decision to start your child on daily medication is often a difficult one. However, medication has been shown to be a highly effective way to improve the ability to focus and reduce impulsivity in children with ADHD. Recognize that medications do not cure this disorder. Medications work by restoring the normal chemical balance in the brain. Medications should be carefully administered, target symptoms should be recognized and evaluated and side effects monitored closely. The doctor will have to choose the dose of medication producing the maximum beneficial effect with minimum side effects.

Common Myths about ADHD Medication

Growth is suppressed

No significant differences in final adult height in studies with patients taking Ritalin compared to those not on Ritalin.

Stimulant medications are addictive

The formulations now available are released slowly into the brain so that a "high" and subsequent addiction is not experienced.

My child will appear to be "drugged"

In the right dose, your child should experience a reduction in his inattention and hyperactivity problems without being sedated or "drugged."

Medications Commonly Used in Treating ADHD

Medication Type	Examples	Common Side Effects
Stimulant	• Methylphenidate (Ritalin, Concerta , Biphentin) • Dextroamphetamine (Dexedrine) • Amphetamine-dextroamphetamine (Adderall) • Lisdeamfetamine (Vyvanse)	• Appetite suppression • Sleep disturbance • Anxiety • Irritability
Non-stimulant	• Atomoxetine (Strattera)	• Appetite suppression • Suicidal thinking
Antidepressants	• Sertraline (Zoloft), Paroxetine (Paxil) • Bupropion (Wellbutrin)	• Restlessness • Agitation • Sleep disturbance • Headache
Alpha-2-agonist	• Clonidine (Catapres)	• Sedation

Behavioral Interventions

Living with and teaching a child with ADHD can, at times, be frustrating and difficult. It is important to remember that children with ADHD are usually not trying to annoy others, but are unable to inhibit their responses. One of the most effective means of preventing loss of self-esteem and subsequent negative consequences is to promote an area of strength in your child — something that makes him happy and gives a sense of accomplishment. This could be a sport, music, art, or any other activity that he enjoys.

Behavior Modification

There are several proven strategies for modifying behavior in a child with ADHD:

- Modifications in the classroom and at home can help minimize distractions and maximize independence.
- Children with ADHD often require organizational aids and reminders. You might pin reminders to his school bag or bedroom door to help him become more independent and prevent a fourth trip to school with something he forgot!
- Preferential seating, for example at the front of the classroom, can help reduce distractions. Increased structure and routine can help.
- Use rewards and appropriate consequences consistently to increase appropriate behavior and reduce targeted inappropriate behaviors.
- Good communication among home, school, and health-care professionals is essential in establishing the success of such management programs.

> **Did You Know?**
>
> **Alternatives**
>
> Alternative therapies for ADHD have not been proven and may even be harmful. Use of megavitamins, essential fatty acids, restrictive diets, eye training exercises, eye glasses, tinted lenses, chiropractic treatments, and biofeedback have not been demonstrated to be effective in carefully controlled trials. Some of these treatments, such as megavitamins and restrictive diets, can even be harmful.

Doc Talk Most children with ADHD can function well when parents, teachers, and siblings are provided an explanation for the symptoms, and the appropriate management is put in place. If your child has more severe behavior difficulties or psychiatric disorders, family counseling and management coordinated with a mental health professional may be of assistance.

Autism (Autism Spectrum Disorder)

What Can I Do?

▶ Because children with autism spectrum disorders respond better to a predictable routine, be sure to plan daily events meticulously using a written and pictorial schedule.

▶ Role playing social situations can be helpful.

▶ Support your school-age child by providing his teachers with an information sheet on his condition and what works best for him.

▶ Build a support network. Parenting a child with autism is frequently frustrating and draining. You may find it helpful to connect with other parents of children with ASD.

❶ What Is Autism Spectrum Disorder?

Did You Know?

New Diagnostic Criteria

Autism spectrum disorder used to have several diagnoses that fell on the "spectrum," including autism, Asperger's syndrome, pervasive developmental disorder not otherwise specified, Rett syndrome, and childhood disintegrative disorder. Recent changes to diagnostic criteria have lumped these diagnoses under one umbrella called autism spectrum disorder, and the subtypes are no longer distinguished.

Children with autism spectrum disorder (ASD) have difficulties with social interaction and communication. They will have some degree of difficulty (with some degree of disinterest) in having meaningful verbal and non-verbal interactions with others. They will also have restricted and repetitive behaviors. These difficulties may be quite mild or very severe, thus the word "spectrum," but in all cases cause some degree of functional impairment.

Autism does not imply abnormal intelligence or IQ (intelligence quotient). Autism is more of a difficulty with EQ (emotional quotient) or "social intelligence." Some children with autism spectrum disorders have severe cognitive delays, while others have a normal or above average IQ.

When should we contact our doctor or local hospital?

Autism spectrum disorder is not an emergency situation. Children with more severe forms of ASD might not talk, play differently, ignore other children, and have repetitive behaviors, such as hand flapping. Children with a milder form of these disorders might speak and interact but, compared with other children their age, can seem unusual in how they converse or have some "odd" behaviors.

Signs and Symptoms

Problems with Communication and Social Interaction

Affected children have difficulties in both verbal (use of spoken language) and non-verbal communication (use of eye contact, pointing, facial expressions, and gestures). They may not speak at all, or talk later than expected, or speak unusually, for example in a high-pitched, song-like voice lacking variation in tone or unusually repetitive. They might use minimal eye contact or none at all. However, it should be noted that many children with autism spectrum disorder can use some eye contact. Pointing at things is frequently delayed.

Children with ASD typically show less interest in playing with other children. They do not share interests with others as you would expect from a child of their age. Imaginative play may be limited compared with other children of the same age. They may have difficulty expressing a range of emotions and recognizing other's emotions.

Fixed or Repetitive Behavior

Typically, children with autism play with toys in unusual ways. They might enjoy watching the wheels of a car spin repetitively. There may be unusual interest in certain sensations, such as the feeling of sand running through fingers, the look of running water, or the sound and sight of a plastic plate spinning. Other children can have an intense dislike of some sensations, such as the feeling of certain clothes or the sound of a baby crying. They might make repetitive movements, such as hand flapping, finger twisting, spinning around, pacing, or jumping.

Diagnosis

There is no single blood test or X-ray that indicates whether your child has autism. The diagnosis is made by gathering information from caregivers and educators and by observing your child directly. A physician or psychologist makes the diagnosis. This person uses the gathered information and decides whether defined criteria are met. A child does not need to have each and every feature on the

Did You Know?

Limited Success

There is no medication that has been found so far to be helpful to treat the basic symptoms of autism. Some children with autism have other associated behavior problems for which medication may be helpful. Treatments such as restricted diets, megavitamins, holding therapy and auditory training have not been shown to be effective and some may even be harmful.

criteria list to be diagnosed with ASD, but symptoms must begin in early childhood and cause functional impairment. Children with a diagnosis of ASD have:

1. Problems reciprocating social or emotional interaction;
2. Problems developing or maintaining relationships;
3. Nonverbal communication problems;

and two of the following:
- Stereotyped or repetitive speech, motor movements, or use of objects
- Excessive adherence to routines or rituals
- Restricted interests
- Unusual interest in sensory aspects of the environment

❷ What Causes Autism?

No one knows for sure. In a small number of cases, there might be an underlying genetic problem, such as fragile X syndrome, that can be determined by a blood test. There does appear to be a genetic basis for autism, because the chance of having a child with autism is increased in families that already have someone diagnosed with ASD.

❸ How Is Autism Treated?

Unfortunately, there is currently no cure available for autism. However, there are treatments that can result in behavioral improvements. Early and intensive interventions are associated with a better outcome. The forms of treatment of autism that are currently felt to be most effective include speech and language therapy and a specific form of behavioral intervention to develop communication, socialization, and play skills, called applied behavioral analysis (ABA) or intensive behavioral intervention (IBI).

Doc Talk

It's 100% certain that it is not your fault! In the past, parents were often blamed for causing or contributing to their child's autism by inadequate or improper parenting; however, research suggests that this disorder is something children are born with. Parenting a child with autism is frequently frustrating and draining. You may find it helpful to connect with other parents of children with ASD to support one another. Allow yourself to be helped by friends and family and be open to assistance from your community.

Backache

What Can I Do?

▶ If your child repeatedly complains of back strain, try a routine of simple but specific exercises that can be obtained from your child's health-care provider.

▶ For acute pain relief, use an ice pack, followed by local heat using a hot water bottle or heating pad.

▶ Be active. Encourage your child to maintain good overall physical fitness.

❶ What Is Backache?

Back pain is a frequent complaint in adults, but did you know that it is also prevalent in older children and adolescents? The spine is a truly remarkable anatomical structure. This flexible column consists of 24 bones (vertebrae) that protect the spinal cord housed inside them. The vertebrae are separated by shock-absorbing discs of cartilage, fastened together by numerous ligaments, and all moved by an array of muscles.

When should we contact our doctor or local hospital?

Common backache is usually described as an aching or stiffness in the middle or lower back that becomes abruptly painful with lifting or arching the back. It tends to resolve gradually after a week or two. Unfortunately, recurrences tend to be common. If it doesn't seem to be getting better or red flag symptoms are present, see your doctor.

⏩ Backache Red Flags

See your doctor right away if your child has:

- Inability to walk
- Extreme pain that is not relieved by analgesic medication
- Back pain with fever, weight loss, or lethargy
- Pain that travels down the back of the leg below the knee
- Pain associated with numbness and tingling
- A major change in bowel/bladder habits
- Appearance of being very sick
- Pain as a direct result of trauma
- Pain that wakes him up at night

> **» Backache Red Flags**

In the following circumstances, you should also consider seeking medical care:

- If the pain is no better after 3 days of treatment
- If your child is younger than 10 years old
- If the back pain is recurrent

❷ What Causes Backache?

The majority of back pain in older children is the result of straining some of the 200 muscles that allow us to move our back or maintain our posture. Usually, the cause can be identified as an injury, overdoing some physical activity, or lifting a heavy object awkwardly. Back strain can result from:

❶ Carrying heavy, improperly packed or positioned backpacks. Backpacks have become the standard device for carrying schoolbooks. If they are not properly fitted, they can cause back strain.

❷ Physical activity and computer usage. It seems that active children are less likely to complain of common backache than sedentary ones. There is also a positive correlation between the number of hours spent at a computer and the frequency of back pain. On the other end of the spectrum, competitive athletes are more prone to back injury. This can be from the stress caused on the back due to hyperextension of the spine (bending far back) as seen in gymnastics, dancing, and diving. Injury in athletes also occurs due to overstretching or contact injury to muscles.

❸ Personality type and underlying mood. Recurrent backache is more likely to occur in children who have a high degree of psychosocial difficulty or previously complained of other pain symptoms, particularly tension headache or nonspecific recurrent abdominal pain. Such individuals seem to respond more intensely to their body' signals.

Backpack Safety

The American Academy of Pediatrics has several tips for backpack safety:

- Distribute the weight properly by using packs with wide padded shoulders and wearing both shoulder straps and a waist strap.
- Tighten the straps so the pack is close to the body.
- Use a lightweight pack with a padded back or one on wheels.
- Pack properly! Avoid overstuffing and distribute the weight evenly by using all compartments.

Other Associated Causes

The list of disorders associated with back pain is quite lengthy. Sometimes, backache can be due to very unusual structural causes, such as spondylolysis (fracture in the vertebrae) or spondylolisthesis (horizontal slippage of the vertebrae). Disc problems are not common in children, but if they occur they usually present as an infection (discitis) and not degeneration of the disc as in older people. The bones of the back can also get infected (osteomyelitis). Rarely, spinal or other tumors cause back pain. Kidney infections (pyelonephritis) or even inflammatory bowel disease are also causes of back pain. Remember, these conditions are very rare, and present with other associated symptoms. Most of the time, muscle strain will be the problem. When in doubt, have your child examined.

Scoliosis

Scoliosis is an abnormal sideways spinal curvature. It may appear as if the child's shoulders are uneven or the hips are not level. The condition is common, especially in pre-adolescent and adolescent females. If a health-care provider suspects scoliosis based on a physical exam, he may order a full X-ray of the spine and try to measure the degree of the curvature. Depending on the severity of the curvature and its progression over time (which can be aggravated by a growth spurt) an orthopedic surgeon will manage scoliosis either conservatively with observation or in more severe cases with a specially designed back brace or surgery.

Did You Know?

Chiropractic Treatment

Chiropractic treatment has been shown to help many adults with recurrent back pain, but its effectiveness for younger patients is less established. Massage certainly can provide short-term pain relief but is unlikely to resolve the problem or prevent recurrence.

Did You Know?

Scoliosis Study

In a large pediatric study of scoliosis, about a quarter of patients reported pain, especially older teenagers and those who had completed their growth.

Doc Talk

The pain of muscle strain is often relieved by simple painkillers, like ibuprofen or acetaminophen. A firm mattress, reinforced with a board if necessary, may help with sleep. Complete bed rest is not usually necessary, but your child should avoid activities that aggravate the pain, especially heavy lifting and jarring sports. The best way to prevent recurrent backache is to maintain good overall physical fitness.

Bed-Wetting (Enuresis)

What Can I Do?

▶ Do not blame or punish your child; rather, support and reassure.

▶ Try a few simple strategies — for example, limit drinking, and encourage going to the washroom, just before bedtime.

▶ See your doctor if your child has been dry for 6 months and is now wetting again.

▶ If treatment is necessary, options include behavioral interventions, alarms, bladder exercises, and medication.

❶ What Is Enuresis?

Most children will become toilet trained between 2 and 4 years of age. However, bed-wetting still occurs in about 40% of 3-year-olds and 20% of 5-year-olds. Boys are more likely than girls to have bed-wetting. Interestingly, there seems to be a tendency for bed-wetting to run in families. If you were a bed-wetter (you will likely need to ask your own parents about this), your child has a 45% chance of following in your wet footsteps. If both you and your child's other parent were bed-wetters, then this likelihood goes up to 77%!

Categories of Bed-Wetting

Not all bed-wetting is the same. Try to distinguish between primary and secondary enuresis.

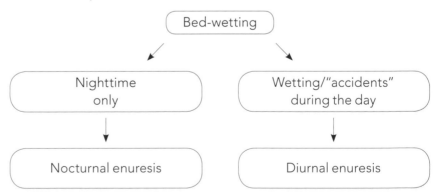

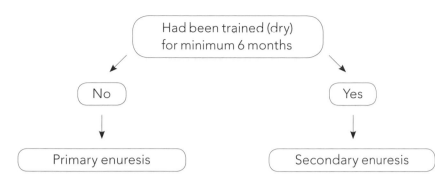

Enuresis and Age

Most parents become concerned about nighttime bed-wetting after the age of 5 or 6 years, although children themselves aren't usually concerned about the issue until 7 or 8 years of age. Daytime wetting may be considered a problem in a child older than 4 years who wets on most days. A child who was previously trained and begins wetting during the day or night has secondary enuresis and should be taken to her doctor to rule out any underlying problem. Children almost always outgrow their bed-wetting, meaning that many will manage well without any specific treatment at all. Only 5% of 10-year-olds and 2% of 16-year-olds will still be bed-wetters.

When should we contact our doctor or local hospital?

Primary Enuresis

Make an appointment to see your child's doctor if you notice these signs and symptoms:

- *Nighttime wetting:* Starts to bother your child, usually by the age of 7 or 8 years
- *Daytime wetting:* Persists from the age of 5 years

Secondary Enuresis

Make an appointment to see your child's doctor, especially if your child presents with these additional symptoms:

- *Frequent urination (urinating more frequently than in the past):* Could be a clue to a bladder infection
- *Polyuria (passing large amounts of urine):* Could be a clue to diabetes
- *Dysuria (burning or pain while urinating):* Could be a clue to a bladder infection
- *Cloudy or smelly urine:* Could be a clue to a bladder infection
- *Constipation:* Can lead to incomplete emptying of the bladder and infection
- *New problems with walking or passing stools:* Could rarely be a spinal cord problem

❷ What Causes Enuresis?

Primary Enuresis

In most cases, bed-wetting is simply a result of a delayed maturation of the parts of the nervous system that control the bladder. Different children are ready for bladder control at different ages. Just like some babies are walking at 9 months and other normal infants only start at 15 months, each individual develops at a different pace. Also, the bladder may not be developed enough to hold urine for a full night. Clues to this lack of readiness include frequent small amounts of urine passed during the daytime or wetness several times during the night. In addition, the child may not be developmentally capable of recognizing that the bladder is full and that she needs to wake up and go to the washroom.

Secondary Enuresis

This can often result from a new stress in the child's life, for example, the arrival of a new sibling, illness, bullying, or a death in the family, even divorce. Very rarely, underlying conditions, such as diabetes or sickle cell disease, can cause secondary enuresis. Constipation and various bladder problems such as infections can also contribute to bed-wetting.

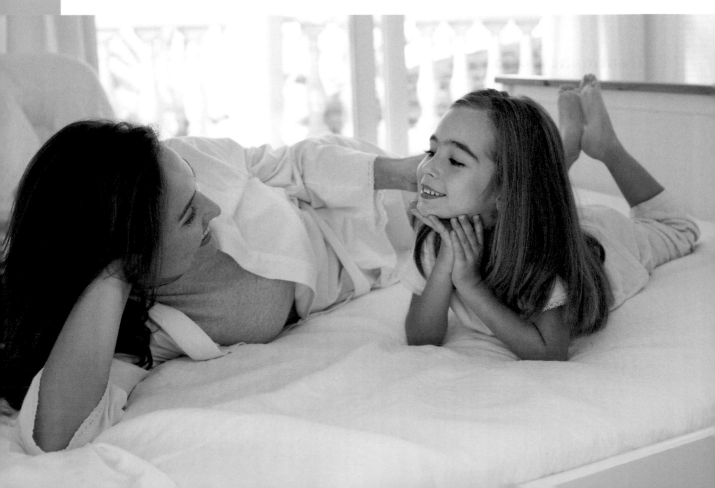

Many of these children display additional symptoms that provide clues to the source of the problem. For example, excess urine production (polyuria) is seen in diabetes. Children with bladder infections might also have pain (dysuria) and frequent urination. They usually need to urinate urgently, and the urine passed may be cloudy and smelly. Constipated children will have very hard, infrequent stools and may also leak some liquid stool (encopresis).

Diurnal Enuresis (Daytime Wetting)

Daytime wetting can be caused by problems with the nerve supply to the bladder (for example, with spina bifida or cerebral palsy). If there is a spinal cord problem, then walking and bowel motions can also be affected. Developmental behavioral issues can also be a factor. One such example includes children with poorly controlled attention deficit hyperactivity disorder (ADHD) who are easily distracted and forget to go to the washroom until it is too late. Other possible causes of daytime wetting include constipation, urinary tract infections, and diabetes.

❸ How Is Enuresis Treated?

Children almost always outgrow their bed-wetting, so many will manage well without any specific treatment at all. When bed-wetting persists, there are several effective treatment strategies.

Treatment Options
- Supportive behavioral interventions
- Bed-wetting alarm
- Bladder exercises
- Medication

Helpful Hints for Managing Bed-Wetting

Enuresis is usually embarrassing for a child and may lead to reluctance to sleep over at a friend's home or go to camp. Some common-sense, simple rules can help.

- Your child should not drink, especially anything containing caffeine, just before bedtime (but do not send a child to bed thirsty).
- Encourage your child to go to the washroom just before bedtime.
- Use a waterproof cover on the mattress.
- If your older child wets the bed, you might want to encourage her to help with changing the bedding. This should not be seen as a

---

Did You Know?

Positive Reinforcement

A calendar on which your child gets to place a sticker after each dry night provides extra motivation. A certain number of stickers is often rewarded with some form of treat or incentive. This is successful in about 20% of children, although some of them do relapse.

punishment, but more as a form of self-sufficiency. Make sure that any other children in the family are also given chores so that one child doesn't feel singled out.

- Encouraging your child to go to bed without diapers when he is not ready is unlikely to help.
- Prevent teasing by other family members: they should be sensitive to the problem.

Bed-Wetting Alarms

Bed-wetting alarms are often recommended with enuresis, particularly for older children who are highly motivated to achieve dryness. There are many different types of alarms. They usually consist of a device for sensing wetness, which is attached to the child's pajamas close to the groin, and a buzzer close by. The first drops of urine will set off the alarm, which wakes the child and stops the urination. The child then shuts off the alarm and goes to the washroom.

Bladder-Stretching Exercises

Some doctors may recommend bladder-stretching exercises, such as encouraging the child to hold on for a few minutes after the initial urge to urinate. This is theoretically helpful in a child with a small functional bladder capacity, but the effectiveness of these exercises is inconclusive.

Medicines

There are a number of medications, such as desmopressin (DDAVP), that are prescribed for the treatment of bed-wetting. Because this is a developmental problem that tends to get better with time, the risks and benefits of these options should be carefully discussed before starting medication. These medications are particularly useful for short-term concerns, such as ensuring dryness on overnight stays with friends or at overnight camp.

Doc Talk The most important thing for you to remember is that enuresis is an unconscious and involuntary behavior. Your child is not trying to make things difficult for you. Most parents do not enjoy having to constantly change and wash the bedding, but resist your feelings of frustration and anger. You need to make sure that your child understands that it is not his fault, that you do not blame him or think he is lazy, and that it will get better with time.

Bee and Wasp Stings

What Can I Do?

▶ Swelling of the lips or tongue, difficulty breathing, or a choking sensation in the throat indicates a medical emergency. Give an epinephrine self-injection pen if available, call 911, and get to the nearest hospital ASAP.

▶ For local reactions, wash with soap and water, remove the stinger if possible, apply a cold compress, and give an antihistamine and pain reliever.

▶ Encourage your child to wear shoes outside and to avoid drinking from an unattended soda pop or juice can when outside. Bees frequently fly inside.

❶ What Are Bee and Wasp Stings?

Bees and wasps usually "sting" in self-defense (or to subdue prey) by injecting venom through a stinger at the end of their bodies. Although honeybees may leave a stinger, wasps and hornets don't. How your child will react to the sting ranges from slight irritation to life-threatening anaphylaxis.

RELATED CONDITIONS

• Anaphylaxis

When should we contact our doctor or local hospital?

A generalized or anaphylactic reaction to a sting is a medical emergency. Follow the procedure for bee and wasp sting red flags.

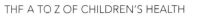

Wasp sting

➤➤ Bee and Wasp Sting Red Flags

A child can react in two ways: locally (at the site of the sting) or generally (when the whole body reacts). A generalized reaction to a bee or wasp sting is an emergency! Give an epinephrine self-injection pen, call 911 to get to your nearest hospital, and give an oral antihistamine (for example, diphenhydramine/Benadryl), if available. Even if your child seems completely recovered, he should still be seen at the emergency room at the nearest hospital. See How to Use an Epinephrine Self-Injection Pen (pages 45 and 46) for instructions.

Reactions

Generally, stings by honeybees, yellow jackets, and hornets produce similar reactions. The particular reaction of any child is governed by his sensitivity, the number of attacking insects, and his age.

Local Reactions

Depending on the child's reaction, a sting can vary from a small, red, itchy raised spot to a larger hive that can measure an inch or more (several centimeters) in diameter. There can be swelling, pain, or itchiness at the site of the sting. Local reactions can be quite dramatic, with a sting leading to swelling of both the hand and arm. While uncomfortable and unsightly, local reactions are not a major concern to your child's immediate health.

Local vs. Generalized Reactions

Type of Reaction	What It Looks Like	What You Can Do
Local	• Red, itchy, painful raised spot • Large hive • Swelling	• Wash with soap and water • Remove stinger ASAP (if there is one) • Apply a cold compress or ice • Elevate the area • Give an antihistamine — for example, diphenhydramine (Benadryl)
Generalized, severe (anaphylactic) — a medical emergency!	• Tingling around mouth or face • Pale, cold, clammy • Dizzy • Swelling of lips or tongue • Difficulty breathing • Choking sensation	• Inject with an epinephrine self-injection pen (if available) • Call 911 • Rush to nearest hospital • Give a steroid (for example, prednisone) • Give an antihistamine — for example, diphenhydramine (Benadryl)

Generalized Reactions

The major concern with stings is the development of a severe, generalized (systemic) allergic response. This is called an anaphylactic or hypersensitivity reaction. Acute hypersensitivity reactions can cause swelling of the lips or tongue, difficulty breathing, or a choking sensation in the throat. The first symptom is frequently a tingling sensation around the mouth or face. This is a true emergency.

❷ How Is a Bee or Wasp Sting Treated?

First Response

- Wash the area with soap and water.
- If there is a stinger, remove it as quickly as possible to reduce the amount of venom released into the skin; it is best removed by a gentle scraping motion or use tweezers if available.
- Treat local reactions with ice or cold compresses to decrease the swelling. You can give your child an oral antihistamine to decrease the reaction and relieve the itch.
- Provide pain relief with acetaminophen or ibuprofen, if needed.
- Be especially alert to the signs of anaphylaxis.

How To: Remove a Stinger

- Identify the stinger.
- Remove with tweezers, if available.
- If tweezers are not available, brush away the stinger with a gentle scraping motion using your fingernail or the blunt side of a knife.

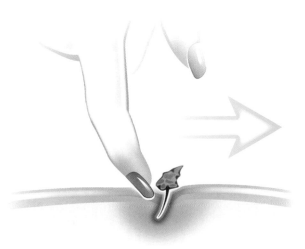

Brush away stinger with gentle scraping motion

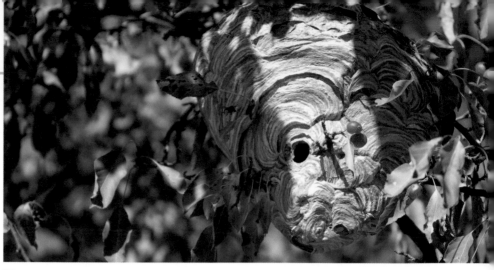

Wasp nest

Prevention

The best treatment is prevention. Here are some simple strategies to avoid bees, wasps, and other stinging insects.

- Don't let your child walk outside in bare feet.
- Stay away and keep your child away from any nests or locations where you see many flying insects gathering at one spot.
- At picnics and when eating outdoors, don't let children drink from opened beverage cans that have been sitting around. Bees frequently fly into sweet drink containers.
- Keep all food covered.
- Cover garbage cans and keep them away from eating areas.
- Avoid using strong perfumes and hair sprays — they attract stinging insects.

Allergic Response

If you know your child is susceptible to generalized reactions, you must have a plan to respond to these situations. Once a child has experienced an anaphylactic reaction to bees, for example, you should have an epinephrine self-injection pen available at all times. Your child should also wear a medical alert bracelet to identify the problem. Fortunately, only about one child in five who suffers an initial systemic reaction from a stinging insect will have a similar response with subsequent stings. You will have to educate your child's teacher and other caregivers about his reaction to stings.

Doc Talk Desensitization injections (allergy shots) have more than a 95% rate of success in preventing a future anaphylactic reaction to a specific stinging insect. Talk to your child's doctor about this option if your child has experienced a life-threatening reaction.

Birthmarks

A B C D E F G H I J K L M N O P Q R S T U V W X Y Z

What Can I Do?

▶ Reassure your child and yourself that birthmarks are harmless and that many will fade with time.

▶ Discuss with your doctor any occasional red flag symptoms.

▶ Take a photo of the birthmark so you can note any changes over time.

❶ What Is a Birthmark?

Birthmarks are very common irregularities on the skin, present in 20% to 40% of infants. Most are present right at birth, with a smaller proportion becoming noticeable in the weeks to months following delivery.

When should we contact our doctor or local hospital?

Most birthmarks are completely harmless and many will fade over time. A small number of birthmarks signify an important underlying medical condition. See the list of red flags for hemangiomas (page 81) and the ABCs of assessment for moles (page 82).

RELATED CONDITIONS

- Freckles
- Hemangioma
- Moles (melanocytic nevi)
- Mongolian spot (slate-gray nevus)
- Port wine stain (nevus flammeus)
- Salmon patch (nevus simplex)

Types of Birthmarks

There are several kinds of birthmarks, and most of them are innocuous — except in a few cases.

Salmon Patch (Nevus Simplex)

One of the most common birthmarks is a salmon patch. As the name suggests, these birthmarks appear pale pink, or salmon-colored, and are flat (if you run your fingers over one with your eyes closed, you cannot feel it). Typically, salmon patches appear on the nape of the neck ("stork bite") or over the eyelids ("angel kiss"). On the face, the patch usually disappears during the first year of life; those on the back of the neck persist.

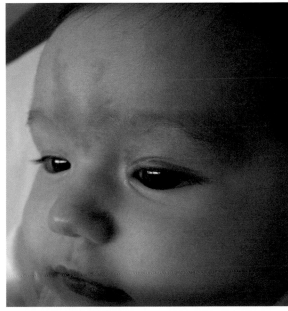

Salmon patch (angel kiss)

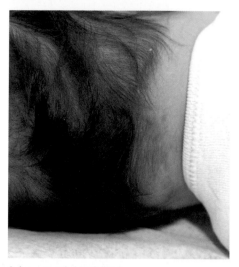

Salmon patch (stork bite)

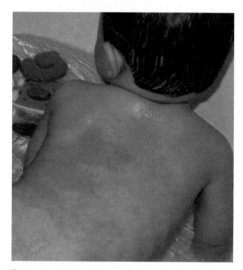

Port wine stain

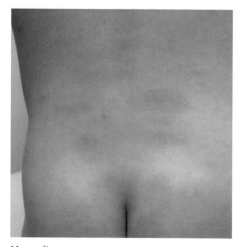

Mongolian spot

Port Wine Stain (Nevus Flammeus)

Port wine stains are flat birthmarks made up of small, abnormal blood vessels (capillaries). They usually appear reddish, pink, or purple. They are uniform in color, with a well-defined border. In the first year of life, some of these port wine stains might become a little lighter in color, but they don't completely disappear. As a child enters adolescence, the port wine stain may become more purple and bumpy. Port wine stains over the eye and upper part of the face may have associated eye and brain abnormalities. These should be evaluated by a dermatologist. Occasionally, port wine stains on the limbs may be accompanied by slightly unequal growth of the affected limb. These should also be evaluated by a dermatologist.

Mongolian Spot (Slate-Gray Nevus)

These birthmarks are flat, bluish-gray areas with wavy and irregular borders. They are most often seen on the lower back or buttocks of darker-skinned babies. They are particularly common in babies of Asian descent. Slate-gray nevi can sometimes be mistaken for bruising because of their color. These birthmarks usually disappear by 3 to 5 years of age and almost all are gone by puberty.

Hemangiomas

Hemangiomas are very common birthmarks caused by the excessive growth of immature blood vessels. They appear as raised red or bluish lumps or clumps of blood vessels ("strawberries") and often feel slightly warm to the touch compared with the surrounding skin. Hemangiomas may not be noticed at birth but can grow rapidly during the first several months of life. After this growth phase, the hemangioma slowly shrinks over several years. In general, about 60% of hemangiomas will disappear by 6 years of age, and 90% by age 9.

Common Hemangioma Concerns

See your health-care provider if your child's hemangioma has either of the following features:

- *Ulcerations:* Hemangiomas do not usually cause problems or discomfort. Occasionally, the skin overlying the hemangioma can open up and form an ulcer. This can be painful. Treatment to prevent infection and scarring, and to speed healing, is often warranted.
- *Bleeding:* Trauma to the hemangioma (picking or scratching) can cause the hemangioma to bleed. Typically, applying constant pressure for 15 minutes can stop any bleeding from the hemangioma. Ongoing bleeding despite pressure, beyond 15 minutes, should prompt a visit to the nearest emergency department.

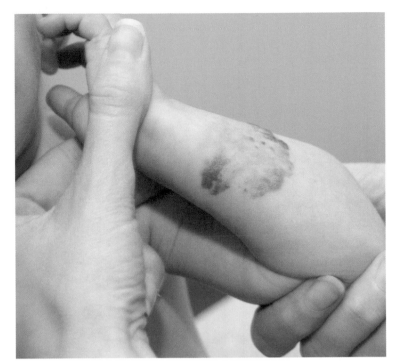
Hemangioma

➤ Hemangioma Red Flags

See your child's doctor about her hemangioma if it appears in any of the following areas:

- Around the eyes: May obstruct vision or prevent the eye from developing properly
- Tip of the nose: Can lead to deformities of the nose
- Lips: Can interfere with eating or ulcerate easily
- Chin or neck: May lead to breathing difficulties
- Diaper area: Humidity and irritation from a wet diaper can lead to ulceration and bleeding

How Is a Hemangioma Treated?

Most hemangiomas eventually shrink over time and require no treatment. However, certain features of hemangiomas warrant treatment with medication to prevent further growth and even promote rapid shrinkage of the birthmark. A very large hemangioma may be disfiguring or make daily activities difficult. See your child's doctor if you are concerned.

Moles (Melanocytic Nevi)

A mole is a type of birthmark made up of cells that create pigment (color) in the skin. These can range from light brown to almost black. Most moles are not problematic unless they are large (greater than $\frac{1}{2}$ inch/1 cm) or are growing rapidly.

The ABCs of Assessing Moles

When a doctor assesses a mole to see if it needs further testing, he uses his ABCs. You can do the same by assessing your child's skin for abnormal moles. Sometimes taking pictures of concerning moles can be helpful so that changes can be assessed over time. Consult your child's doctor if you are concerned that his mole is abnormal.

A	**Asymmetry:** Normal moles are usually symmetrical. If you were to draw a line down the middle of the mole, the two halves should look equal.
B	**Border:** A normal mole has a smooth, clearly defined border. Moles that are jagged or have blurry borders warrant assessment.
C	**Color:** Normal moles are generally uniform in color. New areas of white, black, brown, or red should prompt an assessment.
D	**Diameter:** Moles larger than the tip of your pencil eraser (about $\frac{1}{4}$ inch/5 mm) should be assessed by a doctor, even if all of the other features are normal.
E	**Evolution:** Moles that are evolving or growing, becoming rough to touch, ulcerating or bleeding, or painful deserve assessment.

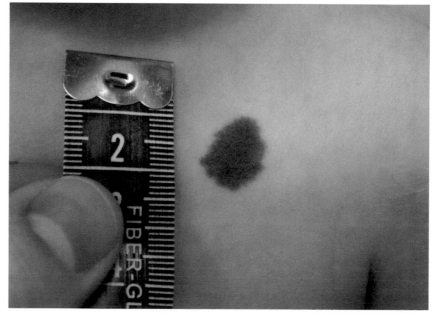

Mole

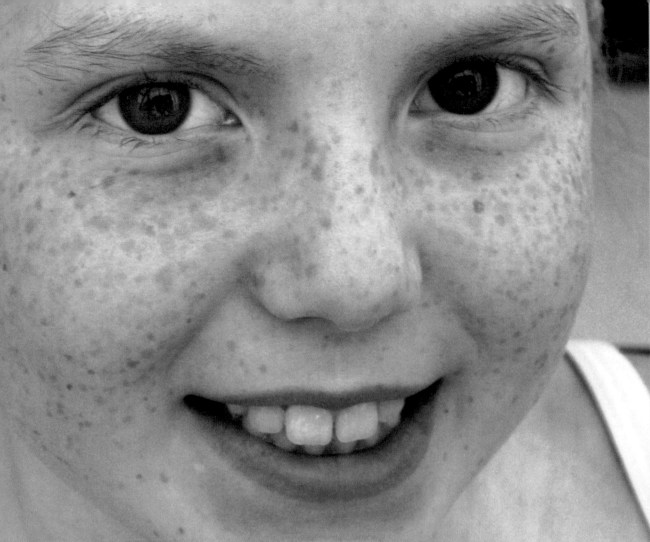

Freckles

Freckles

While they are not technically a birthmark, freckles are small, flat, brown marks on the skin. They are more common in people with lighter skin and eyes, and appear in sun-exposed areas. Freckles often run in families.

Freckles are caused by pigment (melanin) that accumulates in the skin. The sun stimulates the pigment cells (melanocytes) to produce pigment. This is why there might be a seasonal variation in the way freckles look: less noticeable in the winter months, and more noticeable in the summer months. To minimize these color changes, sun protection and sun avoidance is recommended.

> **Doc Talk** In some cultures, children born with birthmarks are honored, not stigmatized. Many birthmarks tend to disappear over time and very few are likely to be problematic.

Bites (Animal and Human)

What Can I Do?

▶ Administer first aid by washing the bite with soap and water, flushing under the tap, applying an antibiotic ointment and giving a pain reliever, if required.

▶ Check your child for signs of the bite becoming infected (red streaks, swelling, and increasing pain) and contact your doctor immediately if this is the case.

▶ Avoid dogs that might bite.

RELATED CONDITIONS

- Infections
- Rabies

❶ What Is an Animal Bite?

Most bite injuries are either scratches or puncture wounds. Claw wounds should be regarded in the same way as bites because the claws can contain saliva and germs. The deeper the wound (for example, when the skin is punctured), the higher the rate of infection compared with superficial lacerations.

When should we contact our doctor or local hospital?

Puncturing of the skin, signs of wound infection, and concern about the possibility of rabies are reasons to seek medical attention.

⏩ Animal Bite Red Flags

You need to either speak to or visit your doctor as soon as possible if:

- Rabies is a possibility (for example, a bite by a raccoon, a fox, a bat, or an unknown animal).
- Skin is split open.
- Wound puncture is deep.
- Your child looks sick or feverish.
- Pain is worse after 2 days.
- Any increase in the extent of the surrounding redness or swelling is noted. If you see red streaks moving outward from the wound, this indicates an infection. Up to 5% of dog bites will become infected, and 20% to 50% of cat bites become infected. If there are no signs of infection after 3 to 4 days, then infection is unlikely to occur.

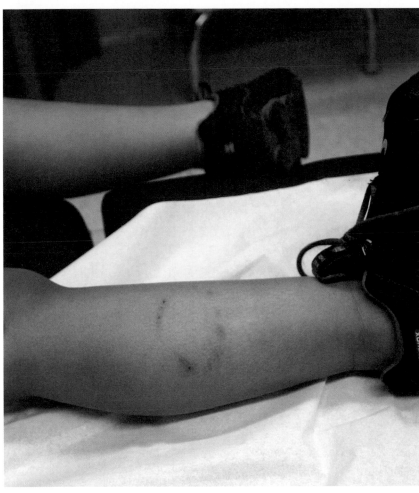

Dog bite on a child's leg

Rabies Alert

Rabies is caused by the rabies virus, which is passed from animals to humans, usually through a bite. Sometimes it can be passed by saliva from an infected animal. Many types of animals can pass rabies to people. Wild mammals — raccoons, skunks, foxes, coyotes, and bats — are the major sources of infection in North America. Dogs, cats, and even cattle can pass rabies to people too. Small rodents, such as hamsters, squirrels, guinea pigs, and rabbits, almost never spread rabies.

Symptoms

In humans, it usually takes from 4 to 6 weeks for the rabies infection to become a disease, but it can also range from 5 days to a year. Children who are infected with rabies become sick with fever and headache. They can then develop neurological symptoms, such as weakness or paralysis. The illness almost always leads to death.

Did You Know?

Who Bites and Who Tends to Get Bitten?

Children can be bitten by a variety of animals, and sometimes by other children! About 90% of all bite injuries are from dogs, cats, and humans. It is estimated that American children incur 4.7 million dog bites, 400,000 cat bites, and 250,000 human bites annually. The majority of dog bites happen to children between the ages of 6 and 11 years. Approximately two-thirds of these attacks occur around the home, and 75% of the biting animals are known to the children. Half of the attacks are said to be unprovoked. Boys seem more prone to dog bites, and girls to cat bites.

Did You Know?

Tetanus Risk
Although the risk of tetanus from an animal bite is extremely low, you should be sure to have your child's immunization records with you if you go to an emergency room to seek care.

Vaccine

After a bite, it is important to thoroughly clean the area with soap and water. A rabies vaccine and rabies immune globulin are available and should be administered after a child has been bitten by a wild or potentially infected animal. The rabies immune globulin is made up of antibodies, which are proteins that help the body fight this infection. The decision to give either or both of these should be made by your doctor, usually in communication with the local public health department.

❷ How Is an Animal Bite Treated?

Prevention of Animal Bites

The best treatment is prevention. Teach your child:

- Not to play with unfamiliar animals.
- Not to put his face near a dog.
- Not to stay alone with a dog, even if he is very familiar with it.
- Not to play around large, potentially aggressive dogs, such as rottweilers, pit bull terriers, and German shepherds.
- Not to tease or torment even a friendly animal.

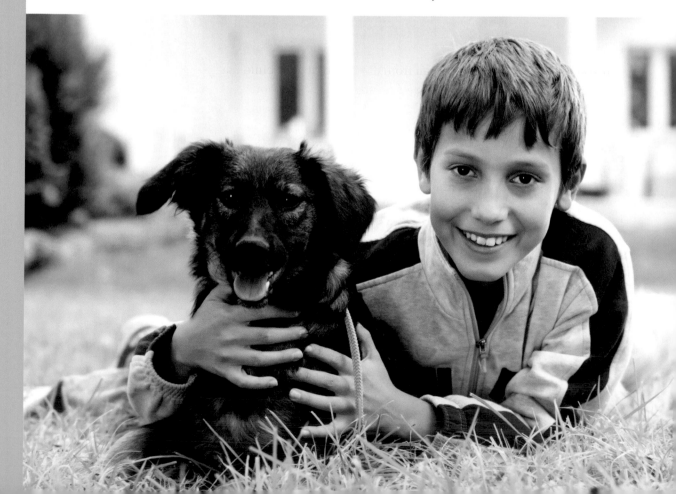

First Aid Treatment for Animal Bites

- Wash all bite wounds thoroughly with soap and water.
- Cleanse and flush the wound under a faucet for at least 5 to 10 minutes.
- Apply an antibiotic ointment.
- Use bandages, as needed.
- Administer pain relievers (optional).

Specific Animal Bite Treatments

Specific treatment will depend on the circumstances of the attack, particularly the type of animal involved.

- Small indoor pet rodents, such as gerbils and hamsters, pose no risk of rabies, and the bite seldom becomes infected. Your child will rarely need medical attention.
- Wild rodents, such as squirrels, mice, and chipmunks, are also considered rabies free, but their bites can cause other types of infections.
- Whenever rabies is a possibility, such as with a bite by a raccoon, fox, or bat, or an unprovoked attack by an unknown animal, your child will need to be seen by a doctor.

Did You Know?

Cat Scratch Disease

Cat scratch disease is a risk following cat bites or scratches. This presents with enlarged lymph nodes above the area of the bite or scratch, as well as a prolonged fever. The glands in the armpit (axilla) are the most likely to be infected. Kittens are more often the culprits than adult cats. A full recovery can be expected.

❸ What Is a Human Bite?

If you get the dreaded phone call from daycare that your child has been bitten by another child or has bitten another child, you are not alone. Children, especially toddlers, sometimes bite as a way of expressing their emotions. Most bites seem to involve the upper limbs or the face, but they seldom actually break the skin. Attention should first be given directly to the victim, not the biter. Biters need to be told that this is unacceptable behavior and will not be tolerated!

Most human bites are from toddlers and they usually do not penetrate the skin. If your child's skin is not broken, you don't have to take him to see a doctor. Simple cleansing and a hug will do.

First Aid Treatment for a Human Bite

If the skin is not broken:

- Wash all bite wounds thoroughly with soap and water.
- Apply a cold compress to the skin.
- Comfort the child.

If the skin is broken:

- Clean the wound under a faucet for at least 5 minutes.
- Apply an antibiotic ointment.
- Observe over the next few days for signs of infection.

➤➤ Human Bite Red Flags

Consult your child's doctor as soon as possible if your child has any of the following symptoms associated with a human bite:

- Skin is widely split open.
- Red streaks or swelling is noted, suggesting infection.
- Your child looks sick or feverish.
- Pain is worse after 2 days.
- Bites to the face, hand, foot, or genitals are more than just superficial abrasions.
- Your child has a bite or bites another child in a way that breaks the skin and is not fully immunized against hepatitis B.

FAQ

Is there any risk of transmission of a serious infection, like HIV or hepatitis B, through a bite from a human?
Transmission of HIV through a biting incident would be extremely unlikely unless there was considerable blood exchange. The same is true for hepatitis B. In some areas, children are immunized against hepatitis B in infancy, so these children would be immune anyway. If your child is not immune to hepatitis B and has been bitten or has bitten another child that breaks the skin, see your health-care provider for a vaccine. The risk of simple bacterial infection is very low.

Doc Talk

Animal and human bites that cause significant damage to the skin or underlying tissues, such as puncture wounds, should be assessed by a physician. Whether your child's doctor prescribes antibiotics to prevent infection depends on the location and nature of the wound. Your child's doctor will decide if he needs stitches. The need is variable and must be assessed on a case-by-case basis. Pets add immeasurably to a child's life. Although animal bites are a concern, you should not let that possibility stand in the way of bringing a pet into your family.

Bloody Stools

What Can I Do?

▶ Try to determine if there is blood in the stool. The blood can be bright red, purple, or tarry black. Use the symptoms guide table on page 90 to see if you can recognize your child's problem.

▶ If any red flags are present, or you are concerned, then seek medical advice.

▶ Help to avoid constipation.

▶ If cow's milk protein is a possible problem, remove it from your child's diet.

❶ What Is Blood in the Stool?

Blood in the stool can take on many different disguises. It can look like small amounts of fresh red blood, as if you had scratched yourself, or it can be plentiful, like a nosebleed. Blood can be just on the outside of the stool or it can be mixed in with the stool. If the blood has been in the intestines for a bit before coming out, it may have a much darker purple or even a tarry, black appearance. Sometimes you may see something red, black, or purple in the stool, that is not blood; it is just related to something that your child has eaten. Who hasn't seen the occasional pea or carrot come out the bottom still relatively intact?

RELATED CONDITIONS

- Anal fissure
- Constipation
- Cow's milk protein intolerance
- Infectious colitis

When should we contact our doctor or local hospital?

If there are no red flag symptoms and your child is well, you can just wait for the next stool to see if it is a single occurrence or a potential ongoing problem that needs attention.

▶▶ Blood in the Stool Red Flags

Seek immediate medical attention if your child has any of the following symptoms associated with blood in the stool:

■ Has more than one episode of significant blood in the stool without constipation.

■ Has a high fever, blood in the stool, and abdominal pain.

■ Appears dehydrated.

■ Is not able to take sufficient fluids to keep up with the loss of fluid in the stool.

■ Appears lethargic.

Symptoms Guide

Use the appearance of the stool and your child's condition to guide you in reviewing this table.

Condition	Stool Appearance	Typical Age	Associated Features
Anal fissure	• Small amount of fresh blood coating the stool or on the toilet paper • Hard stools	Any age	• Constipation
Infectious colitis	• Stool mixed with blood • Diarrhea • Mucus stools	Usually older than 1 year old	• Fever • Abdominal cramps • Recent return from travel • Other family members sometimes affected
Cow's milk protein intolerance	• Streaks of blood mixed in with stool • Diarrhea	Almost always younger than 1 year old	• Bloody diarrhea resolves with removal of cow's milk protein • Poor growth • Fussy with eating

❷ What Causes Blood in the Stool?

Most cases of bloody stools in young children are a result of constipation that leads to a small tear near the anus with the passage of hard stools. Bloody stools can also be caused by different types of infections and by inflammation of the intestines. These infections and inflammation can cause some bleeding, which gets mixed with the stool. Intolerance to cow's milk protein can also cause bloody stools.

Anal Fissures

Anal fissures develop when hard stool is passed through the anal opening, causing a small tear in the lining. It is most common in infants and is almost always associated with constipation. Such fissures are one of the most common causes of bloody stools in infants.

Signs and Symptoms of Anal Fissures

- Fissures and tears can be easily seen when you inspect the anus. It looks like a straight red line or scab radiating from the anal opening.
- Sometimes an extra piece of skin (a skin tag) develops near the fissure.

Did You Know?

Pain Avoidance
A child might avoid passing stool due to the pain of an anal fissure. This retention worsens the underlying constipation and can prevent healing.

- Hard bowel movements that are difficult and/or painful to pass.
- Crying with the passing of stool due to pain associated with the fissure.
- Blood on the surface of the stool.
- Avoidance of passing stool due to pain.

Treatment of Anal Fissures

The successful treatment of anal fissures depends on the successful treatment of the constipation. See Constipation (page 124) Treatment strategies include:

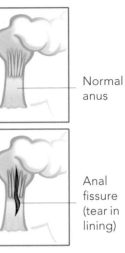

Anal fissure

Large intestine

Rectum

Anus

Normal anus

Anal fissure (tear in lining)

- Giving your child stool softeners.
- Modifying your child's diet by adding more fluids and fiber; this will help prevent the repeated passage of hard stools.
- Lubricating the anal opening with petroleum jelly to help alleviate the pain in the initial few days until the stool becomes softer.

Infectious Colitis

Infectious colitis refers to inflammation of the bowels from bacteria, parasites, or viruses. If the stool is bloody, with slime or mucus, consider a bacterial cause of infection. Bacterial gastrointestinal infections should also be suspected in children who have high fevers and abdominal cramps and who appear unwell.

Cow's Milk Protein Intolerance

Cow's milk protein intolerance or allergy is an adverse reaction by the immune system to one or more proteins from cow's milk. This milk protein can be found in infant formula or in the breast milk of mothers who are eating or drinking any dairy products. This reaction, which usually develops in the first few months of life, results in inflammation of the digestive tract.

Babies with a cow's milk protein intolerance may seem uncomfortable feeding and might even vomit. The inflammation can lead to diarrhea, bloody stools, and poor growth.

Cow's Milk Protein Intolerance Diagnosis

Unfortunately, there is not one sign or symptom that is diagnostic of a cow's milk protein intolerance. A doctor may request certain blood tests to evaluate an infant's general state of nutrition and hydration. If a cow's milk protein intolerance is suspected, your physician may recommend eliminating cow's milk products from the diet.

> **Did You Know?**
>
> **Traveling Bacteria**
> A history of recent travel or exposure to contaminated food or water might also indicate a bacterial infection. Gastrointestinal infections from viruses usually do not cause blood in the stool.

> **Did You Know?**
>
> **Double Intolerance**
> Many infants who are allergic to cow's milk also cannot tolerate soy protein. Infants with this disorder may require a diet free of both milk and soy in order to thrive.

Other Rare Causes of Bloody Stools

Condition	Typical Age	Symptoms	Cause
Intussusception See Abdominal Pain (Acute), page 18	Under 2 years old	• Stool that looks like red jelly • Spasms of severe abdominal pain • Pallor (paleness)	One part of the intestine (usually the small bowel) moves into the segment of adjoining bowel (usually the large bowel) like a telescope; this leads to a blockage of the bowel
Meckel's diverticulum	Young children (most common from birth to 2 years old, but may be seen in older children)	• A sudden gush of fresh, bright red blood from the anus	A tiny piece of tissue left over from fetal development secretes some acid, which causes bleeding from the adjacent intestines
Inflammatory bowel disease (Crohn's disease or ulcerative colitis) See Abdominal Pain (Chronic or Recurrent), page 25	Preteens, teens, young adults (rare in children younger than 5 years old)	• Bloody, mucusy stools • Ongoing diarrhea • Abdominal pain and cramps • Poor appetite • Joint pain • Eye pain • Weight loss • Poor growth • Mouth ulcers • Fevers	Chronic inflammation of the gastrointestinal tract

Cow's Milk Protein Intolerance Treatment

Elimination of food or formula containing both cow's milk protein and soy protein is the mainstay of treatment. If your child is breastfeeding, elimination of these proteins in a mother's diet is essential. Several specialized hydrolyzed formulas are available that do not contain cow's milk or soy protein. This usually leads to an improvement of the diarrhea, bloody stools, and vomiting within a few days. Complete healing can take up to a month. Fortunately, for most affected children, this intolerance seems to disappear by 2 years of age with avoidance of cow's milk or soy protein.

Doc Talk If your child has signs and symptoms of a bacterial cause of bloody stools, she should be assessed by a health-care provider. The stool can then be tested in the laboratory for infection. It is important that your child stays well hydrated. Most cases of infectious colitis will resolve without medication, but your doctor may prescribe antibiotics to treat the infection.

Breastfeeding Problems

What Can I Do?

▶ Be assured that breast milk is best for healthy growth and development.

▶ If your baby is not meeting expectations for weight gain, urination, stooling, or sleep, alert your doctor as soon as possible.

▶ Many parents will have questions and issues, especially early on in the breastfeeding experience. Try to persevere, as almost all of these problems have a relatively simple solution and the benefits of breastfeeding are many! A lactation consultant may be helpful.

❶ What Are Common Breastfeeding Problems?

Parents often worry about whether their baby is drinking enough breast milk. Related to this fear are several physical difficulties the child's mother may encounter: breast engorgement, cracked nipples, and mastitis. In addition, many women have fluctuating emotions after having a baby. This can last 10 days to a few weeks. A smaller percentage of mothers (about 10%) will suffer from postpartum depression. Breastfeeding is no doubt exhausting and difficult at first, but should not make you sad. If you are feeling this way, speak with your health-care provider.

RELATED CONDITIONS

- Blocked duct
- Engorgement
- Leaking nipples
- Mastitis
- Sore or cracked nipples
- Yeast infection

When should we contact our doctor or local hospital?

In most cases, your child will receive enough calories and other nutrients from breast milk for healthy growth and development. Occasionally, your child may encounter problems breastfeeding; see the red flags below.

▶▶ Breastfeeding Red Flags

Consult your doctor as soon as possible if you or your child has any of the following symptoms:

- If your baby does not have enough wet diapers or is not producing stools. See page 97.
- If it is difficult to wake your baby to feed.
- If breastfeeding is painful.
- If you feel persistently sad or teary.

Common Breastfeeding Problems and Their Treatments

Diagnosis	Signs and Symptoms	Common Treatment
Sore and/or cracked nipples	• Red, dry nipples • Visible cracks in nipples; bruising • Pain when breastfeeding, usually most severe when baby first starts to nurse • Nipple is "pinched" when baby comes off the breast	• Ensure that your baby is latching correctly • After feeding, express a few drops of breast milk onto your nipple and let it dry • Use breast pads that breathe • Use a breast shield between feeds, if needed • Apply lanolin ointment to nipples after each feed • Do not apply creams or lotions that need removal prior to feeding • When bathing, use only water (no soap) on breasts
Leaking nipples	• Breast milk leaks out of nipples and onto bra or clothing when baby is not feeding or you are not with baby	• None — this is a natural occurrence for some women • To prevent leakage onto your bra and clothing, use breast pads to collect milk • To prevent complications with dry, cracked nipples, use breast pads that are not lined with plastic
Engorgement (breasts become too full with milk)	• Commonly occurs when milk first comes in or if feedings are missed • Breasts are extremely full and hard • Breasts may hurt when touched • Breasts are very warm • Areola are hard, difficult for baby to latch onto	• Express breast milk frequently to relieve the pressure (preferably with a pump) • Breastfeed more frequently • Apply warm compresses prior to feeding • Apply cold compresses for severe engorgement between feeds • Prior to feeding or expressing, massage your breasts, starting from your armpit and going down to your nipple • Consider pain medication, as required (ibuprofen or acetaminophen)
Blocked duct (one of the ducts that your milk flows through has become plugged)	• One section of the breast is red, hard, and often painful • A lump may be felt	• Feed frequently — your baby's suckling will help unblock the duct • Start feeding on the side that is blocked • Try feeding in a different position • Apply moist heat to and massage the affected area • Monitor a blocked duct very closely; it can lead to mastitis if not treated

Diagnosis	Signs and Symptoms	Common Treatment
Mastitis (bacterial infection of the breast tissue)	• Pain or swelling in the breast, similar to a blocked duct • Fever and other flu-like symptoms	• Try treatments for a blocked duct, but if symptoms persist for more than 24 hours, seek medical attention and treatment with antibiotics • Continue to breastfeed regularly — the infection does not affect the quality of the breast milk, and feeding may help treat the mastitis — abrupt cessation of breastfeeding will exacerbate the problem • To prevent mastitis, avoid pressure on the breasts (for example, from a poorly fitting bra), try to feed your baby regularly, and ensure that she has a good latch and is draining the breast effectively
Yeast infection (may follow antibiotic use in the mother or baby)	• Deep, shooting pain or burning while breastfeeding that lasts for the entire feed • Pain and very sensitive nipples while not breastfeeding — may be worse at night • Breast may not show any physical signs that something is wrong, such as swelling or discoloration • Baby may have white patches (thrush) in her mouth or a persistent diaper rash	• Ensure that your baby is latching correctly — an incorrect latch will increase your pain • Continue to breastfeed regularly — this infection does not affect the quality of the breast milk • Keep breasts dry and, if possible, expose them to the air as much as possible • Do not use breast pads with plastic lining or wear a bra that traps moisture around the nipple • Change your bra daily • If the baby has a pacifier, sterilize it daily • Seek the services of a health-care provider — topical medications for mom and baby may be needed

FAQ

How often should I feed my baby?

Most babies need to be fed 8 to 12 times in a 24-hour period. Once your baby is latching well and beginning to gain weight, she should determine her own feeding and sleeping schedule.

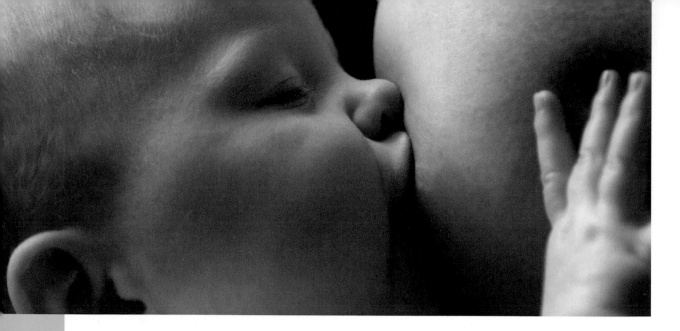

FAQs

Does my baby need to eat or drink anything other than breast milk?
No. Breast milk is the sole source of nutrition required in the first 6 months of a baby's life. If your supply of breast milk is sufficient, there is no need for water, formula, or any other foods until approximately 6 months of age.

Do I need to supplement with vitamin D?
This is a popular question these days. Sunlight exposure on skin is an important source of vitamin D, which is important for the development of strong, healthy bones. For all exclusively breastfed babies in many areas across North America, the lack of year-round sunlight means that breastfed babies require a single daily dose of vitamin D. This dosage is 400 international units (IU) once daily, and if your baby is dark-skinned or lives in a northern community (north of 55 degrees latitude), then she will need 800 IU daily.

Hunger Signs

There are several signs that your baby may be hungry and ready for a feed:

- Your baby awakes stretching and yawning after a deep sleep.
- Your baby may start nuzzling or rooting on your chest or on anyone holding her.
- Your baby may suck on her fist or make sucking motions with her mouth.
- Your baby may cry when she is hungry; however, a crying baby is not necessarily a hungry baby.

Contrary to popular opinion, the duration of each feed, the feeling of fullness in the breasts, and the inability to pump milk are not very reliable ways to determine the adequacy of milk supply.

How Can You Tell if Your Baby Is Receiving Enough Milk?

1. *Weight gain.* A baby who is receiving enough milk will not lose more than 10% of her initial birth weight in the first few days of life, and she will usually be back up to birth weight between 1 and 2 weeks of age.

2. *Stools.* The pattern of stools often changes as babies get more milk. In the first 1 or 2 days, babies pass the newborn stool, called meconium, which is black and tar-like. After a few days, a baby should have regular yellow, "seedy" mustard-like stools. A baby who is still passing meconium stools or no stool at all after the fourth or fifth day should be evaluated by a health-care professional.

3. *Urinating.* A baby who is passing lots of urine is probably receiving enough milk. New babies should urinate at least 3 or 4 times daily. By the end of the first week, many babies are urinating 6 to 10 times daily. With the ultra-absorbent diapers in use today, it can be difficult to tell if there is actually urine present in the diaper. If the diaper feels heavy compared with a new, unused diaper, there is urine present. See Newborn Infant Hydration Red Flags (page 154).

4. *Sleep pattern.* A baby who is receiving adequate amounts of milk will generally settle and sleep for a few hours after a feeding, then will spontaneously awaken to feed vigorously, then fall back to sleep. This must be differentiated from the baby who is too sleepy and does not wake to feed, which may reflect inadequate milk intake.

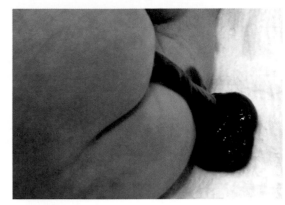
Meconium

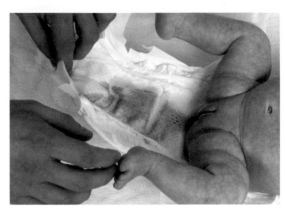
Mustard-like breast milk stools

Did You Know?

Urine Signs

If a baby is not getting enough milk, her urine output will decrease and appear more concentrated (a deeper yellow color). Pink or orange crystals can even be seen in the diaper. In this case, the baby should be seen by a health-care professional to assess hydration.

Doc Talk There are many myths surrounding breastfeeding and breast milk. There is a commonly held misconception that babies who are formula-fed, or babies who receive an early introduction to infant cereal (before 4 or 5 months), sleep longer at night. However, there is no proof for this belief. What is true is that a child's sleep patterns vary widely whether the child is breastfed or formula-fed.

Bruising

What Can I Do?

▶ If your family has a history of a bleeding disorder and your child has an unusual number of bruises, see your doctor.

▶ If the bruise appears unusual — more serious, persists longer, and shows other problematic red flag signs — consult with your doctor immediately.

Case Study

Blair's Bruises

Blair's mother had been noticing some bruises on Blair's shins over the last week. This afternoon when he returned from daycare, she became worried when she saw a big bruise on his upper arm. According to the daycare staff, Blair had been his normal, rambunctious self, with no accidents or falls that they were aware of. Thinking back, Blair had had a bit of a cold the previous week, but otherwise he had been happy, active, and eating well. He had had some minor gum bleeding when he brushed his teeth this week. She called her family doctor's office and made an appointment for later that day.

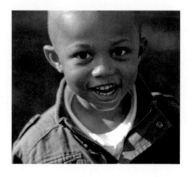

Dr. Fitzpatrick noted that in addition to the large bruise on his arm and multiple small bruises on his legs, he also had some tiny, pink pinpoint spots on his limbs and chest, spots he called petechia, or little bleeds into the skin. A blood test confirmed that his platelet count was only 6,000 (150,000 is normal), and Blair was diagnosed with idiopathic thrombocytopenic purpura (ITP).

RELATED CONDITIONS

- Hemophilia
- Henoch-Schonlein purpura
- Idiopathic thrombocytopenic purpura
- Leukemia
- Von Willebrand disease

❶ What Is Bruising?

Bruises, especially on the shins, are a rite of passage in young children, especially for toddlers who always seem to be on the go. However, if you see bruising that isn't just from bumping against the coffee table or falling while trying to run, it can occasionally signify something more serious, such as:

- Idiopathic thrombocytopenic purpura
- Henoch-Schonlein purpura
- Von Willebrand disease
- Hemophilia
- Leukemia

When should we contact our doctor or local hospital?

In most cases, the bruise is the result of a blow to the skin that heals spontaneously, but see below for red flags that require medical attention.

➤➤ Bruising Red Flags

Consult your child's doctor as soon as possible if your child has any of the following symptoms associated with bruising:

- Bruises that appear without any good explanation (no history of a fall or bump)
- Bruises on soft, protected, or fleshy parts of the body, such as the chest, back, or buttocks, not just over bony prominences, such as the shins or elbows
- Bruises that are excessively large for a minor injury
- Bruising on an infant who is not yet walking
- Multiple bruises
- Bruises that last for weeks
- Bruising that is accompanied by fine pink or red dots that sort of look like freckles and don't go away if you push on them (petechia)
- Bruising with any sign of bleeding (for example, from the gums after brushing teeth, prolonged nosebleeds, or any blood in the urine or stool)
- A family history of bleeding problems

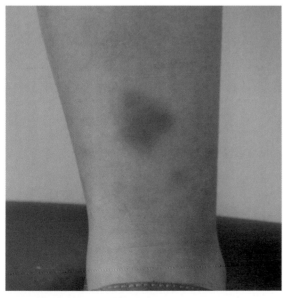

Normal bruising on a toddler's skin

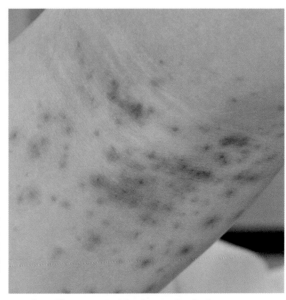

Petechiae (fine pinpoint bleeding in the skin)

What Are Some Other Causes of Bruising?

Occasionally, the bruise may be the sign of a more serious condition.

Symptoms	Possible Condition	Treatment
• Raised bruises in unusual places • Found almost exclusively in boys • Swelling of the joints or muscles due to bleeding • Prolonged nosebleeds or bleeding after tooth extraction or circumcision (in baby boys)	**Hemophilia** • A rare inherited deficiency of clotting factor 8 or 9 in the blood • Inherited on the X chromosome, which is why it is almost exclusively seen in boys	• Diagnosis is made by testing the blood for various clotting factors • Child will need clotting-factor replacement therapy
• Bruising mainly involving buttocks, legs, and feet • Bruises may be a bit raised • Abdominal pains • Painful and/or swollen joints, especially the ankles and knees • May follow a viral illness, such as a common cold • Most commonly affects toddlers and school-age children	**Henoch-Schonlein purpura (HSP)** • HSP is caused by inflammation of the small blood vessels (vasculitis) of the skin, joints, bowels, and kidneys	• Your child's doctor will order a blood count to make sure that your child's platelets are normal (low numbers of platelets are not seen in HSP); she will also examine your child's urine for any abnormality in kidney function • Most children with HSP recover entirely in several days without specific treatment; recurrences can happen • Pain relief is the main treatment, both for the abdominal discomfort and for the joint pain
• Bruising • Pinpoint bleeding spots (petechia) • Nosebleeds or bleeding gums • Recent viral illness, such as a cold • Child usually between the ages of 2 and 6 years	**Idiopathic thrombocytopenic purpura (ITP)** • Bleeding disorder characterized by too few platelets (blood cells that help the blood to clot) in the bloodstream • The immune system attacks the body's own platelets (often triggered by a common viral infection)	• Your child's doctor will perform a blood test that shows a low platelet count with otherwise normal red and white blood cells • If the platelets are only slightly low and your child is not bleeding, your doctor will just monitor the platelet count with serial blood tests • If the platelet count is very low or there are signs of ongoing bleeding, your child may receive intravenous immunoglobulin (IVIG) or steroids • Treatment decisions are based on your child's risk for having a rare but serious bleeding event into the brain — a complication seen in less than 1% of children with ITP • Most children will recover spontaneously within 12 months

Symptoms	Possible Condition	Treatment
• Bruising or skin rash • Pale skin • Decreased energy • Unexplained fevers • Poor appetite/weight loss • Bone pain/limp	**Leukemia** • Cancer of the blood • Most common form of cancer in children • Leukemia occurs when abnormal cancerous cells (called blasts) take over the bone marrow (the blood cell "factory"), impairing normal blood cell production	• Your child's doctor will recommend a blood test to check the numbers of white blood cells, red blood cells, and platelets • If suspicious for leukemia, the doctor will directly examine the bone marrow through aspiration (a needle sampling), and tests will be performed on this specimen to confirm the diagnosis • Leukemia is treated with chemotherapy, a combination of oral and intravenous medications that kill cancer cells • Most children recover from leukemia
• Unusual location of bruising • Abnormal menstrual bleeding • Bleeding from the gums or nose • Excessive bleeding after a tooth extraction • History of bleeding in the family	**Von Willebrand disease** • Inherited disorder that affects the blood's ability to clot properly • Involves a problem with the amount or quality of von Willebrand factor (VWF), which helps the platelets stick to damaged blood vessels	• The diagnosis is made by testing the blood for various clotting factors • Most children require minimal, if any, treatment, unless they have some trauma or are requiring an operation

Doc Talk

At the serious end of the diagnostic spectrum is leukemia. The symptoms of leukemia are mainly related to the decreased number of healthy blood cells. Decreased numbers of red blood cells, a type of anemia, will result in reduced energy and pallor (pale skin). Low platelets will cause easy bruising and a skin rash that consists of small red dots, called petechiae. If the white blood cells are decreased, your child will be more prone to infection. Some children will also have fever and poor appetite. If the leukemia has invaded your child's bones, he might complain of bone pain, limp, or have a swollen joint.

Bullying and Cyberbullying

What Can I Do?

▶ Open the lines of communication with your child and with the school about this issue.

▶ Ask your child directly about bullying, particularly if there has been a change in your child's mood, behavior, or academic performance.

▶ Save and report. Ask your child to save the threatening message and report it to an appropriate adult.

❶ What Are Bullying and Cyberbullying?

Bullying refers to any cruelty or intimidation of the more vulnerable; cyberbullying is bullying using social media technology, such as computers, cellphones, digital cameras, and the Internet.

Bullying may be in the form of either physical assault or emotional cruelty (taunting, ridiculing, humiliating, threatening, intimidating, stealing, or the exclusion of a child from a peer group).

Victims may be afraid of retaliation if they report the event, so it may continue for some time before parents are aware of it. Consequences include poor self-esteem, depression, school avoidance, and occasionally (and tragically) suicide.

Bullies may become overly aggressive adults who have difficulties with social relationships and are at higher risk of criminal behavior and incarceration. Cyberbullying is both public and anonymous, so cyberbullies may be less confrontational and aggressive; they may be shy and quiet, "protected" behind their computers.

The Language of Text Bullying

Text messaging, or "texting," has developed its own language of codes and acronyms:

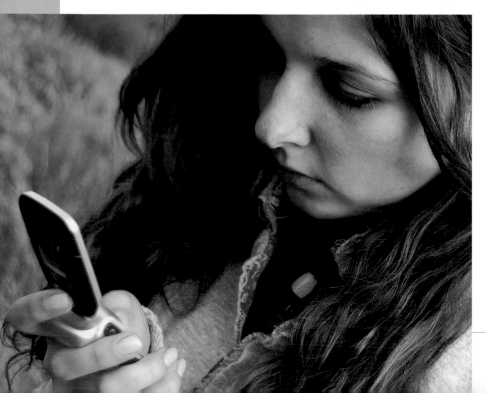

182	I hate you	**MOS**	Mom over shoulder
zerg	Gang up on someone	**PAL**	Parents are listening
P911	Parents alert	**PAW**	Parents are watching
POS	Parents over shoulder	**PIR**	Parent in room
CD9	Code 9 — parents are around	**WYRN**	What's your real name?
KPC	Keeping parents clueless		

Types of Cyberbullying

- *Flaming:* Online arguments using hostile rude language
- *Harassing:* Offensive, insulting text messages or emails
- *Stalking:* Threats made online
- *Outing:* Sharing others' secrets or personal information online to humiliate them
- *Exclusion:* Intentionally excluding someone from a group or list
- *Denigration:* Mean-spirited gossip and hateful comments on websites, blogs, or chats
- *Impersonation:* Posing as someone else (often by using their private passwords) to embarrass them or get them into trouble

❷ How Can Bullying and Cyberbullying Be Prevented?

Anti-bullying programs and clearly articulated policies in schools can be effective if they:

- Provide strategies for victims and for bystanders to safely report bullying
- Communicate clearly the zero tolerance policy, the severe consequences of bullying and enforce them

Did You Know?

Code of Silence
Less than 10% of teens that have been bullied online have told their parents. Some may be afraid of the bully, some are ashamed of the online posting, while others may be afraid of you taking away their cellphone or Internet access.

Doc Talk   Here are a few more basic rules your child can use to prevent cyberbullying behavior:

- Never post or text anything on the Internet that you wouldn't want the whole world to read.
- Never share passwords. Sometimes best friends "turn," and some are simply careless.
- Don't respond. Leave the chat room, online game, social networking site or text chat immediately if a threat is made.
- Block subsequent messages. Use the technology to automatically block texts and emails from the individual.

Burns

❶ What Is a Burn?

A burn is an injury to the skin following intense heat from sunlight, hot water, flames, electricity, chemicals, or a hot element, such as a stovetop gas burner or oven. When injury occurs from hot water or grease, this is typically referred to as a scald burn.

When should we contact our doctor or local hospital?

While most burns are minor, requiring only time to heal, other burns can be very serious, even life-threatening. Most second- and all third-degree burns, as well as burns to the face, hands, feet, genitals, or across a joint, should be seen by your doctor.

⏩ Burn Red Flags

If the burn is significant, call 911 or head to the nearest hospital. Immediately place the burned area under cool running water, if available. Otherwise, cover the area with a clean cloth cooled with water while awaiting help.

Categorizing Burns

Burns are categorized into different degrees based on their depth of damage to the skin.

First-Degree Burn
- Injury to only the top layer of skin
- *Example:* Sunburn

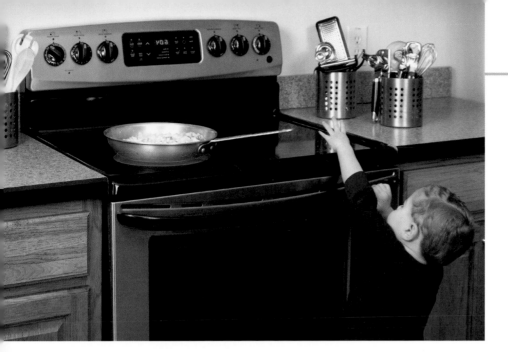

- *Common signs and symptoms:* Redness, swelling, localized pain
- *Healing process:* Resolves within a few days
- *Scarring:* None

Second-Degree Burn
- Injury is deeper, partial thickness (multiple layers) of skin
- *Example:* Hot water, hot element
- *Common signs and symptoms:* Severe pain, redness, blisters that may pop, with redness and wetness underneath
- *Healing process:* 1 to 2 weeks
- *Scarring:* Often

Third-Degree Burn
- Injury involves all layers of the skin (full thickness)
- *Example:* Flame or scald burn
- *Common signs and symptoms:* Often painless because nerves have been burned; black, white, leathery, or charred skin
- *Healing process:* Can take months, may require a skin graft
- *Scarring:* Always

Significant Burns
- All third-degree burns
- All second-degree burns affecting more than 10% of the body surface area
- Any burn affecting the face, hands, feet, genitals, anus, or crossing a major joint
- Burns from electrical current
- Any burn that looks infected (increasing swelling, pain, redness, or creamy discharge, usually at least 24 hours after the burn)

Did You Know?

Burn Size
You can use your child's palm to assess the size of the burn: the inside of your child's palm equals 1% of his body surface area.

❷ How Is a Burn Treated?

Treatment of burns will depend on the degree of the burn, the area involved, and the surface area affected.

Significant Burn Do's and Don'ts
Do
- Call 911 or go to the nearest hospital if you know its location.
- Immediately place burn under cool running water, if available; otherwise, cover area with a clean cloth cooled with water while awaiting help

Don't
- Break any blisters
- Apply any ointments or creams to the affected area
- Remove any burned/charred clothing

Minor Burns Do's and Don'ts
Do
- Immediately place burn under cool running water, if available; otherwise, cover area with a clean cloth cooled with water
- Provide pain relief; give your child acetaminophen or ibuprofen if your child appears to be uncomfortable
- Leave burn either exposed or covered with clean, nonstick gauze
- Change the dressing every few days
- Apply sunblock to skin that has healed following a burn; this should be continued for several months and will prevent worsening of potential scarring

Don't
- Use ice on the area of the burn (may worsen injury to skin)
- Break blisters
- Apply butter or other greasy medications in the initial treatment of the burn (increases risk of infection)

Chemical Burn Treatment
Burns caused by common household products can be extremely damaging to the skin. Chemicals that can cause burns include ammonia, bleach, and other cleaning products. If your child experiences a chemical burn:

- Remove all clothing that was exposed to the cleaning product and that is touching the skin.

- Place the area under running water for several minutes.
- Go to the nearest emergency department for further assessment and treatment.

Prevention

- Do not allow your children to play with matches.
- Lock up all flammable materials safely.
- Watch toddlers constantly when they are near open flames, such as campfires.
- Stoves, hot oven doors, and even the glass screen of a fireplace often cause burns to little hands.
- Beware of the hot steam that emanates from a vaporizer.
- Keep hot liquids away from the edge of the counter.
- Scald injuries from hot water in bathtubs remain a major concern. Lower the setting of your hot water tank to 120°F (49°C) to reduce the chance of scalds.
- Install smoke detectors and plan routes of escape from your home in case of fire.

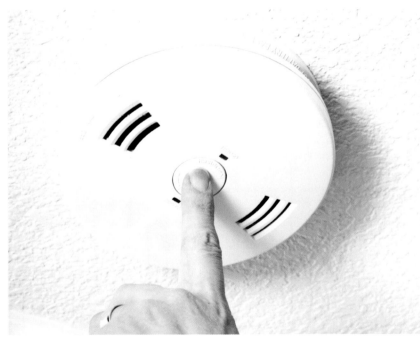

Make sure your smoke detector is working.

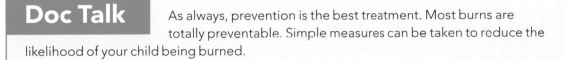

Doc Talk   As always, prevention is the best treatment. Most burns are totally preventable. Simple measures can be taken to reduce the likelihood of your child being burned.

Chest Pain

What Can I Do?

▶ Chest pain can be scary, but be assured that in about half of cases the pain resolves itself quickly, without any harm or a clear cause.

▶ If your child shows any red flags, seek medical attention urgently.

▶ Try rest, heat, analgesics, or specific treatments if, for example, an infection or indigestion is identified.

RELATED CONDITIONS

- Anxiety
- Bruising
- Costochondritis (inflammation of the cartilage in the rib)
- Foreign body ingestion
- Heart problems
- Indigestion and heartburn
- Lung infection
- Muscle strain

❶ What Is Chest Pain?

When most people think of pain in the chest, they worry about a serious heart problem. Although this might sometimes be an appropriate concern for an adult, it is almost never the case in children. Chest pain in children is rarely due to serious illness. Nevertheless, the complaint should be taken seriously because the symptom can be very disturbing, especially in younger children.

When should we contact our doctor or local hospital?

While usually not worrisome, on occasion chest pain can be caused by something that requires medical treatment. See the red flags below.

⏩ Chest Pain Red Flags

Immediately consult your child's doctor if your child has any of the following signs or symptoms associated with chest pain:

- Sudden onset pain at a young age
- Looks unwell
- Significant breathing difficulty
- Fainting or palpitations (feeling like the heart is beating faster or irregularly)
- Possible swallowing of a foreign body
- High fever
- Consistent night pain wakes him up from sleep
- Chest pain accompanied by a dizzy feeling brought on by physical exertion

❷ What Causes Chest Pain?

Chest pain can originate from the muscles and bones of the chest wall, the lungs, the esophagus, or the heart, or it may even be caused by a problem located in the abdomen. This complaint becomes more common after the age of 12, but is not uncommon in younger children. In about one-quarter of the children with chest pain, it will tend to recur for more than 6 months. Interestingly, about half of these children will have a family member with similar complaints.

Causes of Chest Pain in Children

Cause	Suspect If:	Symptoms That Require Emergency Treatment
Muscle strain	• Recent new strenuous exercise • Persistent cough can cause pain due to overuse of the chest muscles	• None
Costochondritis (inflammation of the cartilage in the rib)	• Sharp pain in front of the chest • Tender to touch over breastbone • May be preceded by a cold or exercise	• None
Bruising	• Any injury to the chest	• Any significant blow to the chest
Lung infection	• Presence of cough and some breathing difficulties • Fever	• Significant difficulty breathing (for example, increased rate or effort of breathing)
Indigestion and heartburn	• Often worse after meals or spicy foods	• None
Anxiety	• Common in teenage girls • May experience hyperventilation, tingling of hands and feet, dizziness • May have school or family stresses	• None
Heart problems	• Other symptoms, such as fainting or palpitations • May be worse with exertion • Known history of heart disease	• Fainting, palpitations (heart feeling like it is skipping a beat) • Looks unwell
Foreign body ingestion	• Usually in older babies or toddlers • May have had a choking episode	• Choking episode before pain • Significant difficulty breathing (for example, increased rate or effort)
No underlying cause	• The child is otherwise well	• None

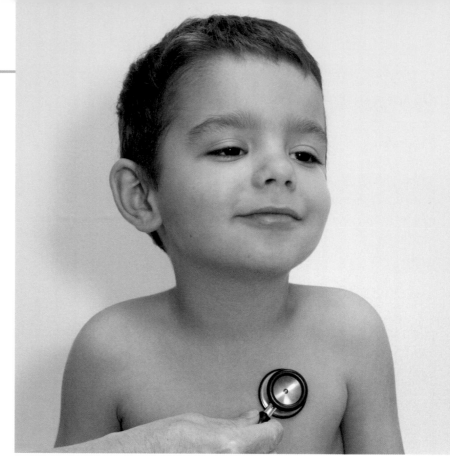

Conditions Causing Chest Pain in Children

Inflammation

Inflammation of the cartilage in the rib, known as costochondritis, is characterized by a very sharp pain in the front of the chest wall. It may also hurt to take a deep breath in. The diagnosis is confirmed by tenderness when pushing over the area where the ribs join onto the breastbone. This problem is sometimes preceded by a cold or exercise.

Infection

Lung infection (pneumonia) or an air leak from the bronchial tubes, called a pneumothorax, may cause pain. Both conditions are accompanied by other signs of breathing difficulty, such as rapid breathing or increased effort.

Indigestion

Esophagitis, an inflamed esophagus due to acid reflux, can cause a burning pain behind the breastbone. Your child will often complain of "heartburn" after meals, particularly if he has eaten spicy foods.

Foreign Body Ingestion

Rarely, in young children, the ingestion of a foreign body, for example, a penny, can lead to pain if the object becomes stuck in the esophagus. This can develop after a choking episode.

Heart Disease

Heart disease is an uncommon cause of childhood chest pain, comprising less than 5% of cases. Abnormal heart rhythms, structural defects, heart-valve abnormalities, and infections of the heart can all cause some discomfort in the chest. This generally happens in a child who is known to have heart disease or who appears significantly unwell at the time. Fainting (syncope), palpitations, and pain with exertion can also suggest that your child's doctor should do a thorough heart exam.

> **Did You Know?**
>
> **Breast Tenderness**
> At the onset of puberty, both boys and girls can have some tenderness of the breasts.

❷ How Is Chest Pain Treated?

Treatment will depend on the likely cause. Comparing your child's symptoms with all possible causes will help to clarify where the pain is coming from. You will need to decide whether to seek medical attention and, if so, how urgently.

Treatment for musculoskeletal problems involving the chest wall includes rest, heat, and analgesics, such as ibuprofen. Chest infections causing chest pain will often need antibiotics. If indigestion is suspected, a trial of antacids is useful. In the latter case, improvement of the indigestion would help confirm your suspicion of esophagitis.

FAQ

What tests will my child need to determine if her chest pain is a serious problem?
If your child has had a direct injury to the chest or there are sufficient clues pointing toward a lung or heart problem, a chest X-ray will likely be necessary. In the rare cases where the heart is potentially the problem, an electrocardiogram (ECG) may be helpful. In the majority of cases, your child's doctor will need a thorough description of the problem followed by a physical examination — and no further testing will be required.

Doc Talk

Up to half of all children complaining of chest pain will have no specific diagnosis. Even after appropriate testing, your child's doctor will not be able to give you a definitive cause for the pain. The good news is that in most of these children, the pain will ultimately disappear without any serious illness ever developing.

Choking and Aspiration

What Can I Do?

▶ If your child is able to speak or cough, calmly encourage him to try to cough the object out.

▶ Stay close to ensure he is breathing adequately.

▶ If this doesn't seem to be working and your child is choking, use standard emergency treatments for choking.

▶ As a preventive measure, learn basic life support (BLS) for babies and young children.

❶ What Are Choking and Aspiration?

Children and even young babies are capable of putting things in their mouth that can cause them to choke. Aspiration occurs when the object goes down the windpipe into the airway instead of down the esophagus into the stomach. Smaller objects can lodge in one of the branches of the airways, which, although not fatal, can cause significant problems that can persist for a long time before being diagnosed. Choking is one of the leading causes of death from injury in the first year of life.

When should we contact our doctor or local hospital?

Most foreign bodies that are aspirated are expelled rapidly by a reflex cough. But if your child does not clear the object, his airway can plug and the event immediately becomes life-threatening. Call 911 if the object cannot be cleared immediately.

➤➤ Choking and Aspiration Red Flags

Choking

■ Unable to breathe

■ Unable to speak or cry

■ Clutching the throat

■ Red in the face, then blue, especially around the mouth

■ Croupy or hoarse cough (occurs when a foreign body is stuck in the voice box, or larynx)

Aspiration (usually after episode of choking)

■ Cough

■ Wheezing

■ Increased rate of breathing

■ Increased effort of breathing

❷ How Are Choking and Aspiration Treated?

Infants Under 1 Year Old

- Lay your baby face down over your forearm or across your lap with his head down.
- Give five short, sharp blows with the heel of your hand between his shoulder blades.

If this doesn't help:

- Turn him over so he is face up.
- Place two fingers just below the nipple line in middle of chest.
- Give five sharp downward thrusts.
- Look in mouth for obvious partially expelled object that might be easy to remove. Do not blindly sweep your fingers through your child's mouth because this can push the object farther down the windpipe.

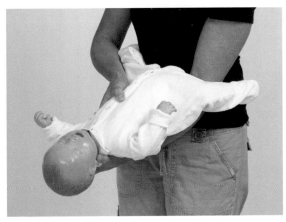

Lay your baby face down.

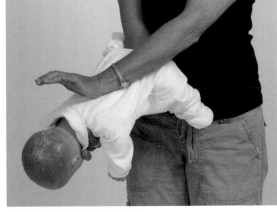

Give five short, sharp blows.

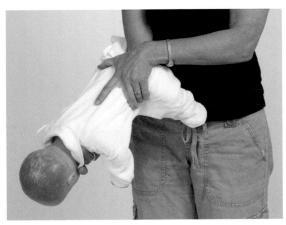

Turn your baby over.

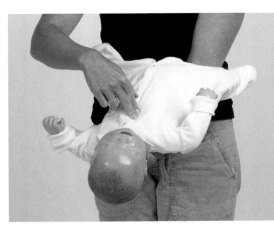

Give five sharp downward thrusts with two fingers.

Children Older Than 1 Year Old

- Kneel or stand behind him (depends on height).
- Wrap your arms around him.
- With a fist, thumb side inward, covered with your other hand, press sharply inward and upward above the belly button (Heimlich maneuver).
- Repeat every 3 seconds until object is dislodged.
- Check inside the mouth for expelled material that can be easily removed, but do not blindly sweep your fingers in a child's mouth — this could worsen the choking event.

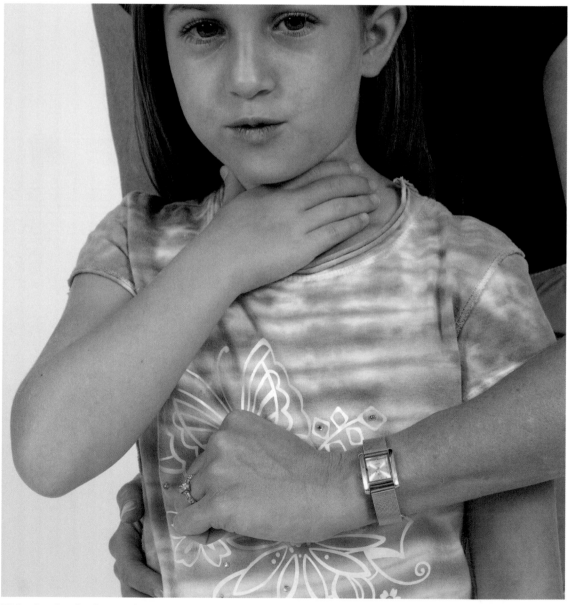

With a fist, thumb side inward, covered with your other hand, press sharply inward and upward above the belly button.

What to Do if Your Baby or Child Becomes Unconscious

- Have someone call 911.
- If you know cardiopulmonary resuscitation (CPR), check the circulation, airway and breathing. If you don't know CPR, ask someone who does to help.
- Start resuscitation with chest compressions.
- Administer rapid (about 100 times per minute) chest thrusts 30 times.
- Administer two breaths, each for one second.
- Repeat this cycle of chest compressions and breaths until professional help arrives or your child is breathing spontaneously again.

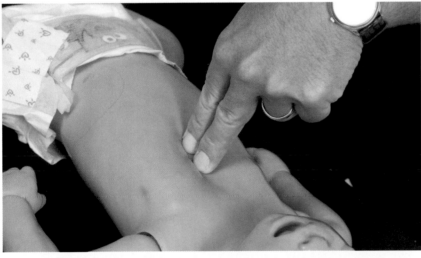

Start resuscitation with chest compressions.

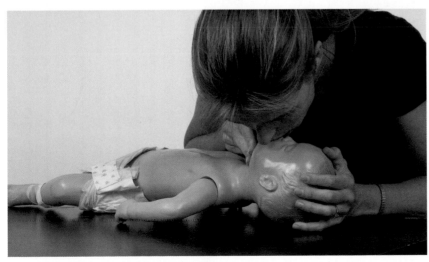

Administer two breaths, each for one second.

Prevention

- Keep small choking hazards and toys with small or loosely attached parts far out of reach of young children; this can be especially challenging when a young child has an older sibling.
- Check that food is appropriate for your child's abilities to chew and swallow.
- Check new toys to make sure they are age-appropriate.
- Do not leave your infant or toddler unattended while eating.
- Children should be sitting down for all meals and snacks. Running with food in the mouth increases the risk of choking.

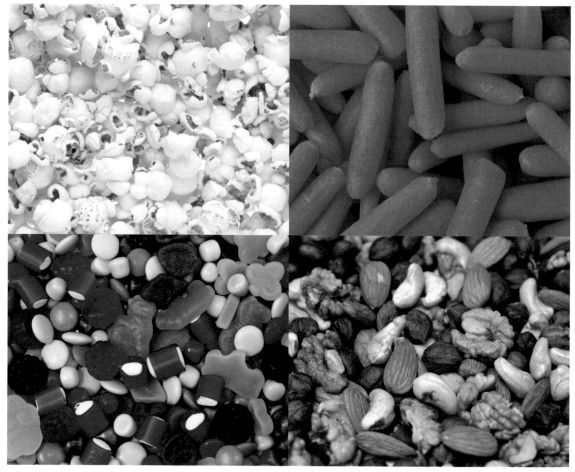

Common choking hazards (popcorn, carrots, nuts and candy)

Doc Talk   New parents are strongly advised to learn basic lifesaving techniques by taking a basic life support (BLS) course that deals with babies and young children. Knowing how to respond to an emergency can help to save a life.

Colic

What Can I Do?

▶ Try to determine if in fact your baby has colic: if your baby is less than 5 months old and has recurrent, somewhat predictable prolonged episodes of inconsolable crying, this is likely colic.

▶ If you think your baby has colic, discuss the various treatment strategies with your doctor. While none of them work for everyone, some of them may be helpful to you.

▶ Be consoled that colic will resolve on its own around the age of 5 months.

❶ What Is Colic?

There are many different definitions of colic. Colic is usually defined as inconsolable crying, often in the evening, for at least 3 hours a day, at least 3 days a week, and at least 3 weeks in a row. During the episode, the baby may scream, turn red in the face, clench his fists, and pull up his legs.

When should we contact our doctor or local hospital?

Crying is a very nonspecific behavior that can be entirely normal in babies or may be a sign of pain or a more serious underlying problem. On the one hand, if crying is recurrent, somewhat predictable, and fits the above description of colic, then you can discuss this with your doctor at a convenient time for you. You don't need to rush into hospital for attention.

On the other hand, if the crying is different than usual, is difficult to settle, or your baby is not interacting appropriately and is just not "himself," then it is best to seek medical advice urgently.

See Crying (page 140).

Did You Know?

Colic and Milk Allergy

Babies with colic who are breastfed may benefit from their mother going on a trial of a strict dairy-free diet for a few weeks to see if there is any improvement in symptoms (if bottle-fed, try a hypoallergenic formula for a few weeks). Dietary manipulations should be under the supervision of your health-care provider.

❷ What Causes Colic?

There is much debate about the exact cause of colic. Some believe it is caused by gas, digestion problems, and abdominal pain. Others feel it is more a result of an immaturity of the nervous system and a difficulty regulating sensory information from both the environment and from within the body. And others wonder if it is a manifestation of individual temperament or personality.

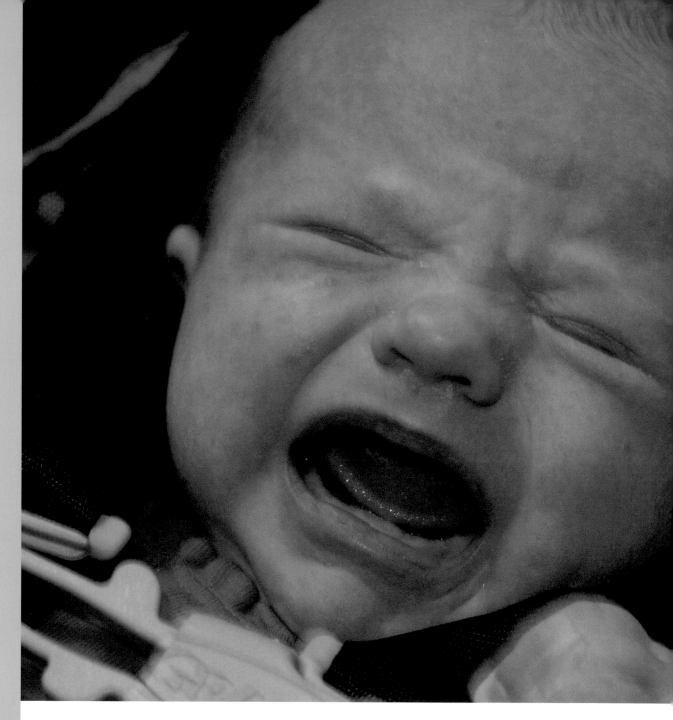

True or False

There are a number of myths associated with colic. The following statements are all not true:

- Colic is worse in bottle-fed babies than breastfed babies.
- Babies with colic are in pain.
- Colic can be fixed with medication.
- Babies with colic are manipulating their parents.
- Colic is the parents' fault.
- Colicky babies will be "difficult" children.

❸ How Is Colic Treated?

Regardless of the cause, no interventions have been shown to reliably treat colic. Babies suffering from colic can be very difficult to soothe, and will often cry no matter what you do. Thankfully, colic will resolve on its own, usually by 3 to 5 months of age. Despite this, colic can be very frustrating for parents. Try soothing your baby with some standard strategies for relief, but know that although some things will work some of the time, you may not find something that will work all of the time.

How To: Calm Your Crying Baby

- *Swaddling:* wrap your baby snuggly in a warm blanket.
- *Swaying:* use rhythmic motion, such as swaying, swinging, bouncing, and vibration.
- *Strolling:* take a walk with baby in the stroller or drive him around in the car.
- *Pacifying:* give your baby a pacifier or a clean finger to suckle.
- *Calming:* reduce stimulation by turning down the lights, reduce noise, or move to a room alone with your baby.
- *Singing and playing:* play calming music, or sing, hum, or dance with baby while making rhythmic "shushing" sounds.
- *Creating white noise:* turn on the clothes dryer, vacuum cleaner, fan, faucet, or a noise machine.
- *Bathing:* give your baby a warm bath or take a shower with your baby.
- *Going outside:* try fresh air to help your baby sleep.
- *Massaging:* slowly and gently rub your little one using baby lotion or oil.
- *Taking a break:* put your baby in a safe place and take a minute for yourself. Call someone you trust for help. Talk about your frustration. Never, ever shake your baby.

Doc Talk Colic has no clear cause and no clear solution. Fortunately, it will resolve on its own, but it can be extremely frustrating for both baby and his caregivers while it lasts. Try to recruit family and friends to give you a break from time to time. Having a colicky baby can feel like running a marathon. You will need to take care of yourself as well.

Common Cold
(Upper Respiratory Tract Infection)

What Can I Do?

▶ Remember that time is the main cure for the common cold — that, combined with a little tender loving care (TLC).

▶ If your child shows any of the red flags for complications of a cold, seek medical advice fairly urgently.

▶ Review the list of do's and don'ts for some tips on how to help your child.

❶ What Is the Common Cold?

RELATED CONDITIONS

- Asthma or bronchiolitis
- Ear infection
- Pneumonia
- Sinusitis
- Strep throat

Although the common cold is a minor and self-limited viral infection, it still can make kids (and adults) miserable. Most colds are the result of common viruses and resolve on their own, usually within about 1 week. However, more serious conditions can result as a complication of a common cold and these may need urgent care.

Signs and Symptoms of a Common Cold

Symptoms are usually short-lived but may persist for 2 weeks in up to 10% of preschoolers.

- Stuffy or runny nose
- Clear nasal discharge, which gradually becomes yellow or green and thicker after a few days
- Sore throat
- Hoarseness
- Fever, often lasting 2 to 3 days but settling before the other symptoms disappear
- Neck gland swelling
- Poor appetite
- Mild headache
- Fatigue

Constant Cold

In the first few years of life, children average eight to nine cold viruses per year! This number can be even higher in families where older siblings may bring home colds from daycare and school. It may seem like your child constantly has a cold!

When should we contact our doctor or local hospital?

Most colds will resolve in time. Occasionally, the virus causing a cold will progress and involve the lungs or develop into a secondary bacterial infection. For these, your child should be assessed by a health-care provider.

▶ Common Cold Complications and Red Flags

Consult your child's doctor as soon as possible if your child has any of the following symptoms associated with the common cold:

- Wheezing
- Rapid breathing or difficulty breathing
- Refusing to drink, or recurrent vomiting after drinking
- Increasing drowsiness
- New onset of fever several days after the cold first appears
- Chest muscles being sucked in with each breath
- Lips looking blue
- Complaining of a severe headache or a stiff and painful neck

Complications of Common Colds

Look for signs of a secondary bacterial infection.

Sign or Symptom	What This Might Mean
Fever for more than 5 days	• Pneumonia • Ear infection
Persistent cold symptoms or fever in child younger than 3 months	• Blood infection • Pneumonia
Ear pain or discharge	• Ear infection
Sore throat with high fever	• Strep throat
Chest pain or difficulty breathing	• Pneumonia
Runny nose for more than 10 days, with greenish discharge	• Sinusitis (uncommon before the age of 10)
Wheezing	• Asthma or bronchiolitis
Stiff or painful neck	• Meningitis

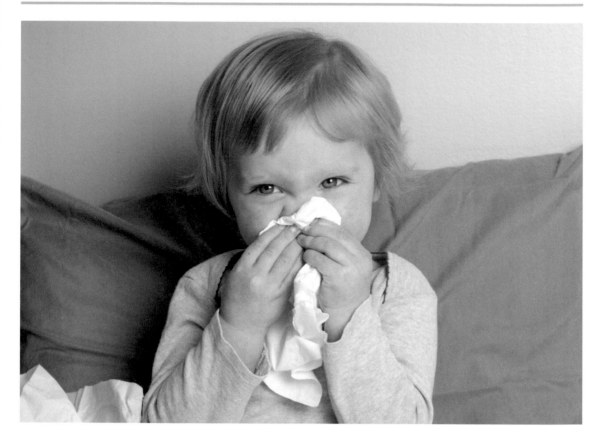

❷ What Causes the Common Cold?

Despite the fact that the common cold is caused by respiratory viruses, many people believe otherwise. Common myths about the common cold (none of these have been scientifically proven!):

- Flu shots cause colds.
- Frequent colds are caused by "weakened immune systems."
- Vitamin C and echinacea prevent colds.
- Drinking milk causes build-up of mucus, so it should be avoided when sick with a cold.
- Being outside in the cold or being chilled causes one to catch a cold.

❸ How Is the Common Cold Treated?

Do's and Don'ts for Managing the Common Cold

Do

- Offer your child fluids to ensure she is well hydrated.

- Try a saline spray for dry nasal passages, or an aspirator to remove mucus from the nose. This can be helpful, especially in young infants.
- Have your child sleep with his head slightly elevated. This can help with postnasal drip, which triggers coughing.
- If he seems to have new aches and pains or is uncomfortable with a fever, you can offer acetaminophen or ibuprofen.
- Humidify the air in your home if it seems to be dry.
- Wash your hands frequently to limit the spread of the virus to others.

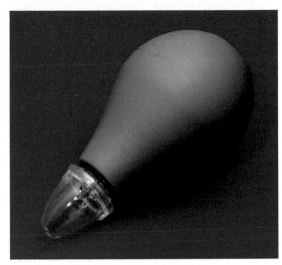

An aspirator to remove mucus from the nose

Don't

- Give your child antibiotics. Because colds are caused by viruses, antibiotics are not effective. In fact, they can cause harmful side effects if used inappropriately.
- Give your child over-the-counter cough and decongestant medicines. Studies have actually found them to be ineffective. In particular, in children younger than 6 years old, over-the-counter cough and cold medicines should be avoided because of potentially dangerous side effects. These preparations often contain chemicals that can cause harmful effects on the heart and interfere with breathing in young children
- Expose your child to irritants, like smoke or fumes.

Decongestants and Antibiotics

Oral decongestants and other over-the-counter cough and cold remedies are not recommended for children, especially those younger than 6 years of age. They are not particularly effective and can do more harm than good. Antibiotics are likewise not effective in treating a viral infection, such as the common cold.

Doc Talk

Time is the main cure for the common cold — that, combined with a little tender loving care. Children cure themselves. You can use acetaminophen or ibuprofen for relief of pain, aches, or fever, but avoid aspirin (acetylsalicylic acid) because it can lead to liver damage (Reye's syndrome). Coughing and congestion due to cold viruses usually resolve within 2 weeks. If symptoms are persistent, your child should be checked by a doctor.

Constipation

Case Study

Claire's Constipation

Claire is a 2½-year-old toddler, a healthy and independent little girl. She used to have soft bowel movements once daily until a few months ago when her dad noticed she was only going every few days. She was toilet trained at 2 years old. Recently, she has been avoiding going to the potty to have a bowel movement, and when she does go, boy, is it a battle! She usually ends up in tears and occasionally there is a bit of blood on her toilet paper. Claire is a picky eater and she has made it clear to her parents that she doesn't like fruits and vegetables. She would much rather have spaghetti or peanut butter sandwiches on white bread for all of her meals. Needless to say, Claire and her parents have become frustrated, both with meals and potty time.

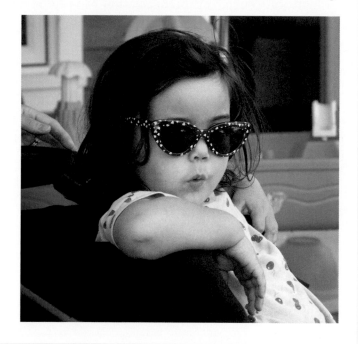

❶ What Is Constipation?

Constipation in children refers to a pattern of infrequent bowel motions associated with hard stools, straining, and discomfort. There is a wide variation in the frequency with which children pass stools. Some children will go three times daily, and others go every 3 days.

Both patterns may be normal. It is not so much the frequency of stools that makes the diagnosis but rather the associated symptoms of pain, hard stools, and straining.

When should we contact our doctor or local hospital?

Consult your child's doctor if your child has any of the following symptoms associated with constipation:

- History of failing to pass meconium (the first stool; a dark greenish black color) within 24 to 48 hours after birth
- Decreased appetite with weight loss
- Frequent bloody stools
- Constipation in infants younger than 4 months
- Pain with urination or frequent urination; this could suggest a urinary tract infection

⏩ Constipation Red Flags

Seek urgent medical attention if your child has any of the following symptoms associated with constipation:

- Vomiting, especially if vomit is green. See Vomiting (page 415).
- Severe abdominal pain. See Abdominal Pain (Acute) (page 18).

Signs and Symptoms of Constipation

- Fewer than three bowel movements weekly (infants younger than 6 months may only have a bowel movement once weekly)
- Fecal incontinence (soiling) in a previously toilet-trained child
- Retentive posturing or stool-withholding behaviors; a child may refuse to sit to have a bowel movement or may dance around or tip-toe, trying to hold in the stool
- Hard (pellet-like or well-formed) stools
- Painful bowel movements
- Large-volume stools that may block the toilet
- Tears in the pink lining of the anus (anal fissures), resulting from the passage of hard stools (see Bloody Stools, page 89)
- Blood on the toilet paper or the surface of the stool from an anal fissure
- Urinary tract infections, especially in toddlers; constipation may prevent the normal emptying of the bladder, leaving urine in the bladder, which can get infected

② What Causes Constipation?

More than 95% of childhood constipation cases are due to chronic functional constipation, which means that no identifiable disease is at fault. Rather, a number of factors can be involved. Rarely, a true pathological condition may be causing a child's constipation. Hirschsprung's disease, which is associated with faulty neurological development in the large bowel, can produce constipation from birth.

Functional Causes of Constipation

- Inherited tendency toward slow movement of the feces through the bowels
- Too little fiber from fruits, vegetables, and whole grains in the diet
- Not enough fluid daily
- Ignoring the need to have a bowel movement, such as when a child doesn't want to interrupt play or ask a teacher to use the toilet
- Psychological issues, such as too much pressure to become toilet trained or a fear of public bathrooms
- Avoidance of painful defecation caused by huge bowel motions, which leads to further stool retention

Pathological Causes of Constipation

- A history of the baby not passing meconium in the first 24 to 48 hours of life
- Any suggestion of an abnormality of the spinal cord, such as problems with the movement of the legs or passing urine
- Some hormonal or electrolyte disorders, such as a low thyroid hormone (hypothyroidism) or high blood calcium (hypercalcemia)

Did You Know?

Challenge
Constipation is one of the most common and challenging problems of childhood for doctors and parents alike. Unfortunately, it is also one of the most undertreated problems in children. Because it often goes unrecognized, children suffer, unnecessarily, from recurrent tummy pains, the painful passing of stools, decreased appetite, fecal incontinence, and interference with family routines.

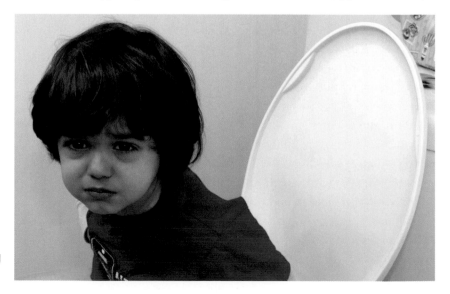

Retentive posturing from constipation

Behavioral Causes of Constipation

Some children develop significant stool-withholding behaviors that lead to constipation. These behaviors often arise around the time of toilet training. Some children fear having a bowel movement on the toilet. Others are fearful of passing large, painful bowel movements, further contributing to constipation. Children who are fearful of having bowel movements will often withhold stools for several days, creating a cycle of infrequent, large, painful bowel movements. This stretches out the bowel wall, which in future will make it more difficult for the child to know when they actually need to empty their bowels. This cycle must be broken to prevent long-term problems with constipation.

Onset

Although the majority of constipation occurs gradually over time, there are some very predictable times in a child's life when parents are more likely to notice constipation becoming a problem.

- During the introduction of solid foods at 4 to 6 months
- When transitioning from breastmilk or formula to cow's milk
- During changes in normal routine, such as at the start of school or when traveling
- While toilet training
- During acute illness, such as the flu, when a child might have vomiting, fever, and dehydration

❸ How Is Constipation Treated?

Because the causes of constipation are often multifactorial, treatment plans for constipation ideally target behavioral, dietary, and physical influences for constipation. Any treatment should be in place for a minimum of 6 months to allow the bowel time to get back to normal. Treatment of constipation will also differ between infants, toddlers, and children.

Dietary Strategies
Infants Younger Than 4 Months

Infants at this age generally do not have constipation. If you are worried that your infant is suffering with her bowel movements, see your doctor. Do not switch your baby's formula or breast milk to remedy the problem. Prior to giving any medication for constipation, see your child's doctor.

Infants 4 to 12 Months

After your infant has started on solids, you can feed her high-fiber foods that have been strained. Examples include peaches, pears, plums, prunes, apricots, beans, and cereals.

Toddlers and Children

- Ensure your child drinks adequate amounts of fluids. Adequate fluid intake is based on your child's weight. Daily fluid intake should be at least 32 ounces (1 L) in a 22-pound (10 kg) child, 48 ounces (1.5 L) in a 44-pound (20 kg) child, and 64 ounces (2 L) in an 88-pound (40 kg) child.
- Give your child at least 4 to 6 servings of fruits and vegetables daily.
- Add bran to your child's food; bran is very high in fibre and acts as a natural stool softener.
- Limit foods that contribute to constipation, such as bananas, rice, white bread, white pasta, peanut butter, and junk food.

How To: Increase Dietary Fiber

Foods to Choose

- Whole-grain breads and pastas
- High-fiber fruits and vegetables, such as plums, peaches, prunes, and apricots — with the peel on
- Fresh baked goods with wheat germ, or sauces (for example, spaghetti sauce) with bran
- High-fiber cereals, such as bran, shredded wheat, whole grains, and oatmeal
- Unbuttered, unsalted popcorn (if child older than 3 years)
- Up to 16 ounces (500 mL) a day of milk and the remainder of fluids given as water

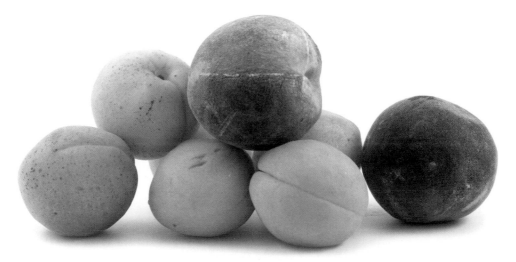

Foods to Avoid or Restrict

- White breads and pastas
- Constipating fruits and vegetables, such as bananas and cooked carrots
- Processed baked goods high in sugars and low in fiber
- Low-fiber cereals, such as corn flakes cereal or crisp rice cereal
- Potato chips, crackers
- More than 16 ounces (500 mL) a day of milk with limited water intake

Behavioral Strategies

- Encourage your child to sit on the potty, just for a few minutes, after meals and at bedtime. This should be unhurried.
- On the potty, your child's feet should be flat on the floor (or on a stool if sitting on the toilet). This helps a child "push down" and pass stool more easily.
- If going to the toilet to have a bowel movement is a battle, consider a reward system, such as a sticker chart for attempts to sit on the toilet. Lack of success should not be punished.
- Apply a small amount of petroleum jelly around the opening of the anus if you ever see a small amount of fresh blood in the stool. This may indicate a small tear in the anus.
- If you are in the process of toilet training and your child is withholding stools, consider delaying toilet training until she is more ready and the constipation is under control.
- See your health-care provider if your child is exhibiting stool-withholding behaviors— the earlier these behaviors are addressed, the easier they are to fix.

Medication Strategies

Medication is a major component in the treatment of chronic constipation, both for relieving the constipation and for maintaining soft, regular stools. Many parents will want to treat constipation naturally, but even the most optimal diet and adherence to behavioral strategies are often insufficient. Some children just need a little extra help! Children should be treated for several months to help restore normal rectal tone and stool evacuation.

There are several different types of laxatives given by mouth (orally) and in the rectum (suppository or enema). Some act as lubricants, others act to increase the water content of stool, and others increase the muscle tone of the rectum, helping to stimulate the stool to move forward. Medication for constipation is best used in consultation with your health-care provider, who can offer support and guidance.

Medications Used to Treat Constipation

Consult with your child's doctor before using any medication to treat constipation.

Medication	Dose	How It Works	Comments
Polyethylene glycol 3350 (PEG 3350, Lax-a-Day, MiraLAX, ClearLax)	0.4 to 1 g/kg/day up to 17 g total/day; may occasionally be used in higher doses with physician's guidance	Increases stool water content	• Safe, very well tolerated • No long-term dependence • Tasteless, colorless, and odorless
Mineral oil	1 to 3 mL/kg daily	Acts as a lubricant laxative	• Not for young infants • Never force-feed: it can cause damage to the lungs if it goes down the wrong way by accident • Unwanted oily seepage in underwear
Lactulose	1 to 3 mL/kg daily, in divided doses	Increases stool water content	• Safe and well tolerated • May cause some gas and bloating • Good choice for infants
Sorbitol	1 to 3 mL/kg daily	Increases stool water content	• Safe and well tolerated
Senna (Senokot)	1 to 5 years old: 5 mL once daily; 5 to 12 years old: 5 mL twice daily	Acts as a stimulant laxative	• Used for disimpaction (removal of very hard, large, stools that are difficult to pass) • Don't use if severe cramping present
Bisacodyl (Dulcolax)	5 mg orally, or 5 to 10 mg rectally daily	Acts as a stimulant laxative	• Used for disimpaction • Give at bedtime to reduce cramps
Docusate (Colace)	2 to 3 mL/kg daily in divided doses	Acts as a stool softener	• Safe but don't use in combination with mineral oil because oil absorption is increased
Glycerin suppository	1 infant suppository daily	Acts as a lubricant	• Used for disimpaction • Good choice for infants
Phosphate enema (Fleet)	2 to 12 years old: 60 mL as a one-time dose	Increases stool water content	• For disimpaction only • Use only with medical advice

FAQs

My 3-month-old son strains and becomes red in the face while passing stools. His stools are still soft. Is he constipated?

Probably not. Infants have not yet learned how to coordinate relaxation of the pelvic muscles with pushing to evacuate their bowels. This appearance of straining is the result of this lack of coordination. If the stool is soft, your son is by definition unlikely to be constipated. If you notice hard stools or a fissure developing at the opening of the anus, your child is likely constipated and may need a stool softener.

My child often has small bits of diarrhea followed by larger pellet-like stools. Is this still constipation even though he is having diarrhea?

Yes! This is likely overflow stool. This often happens with chronic constipation when the bowel wall has become stretched out and lost its tone. Stool builds up in the enlarged rectum, blocking the exit. Sometimes looser stool from higher up in the bowel seeps around the large fecal mass sitting in the rectum and comes out as diarrhea.

I keep hearing that my son needs to use constipation medication for several months. Is it safe to use them for so long? Why can't I just stop them when the stools are back to normal?

Many studies have shown that medications such as PEG 3350 and lactulose are very safe for children for long periods of time, with no known long-term adverse effects. Children need to be continued on medications to keep their stools soft so that the bowel can return to normal size and regain its normal tone. This process takes several months.

My daughter is showing signs of toilet-training readiness but she is constipated already. Is it too early to start toilet training?

Treating the constipation before trying to toilet train your daughter is critical. This will make the training much easier and prevent worsening of the constipation with the added pressure of mastering the potty.

Doc Talk Chronic constipation takes a really long time to treat because the bowel wall becomes very stretched out. The bowel wall muscles need to be "retrained" so that they can regain their tone. Treatment should be for a minimum of 6 to 12 months.

Cough

What Can I Do?

▶ Be reassured that most coughs will resolve in a matter of days.

▶ Review the list of red flags to see if your child needs urgent medical attention.

▶ Do not use over-the-counter cough medications in children under 6 years of age; they can cause more harm than good.

❶ What Is a Cough?

RELATED CONDITIONS

- Allergic rhinitis
- Asthma
- Bronchiolitis
- Choking
- Common cold
- Croup
- Pertussis
- Pneumonia

Coughing is one of the most common reasons for a child to be seen by his health-care provider. Coughing is a protective reflex that helps clear the airways of mucus and secretions. This helps the body prevent and recover from infections. Naturally, parents may worry and wonder if their child's coughing is just a simple cold, something more serious (such as pneumonia), or if their child has asthma.

Coughing is rarely an isolated symptom but rather is accompanied by other symptoms, such as congestion, fever, wheezing, or difficulty breathing. These other symptoms provide clues to the correct diagnosis and treatment.

When should we contact our doctor or local hospital?

In most cases, coughing will resolve in time, but occasionally the cough will indicate a more serious cause that may require attention and treatment. If red flags are present, seek medical attention.

➤➤ Coughing Red Flags

Consult your child's doctor as soon as possible if your child has any of the following symptoms associated with coughing:

- Breathing becomes faster than normal
- Chest muscles are sucked in with every breath
- Disinterest in feeding or in drinking (expect appetite to be a bit lower than normal)
- Not as interactive as you would expect with a simple cold
- Bluish color around the mouth
- Persistent cough lasting more than a couple of weeks

Cough Symptoms and Causes

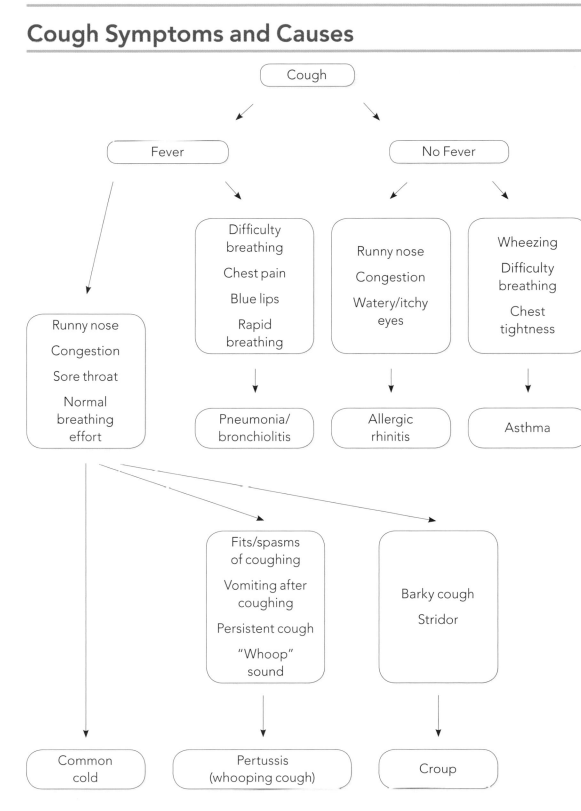

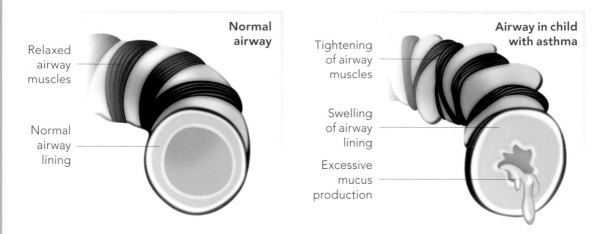

Normal airway

Relaxed airway muscles

Normal airway lining

Airway in child with asthma

Tightening of airway muscles

Swelling of airway lining

Excessive mucus production

Common Conditions Causing Cough

- Asthma
- Bronchiolitis
- Croup
- Pneumonia
- Common Cold
- Choking
- Pertussis

Asthma

Asthma is one of the most common chronic conditions of childhood, diagnosed in as many as 1 in 10 children.

Signs and Symptoms of Asthma

- Wheezing
- Coughing, especially at night
- Prolonged cough that won't go away
- Chest tightness
- Shortness of breath
- Tires quickly or coughs while playing or exercising
- May cough for longer than expected after a common cold

Common Asthma Triggers

- Viral upper respiratory tract infection (common cold)
- Smoke
- Dust
- Pollen
- Cold weather
- Humid weather

Did You Know?

Genetic Predisposition

A combination of genetic factors (asthma tends to run in families) and triggers in the environment predispose a child to asthma. It is also more common in children with eczema and children with food or environmental allergies.

- Air pollution
- Strong odors or perfumes
- Exercise

Causes of Asthma

Asthma is caused by a narrowing of the small airways in the lungs. This makes it difficult for air to move in and out. Three processes can occur in a child with asthma to make this happen. First, the lining of the airways becomes inflamed, resulting in thickening and swelling. Second, the muscles lining the airways tighten, causing the airways to narrow, a process called bronchoconstriction. Third, the airways produce excessive amounts of mucus, which blocks air from flowing out of the lungs easily.

Diagnosis

Asthma is diagnosed based on a cluster of signs and symptoms:

- Repeated episodes of wheezing
- Persistent cough or breathing difficulty in response to common triggers
- Often appearing well between episodes
- May also have eczema and/or allergies
- Others in the family have asthma or allergies
- In older children coordinated enough to cooperate (usually around 6 years old), lung-function testing can be helpful in diagnosing asthma

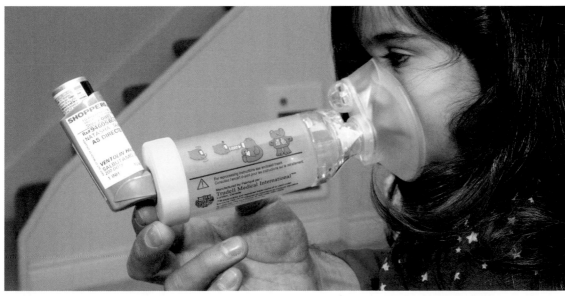

A child using an aerochamber and metered-dose inhaler (MDI)

Treatment

Treatment of asthma involves both managing the symptoms and reducing underlying inflammation as well as avoiding any known triggers. It is sometimes helpful for children to undergo allergy testing to learn about potential triggers that might go under-recognized. Some children tend to "outgrow" their asthma as they get older. For others, although their asthma may be chronic, it can be effectively controlled with medication and education.

Medications

Two types of medications are used to treat asthma: reliever and anti-inflammatory medications. Reliever medicines — for example, albuterol or salbutamol (Ventolin) — act quickly to help when symptoms (wheezing, cough, shortness of breath) are present. This medicine helps relax the muscles around the airways, allowing air to flow more freely. Anti-inflammatory medications — for example, fluticasone (Flovent), budesonide (Pulmicort), and ciclesonide (Alvesco) — can be used on a regular basis to prevent inflammation and are sometimes called "preventers."

Croup

Many children will experience what appears to be a run-of-the-mill common cold followed by the sudden onset of a loud, barking cough that can sound like a seal or foghorn. It frequently develops out of the blue, often in the middle of the night. This is the typical description of croup, which is caused by swelling of the upper windpipe and voice box due to a viral infection. It usually affects toddler-age children, most commonly in the fall.

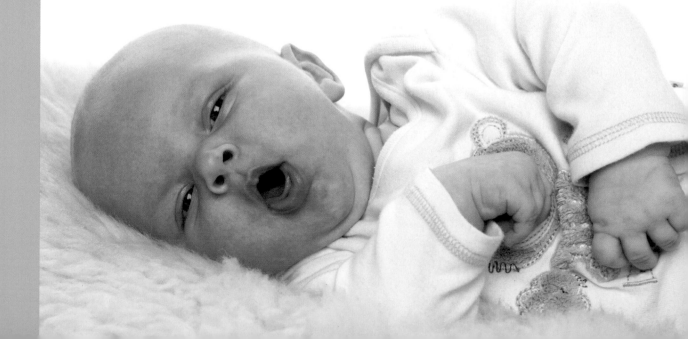

Signs and Symptoms of Croup

The loud coughing can be very alarming, but the bark is usually worse than the bite! If your child only has the loud coughing but is otherwise well, there is no cause for alarm. Signs and symptoms of worsening croup requiring medical attention include:

- A harsh, high-pitched breathing noise that is most noticeable when a child breathes in (called stridor)
- Breathing appears rapid
- Muscles in the chest or neck become noticeable as more effort is used for breathing
- Bluish color appears around the mouth
- Not able to eat or drink, or disinterested in food and drink

Treatment

Most mild cases of croup resolve on their own, without the need for any treatment. When the onset is sudden, some children will find it comforting to be exposed to either colder air by taking them outside on a cool night or to humidity in a steamy bathroom. Your doctor might prescribe a dose of oral liquid steroid medication if the symptoms are more persistent. Children with more severe symptoms will need to be seen in the emergency department, where other medications, including aerosolized inhalations, may be advised.

Pneumonia

Common upper respiratory tract infections usually resolve on their own over a week, and the last few days are typically better than the beginning of the illness. If fever is persistent and the cough and other symptoms seem to be getting worse rather than better over the course of the week, this may be a sign that the infection is now involving the lungs and small breathing passages (pneumonia) rather than the upper airway (ears, nasal passages, and throat). Pneumonia is one of the most common infections in children. Pneumonia is most commonly caused by viral infections in young children (younger than 3 years old), with bacterial infections being more likely in older children.

Signs and Symptoms of Pneumonia

- Persistent/worsening cough or fever
- Rapid breathing
- Abdominal or chest pain
- Visible use of chest muscles in an effort to breathe

Any of these signs should prompt a visit to the doctor. Antibiotics are usually prescribed if bacterial pneumonia is suspected.

Common Cold

The common cold is one of the most common causes of coughing in children. It tends to be associated with fever, runny nose, and congestion. See Common Cold (page 120).

Pertussis (Whooping Cough)

If your child has coughing spasms that make her go red in the face and seem to last forever, she may have whooping cough. Infants are routinely immunized against pertussis beginning in the first few months of life. Unfortunately, infections and outbreaks still occur, even in children who have been immunized (though in a much milder form compared with unvaccinated children). In some parts of the world, this infection is known by the aptly named "100-day cough."

Signs and Symptoms of Pertussis

Pertussis may start out appearing as a common cold, but then may evolve into persistent and prolonged spasms of coughing. The name whooping cough is derived from the high-pitched sound made when catching one's breath following a prolonged coughing fit. Young infants are most susceptible to getting severely ill from pertussis. Other signs and symptoms include choking, vomiting after fits of coughing, burst blood vessels in the eyes from forceful coughing, blue spells, breath-holding, and frank stopping of breathing (apnea).

Diagnosis

If your doctor suspects pertussis, testing using a swab from the nose and throat may be suggested. Antibiotics are given to lessen the spread of infection to other people, but they do not shorten the course of the illness.

Choking

As young children begin to explore, they inevitably will put things into their mouths. They are at risk for choking on food or other objects that may end up lodged in the windpipe (trachea) or large airway (bronchus). Children younger than 3 years old are at the greatest risk of choking. The aspiration (inhaling) of an object into the large airways may cause immediate symptoms, such as choking, obvious breathing difficulty, or stridor. However, sometimes the symptoms are more subtle, and caregivers might not recall or have witnessed a choking event. If it has lodged in a smaller airway, a foreign object may cause persistent coughing or wheezing (a high-pitched noise heard when breathing in and out).

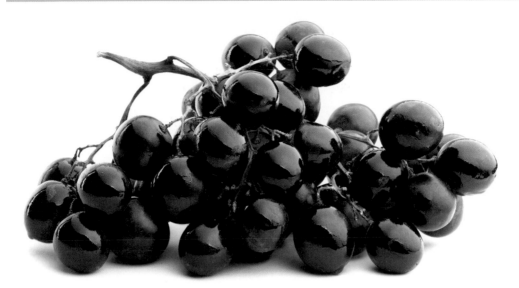

Common food objects leading to choking:

- Hotdogs
- Peanuts
- Uncut grapes
- Hard candies
- Popcorn
- Marshmallows

Some toys — such as marbles, small balls, or anything than can lodge in the breathing passages (generally less than $^3/_4$ inch/2 cm in diameter) — are common choking hazards.

Treatment

If you are worried that your child may have choked on something, consult with your doctor. Sometimes an object or other clues of an aspirated object can be seen on an X-ray, but unless it contains metal, it will not usually be seen. Other procedures may be necessary if an inhaled foreign object is suspected. See Choking and Aspiration (page 112) for the emergency management of a choking child.

Doc Talk

The information in this section can serve as a general guide, but please remember that children don't always follow the "textbook"; for example, in the algorithm on page 133, one child may get the common cold with absolutely no fever, and another may have asthma with a fever if their asthma attack was triggered by a viral cold.

A
B
C
D
E
F
G
H
I
J
K
L
M
N
O
P
Q
R
S
T
U
V
W
X
Y
Z

Crying

What Can I Do?

▶ Try to assess the 12 common options that may be causing your baby's crying.

▶ Address the appropriate cause using the strategies provided.

▶ If none of them provides the solution and you are concerned that your baby may be in pain or be sick, seek medical advice .

❶ What Is Crying?

Did You Know?

Crying Time
Some babies cry very little, as little as 1 hour daily or less (lucky parents!), and others can cry up to 5 or 6 hours daily. Crying increases over the first few weeks of life, reaching a peak at about 6 weeks. Crying then gradually decreases over the next few months.

Babies cry to communicate what they need because they can do little for themselves. As your baby gets older, she will learn to use other sounds, facial expressions, and gestures to communicate her needs. Realistically, however, she will continue to cry from time to time anyway.

Crying is perfectly normal, but there is a wide range of "normal." As parents, we are often sleep-deprived and worried, which makes interpretation very challenging at times.

When should we contact our doctor or local hospital?

Some crying is natural. It is a way for your child to communicate her needs. However, crying can indicate pain and discomfort that your child cannot resolve without medical assistance. If your baby is not acting normally, for example not interacting appropriately, not "herself," or not feeding as you would expect, and you are concerned that she may be sick, see your doctor.

❷ What Causes Babies to Cry?

There are many reasons babies cry. Often it will take a bit of trial and error to sort out the cause and to find a working solution. Try using these questions to communicate with your child. Rule out causes one by one.

Are You Hungry?
Most babies will cry when they are hungry. Your baby may put her hand to her mouth, suck vigorously on a finger or pacifier, smack her lips, or root. Try offering your baby a feed.

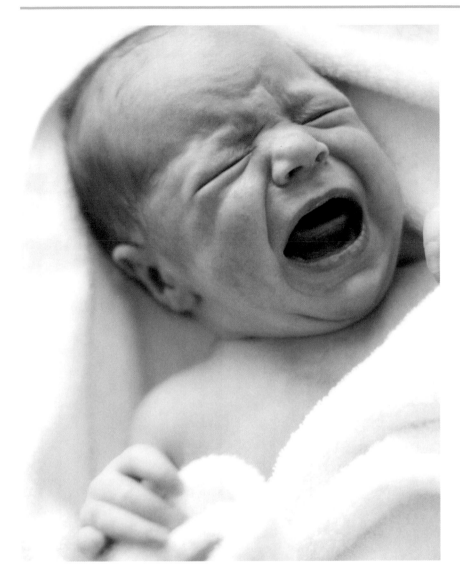

Do You Need a Diaper Change?

Babies vary in how long they will tolerate a wet or soiled diaper. Some will want to be changed right away, but others don't even seem to notice. A clean diaper will quickly solve crying as a result of a dirty bottom!

Are You Tired?

Babies need a lot of rest, but often have difficulty soothing themselves to sleep. They will often fuss, cry, and become agitated or inconsolable when they need to sleep, especially if they are overtired. A young baby may need your help falling asleep; removing stimulation and providing a calm, dark, and quiet environment may help. Some babies may also need to be rocked, swaddled, or otherwise soothed to sleep.

A B C D E F G H I J K L M N O P Q R S T U V W X Y Z

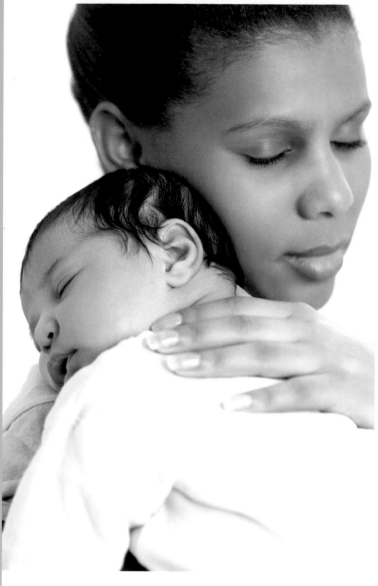

Do You Want to Be Held?

Babies love to be held close in order to feel, hear, and smell their caregivers. Many people worry about spoiling a baby by carrying them too much, but you cannot spoil a baby with attention in the first few months of life. If your baby wants to be held all the time, you may find an infant carrier helpful and convenient.

Is Your Tummy Bothering You?

Gas can make an infant uncomfortable. Infants may pull up their legs, pass gas, or strain and grunt when passing stool. Try placing your baby on her belly, moving her legs back and forth in a bicycling motion, or give a gentle tummy massage. There are many over-the-counter medications for gas. They have not been scientifically proven to work, but, on the other hand, they are generally not harmful. If you suspect this is the source of your baby's crying, you should discuss these options with your doctor. More serious causes of abdominal pain, such as milk allergies, blockages, and infections, will also require your doctor's help to sort out.

Do You Need to Burp?

Crying that occurs during or after a feed can be due to gas or liquid and stomach acid traveling back up the esophagus. Babies can swallow a lot of air while breast- or bottle-feeding and may need to burp during or after feeding. Some babies burp spontaneously, but others need help to do so. Some strategies to help a baby burp include patting her back or putting gentle pressure on her stomach by holding her over your shoulder or knee.

Are You Too Warm or Cold?

Babies may feel too hot or too cold, and are very sensitive to being over- or underdressed. Generally, one light layer more than what an adult is wearing will keep a baby comfortable.

Are You in Pain?

Little things that can be hard to spot may be causing your baby pain. Small cuts or abrasions may be difficult to see, or a rough tag or stitching on clothing may be causing discomfort. If you can't find any obvious reason for your baby's crying, undress her completely and give her a good once-over.

Are You Teething?

In general, the first tooth arrives between 6 and 10 months, but there is huge variation. A teething baby may drool or mouth objects more than usual. Her gums may appear red or swollen, and you may be able to feel or see a hard white bump under the gums or breaking through. Teething pain may be relieved by over-the-counter pain medication, including acetaminophen or ibuprofen, or by providing a cool, clean cloth or teething ring for baby to chew on.

Do You Need a Break?

The sights, sounds, sensations, and smells of the world outside the womb are all new to a baby. Sometimes a baby may want to experience more of what is around her and she'll cry to tell you she needs more stimulation. Other times, a baby may cry to tell you that there is too much going on and she needs a little break. Finding the right amount of stimulation for your baby is a learning process and will change as your baby grows.

Are You Sick?

Babies may cry to tell you they are feeling sick. A sick baby may be less active, may not want to feed or feed less, or may have a fever. Trust your instincts, because you know your baby best. If you suspect your baby is sick, you should talk to your doctor.

Do You Have Colic?

Read the discussion on Colic (page 117).

| **Doc Talk** | Crying is your baby's way of communicating with you. It can be hard to work out why your baby is crying, but in time, you will learn to recognize what your baby is trying to tell you. |

Cuts (Lacerations), Scrapes, and Wounds

What Can I Do?

▶ Learn basic first aid and keep a fully stocked first aid kit available.

▶ Aim to stop the bleeding by keeping steady pressure on the cut or wound for at least 5 minutes without constant peeking.

▶ Remember to compress, elevate, clean, and dress the wound.

❶ What Is a Laceration?

Very few children will grow up without suffering a cut or laceration, and minor scrapes can seem like a way of life for the accident-prone child. In most cases, a bandage to stop the bleeding and some Polysporin to prevent infection will do the job. Deep cuts and serious scrapes may require serious medical attention to stop the bleeding and help with the healing process.

When should we contact our doctor or local hospital?

Children frequently sustain minor cuts and lacerations. While most will heal by themselves, others require medical attention if the bleeding persists, if the wound is deep and gaping, or if the cut looks to be infected. Any cuts that you think may require stitches, glue, or staples should be assessed as soon as possible after the injury, ideally within 6 to 8 hours. Beyond 12 hours, most cuts cannot be closed with these techniques.

⏩ Cuts and Scrapes Red Flags

Seek medical treatment if:

- The bleeding does not stop on its own after applying firm pressure for 5 minutes

- The cut is deep (there may be damage underneath the skin)

- The cut looks infected, with redness or pus around the site

- Your child cannot completely bend or straighten his finger, arm, or leg without reopening the cut

- The laceration is from an animal bite

- You suspect that there is any foreign material in the wound, such as dirt, glass, or wood

Signs that the wound may be infected:

- Increasing redness around the wound
- Increasing swelling around the wound
- Creamy yellow discharge (pus) from the wound

❷ How Are Cuts and Lacerations Treated?

Compress

Apply direct firm pressure with clean gauze or even clean paper tissues, if nothing else is available.

Elevate

Elevate the area if practical — for example, if it is a finger or toe, make sure that it is raised above the level of the heart (in the case of the toe and leg this will require lying down!)

Clean

The most important factor in healing is to ensure the wound is clean. You need to determine whether there is any dirt or foreign material in the cut. This might include bits of sticks or stones and gravel and will increase the risk of infection. To eliminate or minimize bacterial contamination, rinse a potentially dirty wound with clean water. This may involve washing the area under a running faucet or placing the cut/scraped area in a bowl of warm soapy water. After the wound is cleaned, pat it dry.

Dress

Many health-care providers will recommend using a topical antibiotic ointment (for example, Polysporin) once or twice a day, especially if there is concern that the wound is at risk of getting infected. If there are any signs of infection, then it is an indication to seek further help.

> **Did You Know?**
>
> **Steady Pressure**
> A common error in treating bleeding from a cut is to constantly be checking to see if it is still bleeding. The best approach is to maintain a steady pressure for 5 minutes before checking to see if the bleeding has stopped. With this approach, almost all bleeding will stop!

> **Did You Know?**
>
> **Sun Damage**
> Sun damage to fresh skin where a scar has formed can damage the skin further. Keep all wounds covered with clothing and sun block for several months after the injury.

FAQ

Does the cut need to be closed?
Most wounds benefit from being closed to prevent infection, to speed healing, and to decrease scarring. However, cuts inside the mouth or on the tongue, for example, from falling and biting the cheek or tongue, usually don't have to be closed unless they are bleeding excessively.

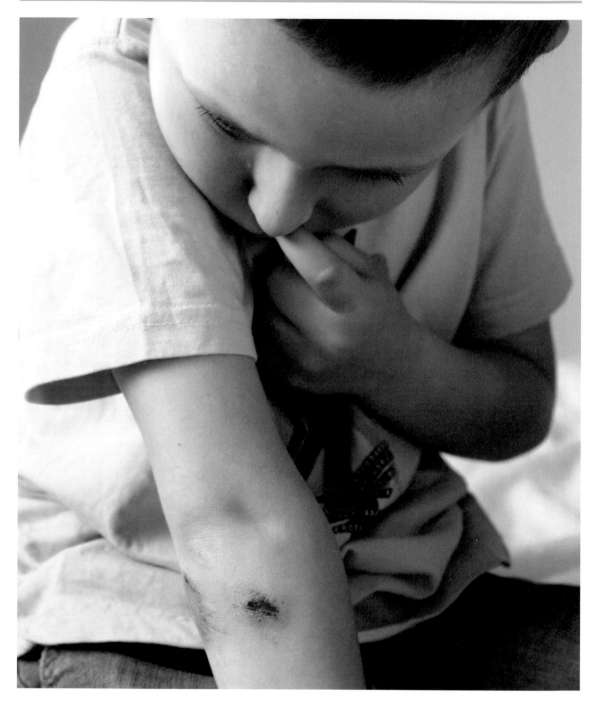

Types of Closure

The type of closure used will depend on the depth, location, and type of wound. If your child has a deep wound, you might have to take him to an emergency room for stitching, staples, or gluing to obtain the best result. Generally, the time interval between the laceration and the repair should be as short as possible. Lacerations should be closed within 6 to 8 hours of injury.

Type of Closure	When Is It Used?
Sutures/stitches	Deep cuts, jagged edges, areas that are stretched (over the elbow, around the knee)
Glue	Medium to deep cuts with smooth edges, areas with minimal tension (face)
Staples	Deep cuts, jagged edges, areas with a lot of bleeding (scalp)
Steri-strips	Shallow to medium cuts with smooth edges
Adhesive bandage	Shallow/superficial cuts anywhere

Did You Know?

Stitches and Staples

Stitches and staples usually come out after 7 to 10 days, although a bit earlier if they are on the face. This is usually done at the doctor's office or clinic.

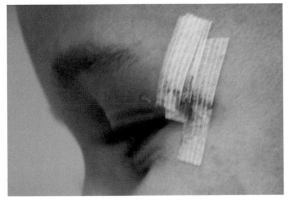

Sutures/stitches

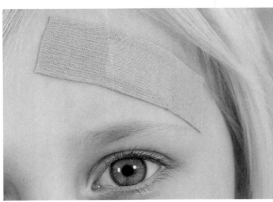

Staples

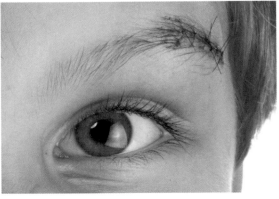

Steri-strips

Adhesive bandage

Doc Talk If possible, take your child's immunization record to the emergency room. His tetanus status must always be checked. A tetanus booster is required every 10 years, although after a potentially contaminated laceration, a booster should be given after 5 years.

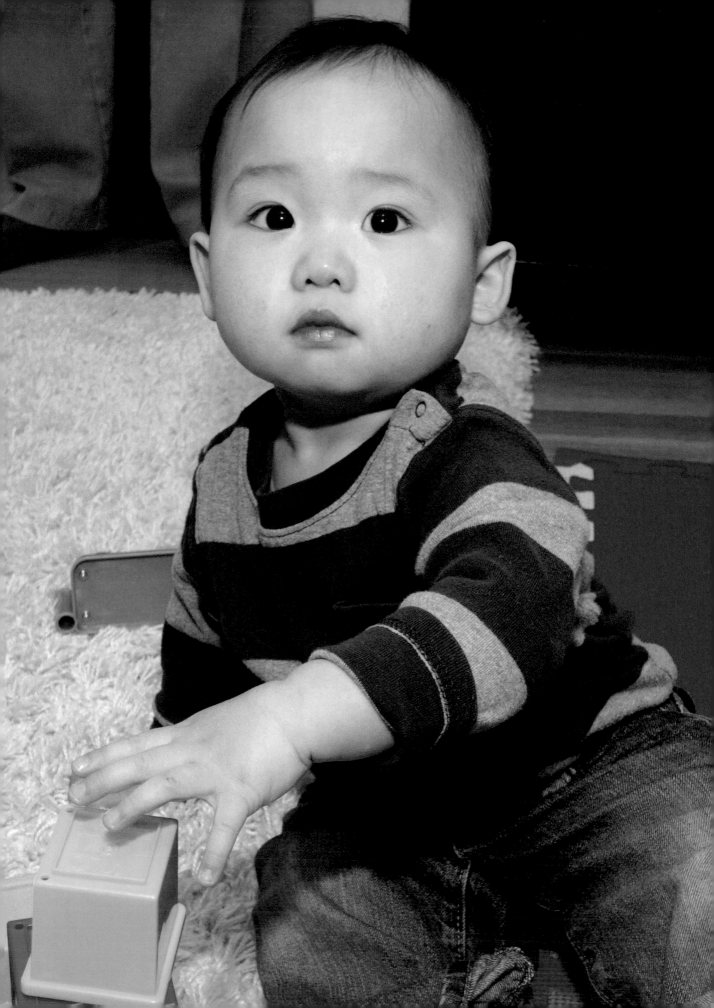

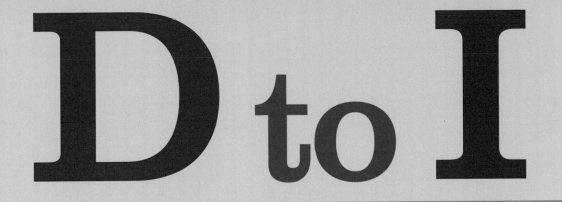

D to I

Dehydration

What Can I Do?

▶ If your child shows mild signs of dehydration, provide small frequent amounts of fluids. Oral rehydration solutions work best.

▶ See the algorithm on page 152 for some guidance about how much and how fast to give fluids.

▶ To determine if your infant or child is receiving enough liquids, monitor how much she is urinating by either checking her diaper or keeping an eye on how frequently she takes trips to the bathroom.

❶ What Is Dehydration?

Dehydrated infant with sunken eyes, absent tears, and dry mouth

Dehydration refers to the loss of water and salts from the body. These can be lost from vomiting, passing stools, voiding (peeing), sweating, and breathing. We replace this lost fluid by eating and drinking. Our body normally regulates the fine balance of gaining and losing fluid

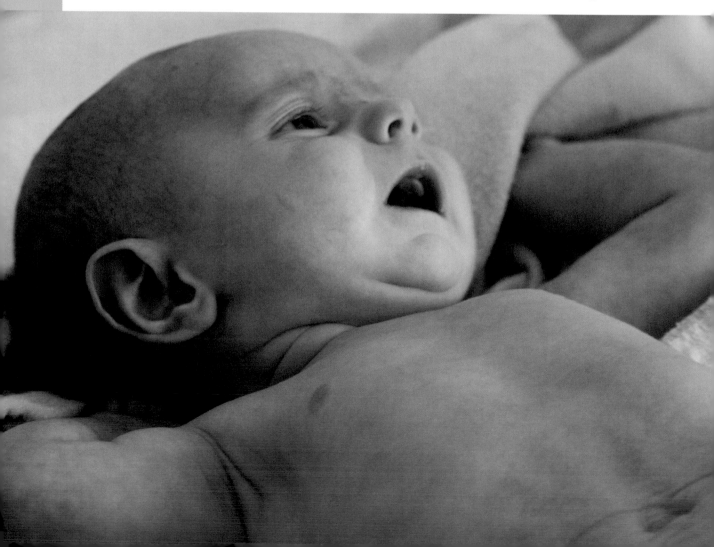

very well. However, when we are sick, this tightly regulated process can become unbalanced and we need to actively replace our lost fluid.

Signs and Symptoms

- Dry eyes, with decreased or absent tears
- Dry, sticky mouth and tongue
- Sunken eyes
- Sunken soft spot (fontanelle) in infants
- Decreased energy, lethargy, lack of interest in surroundings, irritability
- Decreased urine output
- Dark, concentrated urine
- Increased thirst

When should we consult our doctor or local hospital?

In most cases, dehydration can be managed simply by providing your child with plenty of fluids. Sipping fluids from a glass works just fine. In some cases, you may need help in rehydrating your child. If you are not able to improve symptoms, seek medical attention.

⏩ Dehydration Red Flags

Seek urgent medical attention if your child has any of the following symptoms associated with dehydration:

- Inability to keep down fluids for more than a few hours
- Lethargy, lack of interest in surroundings
- Dry mouth, without saliva
- Dry, sunken eyes, with absent tears
- Lack of urine
- Sunken soft spot (fontanelle)

❷ What Causes Dehydration?

The most common causes of dehydration in children include:

- Excess fluid loss from vomiting or diarrhea
- Decreased fluid intake when a child is feeling unwell
- Increased fluid loss from the skin with fever and sweating

How Much Fluid Do I Give and How Fast?

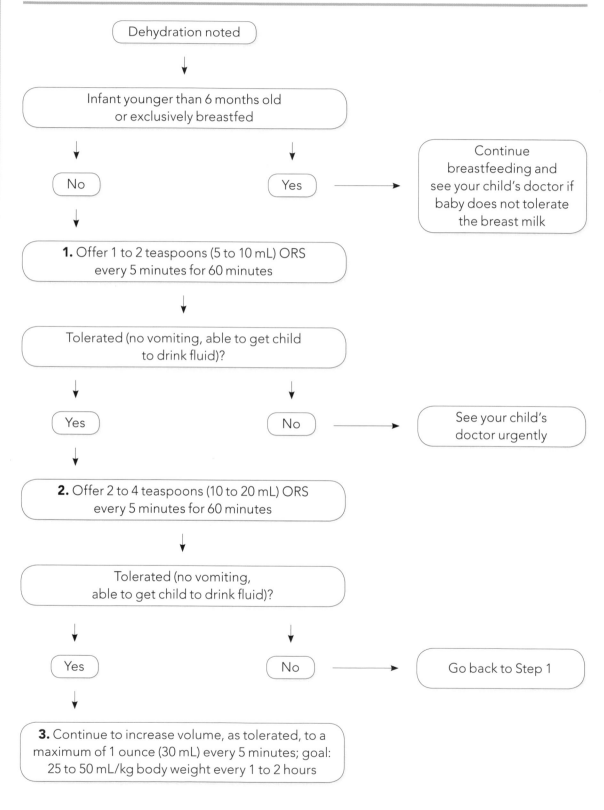

Dehydration noted

↓

Infant younger than 6 months old
or exclusively breastfed

No → **1.** Offer 1 to 2 teaspoons (5 to 10 mL) ORS
every 5 minutes for 60 minutes

Yes → Continue breastfeeding and see your child's doctor if baby does not tolerate the breast milk

↓

Tolerated (no vomiting, able to get child
to drink fluid)?

Yes → **2.** Offer 2 to 4 teaspoons (10 to 20 mL) ORS
every 5 minutes for 60 minutes

No → See your child's doctor urgently

↓

Tolerated (no vomiting,
able to get child to drink fluid)?

Yes → **3.** Continue to increase volume, as tolerated, to a maximum of 1 ounce (30 mL) every 5 minutes; goal: 25 to 50 mL/kg body weight every 1 to 2 hours

No → Go back to Step 1

❸ How Is Dehydration Treated?

Mild dehydration can be managed at home, whereas significant dehydration often needs to be treated in hospital. Children should be offered a commercially prepared oral rehydration solution (ORS), for example, Pedialyte, Enfalyte, or Gastrolyte. These are available, without prescription, at most drugstores. These solutions taste a little bit salty, so flavored solutions often work best. If your child is not willing to drink from a cup or bottle, try feeding with a spoon or a syringe, or perhaps try the frozen ice-pop option. The fluid can be served at any temperature.

How To: Get Your Child to Take an Oral Rehydration Solution

Getting your child to drink extra fluids when he is sick is inevitably challenging. His fussiness from feeling unwell and your sleep deprivation from being up all night with him certainly don't help the matter! Try these simple solutions to prevent or treat dehydration in your child.

- Try different flavors of oral rehydration solution. Pedialyte comes in strawberry, grape, apple, fruit punch, and bubble gum. It may take going through all of the flavors to find the one your child accepts.
- Oral rehydration solutions come in powders, ice pops, and ready-to-serve liquids. Find the one your child likes best.
- Oral rehydration solutions can be served at any temperature. Sometimes children will prefer a cold drink, and others may like it best at room temperature.
- If your child won't take a cup or bottle, try giving fluids using a spoon or a syringe.
- Offer your child oral rehydration solution as soon as you notice vomiting, diarrhea, or decreased fluid intake. Getting fluids into your child early will not only prevent dehydration, but it is often much easier when your child is feeling a bit better and less sleepy.
- Give your child acetaminophen or ibuprofen if he is uncomfortable from fever or pain. This will make getting any fluid into him easier.
- If your child is having difficulty keeping fluids down, talk to your doctor about medication for reducing nausea and vomiting. dimenhydrinate (Gravol) and ondansetron (Zofran) are two commonly used medications to treat a child who is vomiting from gastroenteritis. These should not be used without consulting with your doctor first.

Did You Know?

Rehydration Solution

A commercially prepared oral rehydration solution provides optimal amounts of sugars and salts to treat dehydration. Other solutions, such as flattened soft drinks, juice, tea, and soup, do not have the right mix of sugar and salt. These should not be used to treat dehydration.

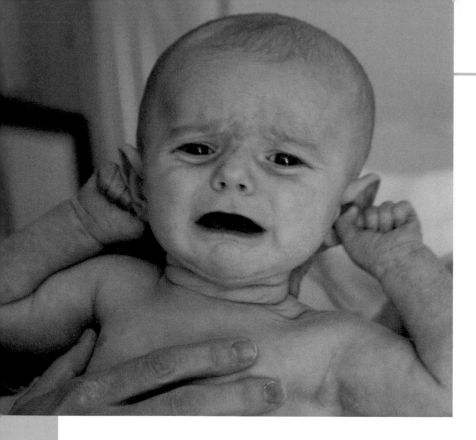

Dehydration in Newborn Infants

Newborn infants can become dehydrated very quickly after birth. The easiest way to tell if your newborn is dehydrated is to assess how well he is feeding, how many wet diapers he is having, and his weight. Below are guidelines for assessing if your newborn is adequately hydrated. If any red flags are present, see a health-care provider urgently.

Newborn Infant Hydration Red Flags

Day	Frequency of Feeding	Minimum Urine Output	Red Flags
1	Minimum 6 to 8 times in 24 hours	1 wet diaper in 24 hours	• No urine output
2	Minimum 8 times in 24 hours	2 to 4 wet diapers in 24 hours	• Decreased urine output
3 to 6	Minimum 8 times in 24 hours	4 to 6 wet diapers in 24 hours	• Decreased urine output • Baby too sleepy to feed • Weight loss greater than 7% of birth weight
7	Minimum 8 times daily; every 2 to 4 hours (baby satisfied between feeds)	6 or more wet diapers daily; urine is pale yellow	• Decreased urine output • Baby too sleepy to feed • Weight loss greater than 10% of birth weight

Adapted from Toronto Public Health with permission.

Doc Talk Take hydration seriously. While water is usually the best form of hydration in older children, in cases of dehydration they will need to replace the sugars and salts in addition to the water that has been lost. This is most completely achieved by using an oral rehydration solution.

Developmental Delay

What Can I Do?

▶ Remember, there are average ages at which children reach developmental milestones, but there is also a wide range of what is still considered normal.

▶ If you suspect that your child has a developmental delay, especially if you see any red flags, consult with your doctor to rule out any condition that may be affecting normal development.

▶ Be sure that school expectations, programming, disciplinary measures, and safety-proofing of the home are appropriate for your child's developmental level, rather than his actual age.

❶ What Is Developmental Delay?

Developmental delay refers to a failure of a child to reach their expected developmental milestones in one or more spheres. These can include:

- **Gross motor development** — How your child moves the large muscles of the body.
- **Fine motor development** — What your child can do with his or her hands.
- **Expressive language development** — How your child communicates with others.
- **Receptive language development** — How your child understands others.
- **Social development** — How your child interacts with others.

When should we contact our doctor?

Parents are often concerned about the pace at which their child is developing. "Normal" and "abnormal" are broad terms, but milestones have been established in response to this question to reassure parents and to alert caregivers if there is a developmental problem. If a particular milestone is not reached by the upper limit of the normal range, then a developmental delay in that category of development should be considered. If your child has not reached any of the milestones on page 156, see your doctor for evaluation.

Did You Know?

Average or Normal

The average age to reach a developmental milestone and the normal range are two different things. The average age for beginning to walk is 13 months old, but the normal range for the mastery of walking independently is 9 months to 18 months old. Kids who walk earlier than others may often simply be less cautious rather than more clever.

Developmental Delay Red Flags

Area of Development	Warning Sign
Gross motor development	• Not walking by 18 months
Fine motor development	• Holding hands tightly in fists for most of the time at 3 months • Preferring left or right hand before 18 months
Expressive language development	• Not using three words by 15 months • No pointing by 12 months • Words spoken are difficult to understand at 3 years
Receptive language development	• Not responding when name is called at 18 months • Not able to identify body parts by 2 years
Social development	• Not interested in other children at 2 years • No imaginary play at 2 years

Gross Motor Development

Gross motor development refers to the way a child uses large muscles to move and balance. Milestones have been established to gauge your child's development month by month during the baby and toddler years.

Activity	Average Age	Description
Lifting head	2 months	Most babies are able to lift their heads when placed lying on their stomach by 2 months of age
Rolling over	4 to 5 months	Babies typically roll over by 4 to 5 months
Sitting up	6 to 7 months	Most babies sit unsupported by 6 to 7 months
Standing	9 to 10 months	Infants are often able to pull themselves up to a standing position by 9 to 10 months
Walking	13 months	On average, babies are able to walk at 13 months
Playing	2 years	Many 2-year-old toddlers can run, climb onto furniture, throw a ball, jump, and walk up the stairs holding onto the railing or an adult's hand
Cycling	$3\frac{1}{2}$ to 6 years	Toddlers can peddle a tricycle, progressing to a bicycle with training wheels around 4 years old, then riding alone between 5 and 6 years old.

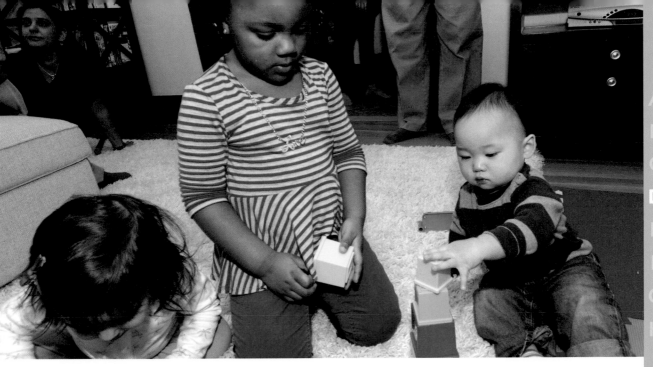

Fine Motor Development

Fine motor development refers to the mastery of the smaller muscles, such as those in the hands. Infants who are 4 months of age reach for and grasp objects, such as a block or rattle; by 6 months, they have learned to pass the object from one hand to the other. On average, infants who are 9 or 10 months old are able to pick up small objects with the thumb and forefinger and can bring food (and other objects!) to their mouths. By 18 months of age, most children can hold a crayon and scribble with it, and they can begin feeding themselves with a spoon. Two-year-olds can often remove their shoes and are typically able to draw straight lines; by 3 years, circles. By 4 years, children can often dress themselves, but need help with buttons and zippers, often until they are 5 years old. Tying shoelaces is a skill usually learned around 6 years old.

Language Development

Language development is usually divided into expressive language — what your child says — and receptive language — what your child understands. Cooing sounds are vowel sounds, such as "ooh" and "ah," and are normally heard before 6 months. By that age, most infants are able to babble, using vowel-consonant combinations, such as "babababa" and "lalalalala." The first word used with meaning, which is typically "dada," is usually spoken at about 1 year of age.

By 18 months, toddlers usually understand words for their body parts and can point to their head, hair, eyes, nose, mouth, ears, belly button, and toes. At 2 years old, children generally use between 20 and 50 words, and are starting to put two words together, such as "more milk" or "my chair," although up to half of these words might

Did You Know?

Slow to Talk

If a child is slow to talk (delayed expressive language) but understands a level of language that is appropriate for his age (normal receptive language), there is generally much less to worry about. Kids who have normal receptive language and normal social development tend to do just fine.

Did You Know?

Autism Symptoms

Children who have delays in both social development and language development may have autism. Encouraging findings from research indicate that early behavioral interventions for kids with autism can be very important to achieving maximum potential. See Autism (page 64).

only be understood by people who know the child well. At this age, children can usually understand and follow simple instructions, such as "Go get your shoes, please." By 3 years old, children can speak three-word phrases and in full sentences. By 4 years old, almost all of a child's language can be understood by a stranger. Most 3-year-olds can identify colors, and by age 4 or 5, letters of the alphabet. Most 4- and 5-year-olds can identify letters and print their name. Reading typically begins between 5 and 6 years old. See Speech and Language Problems (page 375).

Social Development

Social development refers to the way children learn to interact and behave. Around 6 weeks of age, babies start to smile in response to a parent's smile. By 4 to 5 months, babies are often laughing, and at 9 months, infants begin to enjoy playing peekaboo. By 12 months, most infants can imitate clapping hands and waving good-bye. Toddler temper tantrums are typical in 2- to 3-year-olds. Children of this age are starting to use some imaginary play, such as pretending to talk on the telephone or putting a stuffed animal to bed. By the age of 3 years, many children participate in more interactive play and understand simple rules in games, such as tag and hide-and-seek. Toilet training has a wide range of normal, from 18 months to 4 years, after which accidents are still not uncommon, particularly at night.

FAQ

When should I be worried about my child's development?
A delay in achieving just one developmental target does not automatically indicate a problem. This might make it difficult for you to know when to be concerned. In general, if you are worried about your child's development, you should discuss your concerns with your child's physician.

❷ What Causes Developmental Delays?

In many situations, particularly when there is a single area of delay and the delay is mild, the cause may be unknown. When there are physical differences in appearance or there are associated health problems, or when the delay is more severe, a medical cause is often identified.

If you suspect your child has a developmental delay, discuss this with your child's doctor as soon as possible. In most cases, unless there are significant global developmental delays (meaning that two or more areas of development are affected), few, if any, tests are necessary or helpful. If there are specific medical signs, your child's doctor might discuss the options of genetic blood tests or radiological imaging of the brain (a CT scan or magnetic resonance imaging/MRI). However, in most cases, these tests are not necessary and the focus is on management.

❸ How Are Developmental Delays Treated?

Motor Development Delays

Rehabilitation specialists, such as physiotherapists and occupational therapists, can provide further assessment and recommendations.

Language Development Delays

A speech and language therapist should be consulted to assess your child and make specific recommendations. The most effective form of speech and language therapy for young children is provided by their caregivers, who are with them regularly, rather than provided directly by a therapist, who can typically offer service only once per week or less.

Social Development Delays

Psychologists or pediatricians specializing in developmental disorders can provide further assessment for possible autism spectrum disorder, for example. If identified, your child has the opportunity to respond to specific behavioral management interventions and social skills training — the earlier the better.

Consider meeting with the school principal in the winter or early spring of the year before your child begins school. Careful planning will be important to ensure adequate support is available and that appropriate programming is thoughtfully planned.

| Doc Talk | The underlying cause of a developmental delay among kids who are otherwise healthy will frequently remain unknown, despite medical investigation. Although it is frustrating to not know the source of the delay, these kids often have a better developmental outcome than do the children who have identified causes, with abnormal findings on test results. Early intervention for any developmental delay is key to helping your child reach his full potential. |

Diaper Rash (Diaper Dermatitis)

What Can I Do?

▶ Change your child's diaper regularly to keep him clean and dry, especially if stools are loose or frequent.

▶ Apply a very generous layer of zinc oxide–based cream or petroleum jelly as a barrier at each diaper change.

▶ See your doctor if the diaper rash is not improving after 3 days of frequent diaper changes with regular application of a barrier cream.

▶ Leave open to the air when possible.

❶ What Is Diaper Rash?

Almost every infant has at least one episode of diaper rash before she is toilet trained. The most common cause of diaper rash is irritation of the baby's skin due to contact with urine and feces. Besides irritant dermatitis, there are other common causes of diaper rash, such as yeast (candida) infection and seborrheic dermatitis. Bacterial infection is a less common cause of diaper rash in infancy.

Kinds of Diaper Rash

- Contact or irritant dermatitis
- Yeast infection (*Candida albicans*)
- Seborrheic dermatitis
- Bacterial infection (staphylococcus/streptococcus)

When should we contact our doctor?

A diaper rash is not an emergency. However, early treatment with frequent diaper changes and application of a barrier cream is essential to prevent worsening of the rash. Any diaper rash that is not showing signs of improvement after 3 days should prompt a visit to your primary care provider.

What Are the Causes, Symptoms, and Treatments for Diaper Rash?

Causes	Description	Symptoms	Treatments
Contact or irritant dermatitis	• Skin becomes irritated and inflamed after prolonged contact with acidic urine or feces. • Made worse by wet or soiled and poorly absorbent, tight-fitting diapers. • Very commonly occurs in infants with a diarrheal illness where their bottoms are repeatedly exposed to irritating feces.	• Redness around the labia and anus but sparing in between the skin creases in the groin. • Redness can progress to painful, shallow ulcerations.	• Change your child's diaper frequently to avoid contact with urine and feces. Leave the skin open to fresh air whenever practical. • Apply a very generous layer of zinc oxide–based cream or petroleum jelly (Vaseline) as a barrier with each diaper change. • Avoid aggressively removing the barrier cream at the next diaper change; this may cause further abrasion. Gently remove soiled diaper and apply more protective barrier cream. Use a warm, wet cloth, if possible. • A mild corticosteroid cream may be prescribed by your doctor to help if the rash is severe.
Yeast infection	• Infection of the skin by the yeast that generally lives in the gastrointestinal tract. • This commonly occurs when the skin is already damaged from a preceding irritant in diaper dermatitis. • Yeast grows especially well in warm, moist areas, such as the groin creases. • Risk factors for yeast overgrowth include recent use of antibiotics or recent diarrheal illness.	• Redness with white, scaly edges primarily affecting the anal area. • Small satellite lesions are usually found away from the perianal area, on the periphery of the rash.	• Any diaper rash that is not improving after 3 days of frequent diaper changes with regular application of barrier cream should be assessed by your doctor. • Your doctor may prescribe an antifungal topical preparation that may be combined with topical corticosteroid.

Causes	Description	Symptoms	Treatments
Seborrheic dermatitis	• Inflammation of the oil-producing glands of the skin.	• Yellow, greasy scales and red bumps. • Rash may also appear on the scalp and face.	• Your doctor may prescribe a mild steroid cream.
Bacterial infection (staphylococcus/ streptococcus)	• A disruption in the natural balance of bacteria on the skin, such that certain bacteria will multiply, leading to infection. • Commonly occurs where skin breakdown has already occurred from irritant diaper dermatitis.	• Small pimple-like lesions on a red background that occasionally progress to large blisters. • Blisters may slough off and leave a raw, red background.	• Bacterial infections can be more serious. A topical antibacterial agent may be useful. • You will have to take your child to see her doctor, especially if she appears sick. • Treatment with oral antibiotics may be necessary in more severe cases.

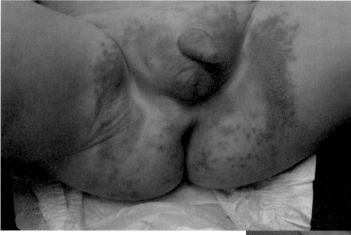

Irritant diaper rash (note sparing of the skin creases)

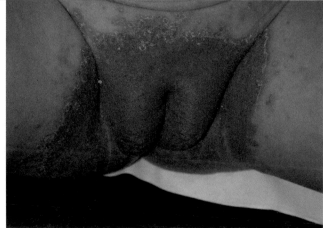

Candida diaper rash (note involvement of the skin creases)

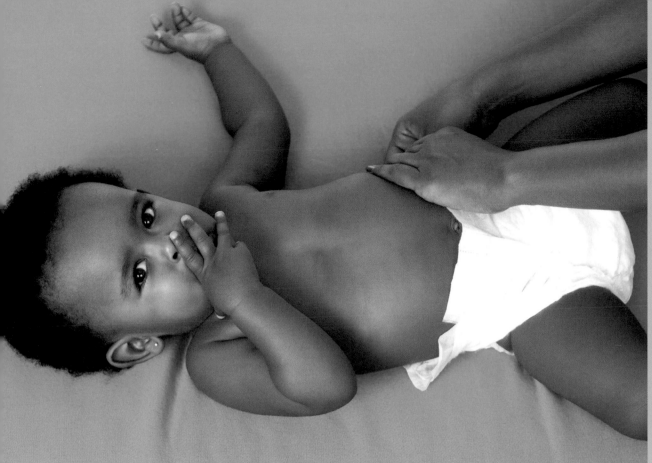

How To: Manage Diaper Rash

1. The key to the management of irritant diaper dermatitis is prevention! No diaper, no rash. Unfortunately, it is not very practical for babies to roam diaper-free. Therefore, try to change your baby's diaper frequently, and routinely use zinc oxide or petroleum jelly as protective agents.
2. Avoid fragrances and alcohol-based wipes to prevent diaper area irritation.
3. Avoid tight-fitting diapers. Super-absorbent synthetic diapers, although perhaps less environmentally friendly than cloth diapers, appear in recent studies to be superior in preventing diaper dermatitis because they draw water away from the skin into a gel matrix.
4. When using a steroid preparation topically, use only as frequently as recommended (usually twice daily) and apply a small, thin layer.

Did You Know?

Potency Caution

Creams marked as having the same percentage of steroid but with different names may have very different potencies. Do not use cream or ointment that was not prescribed for your baby's diaper rash.

Doc Talk Do not despair — some babies just have sensitive bottoms, and diaper rash will happen despite caregivers' best efforts. With age and toilet training, this will disappear!

A B C D E F G H I J K L M N O P Q R S T U V W X Y Z

Diarrhea

What Can I Do?

▶ Monitor your child for signs of dehydration or blood in the stool. Seek urgent medical attention if these symptoms appear.

▶ Be sure everyone in your household washes their hands regularly to prevent the spread of infectious diarrhea.

▶ If diarrhea lasts more than 2 weeks, see your doctor.

❶ What Is Diarrhea?

RELATED CONDITIONS

- Constipation
- Cystic fibrosis
- Gastroenteritis
- Inflammatory bowel disease (Crohn's disease and ulcerative colitis)
- Lactose intolerance
- Milk protein intolerance
- Toddler's diarrhea

Diarrhea is the passage of stools that are more frequent and loose than usual. In order to decide whether or not your child has diarrhea, it is necessary to compare his current bowel pattern with his typical bowel pattern.

Diarrhea can be described as either acute or chronic, depending on its duration. Anything less than 2 weeks is referred to as acute diarrhea; more than 2 weeks is chronic diarrhea.

Normal Stooling Pattern

A child's stool frequency and consistency depend on his or her age and diet. For example, the stool of a breastfed infant is typically mustard-colored, watery, and seedy. Some healthy breastfed babies will have 10 stools a day, but others are equally happy producing one or two stools per week. By the age of 18 months, most children have one or two formed stools a day. The water content of the stool is what determines its consistency. Normally, much of the liquid present in stool is reabsorbed through the lining of the large intestines, resulting in a solid bowel movement. However, when the intestines are irritated (for example, during an infection), the stool rushes through the bowel, quickly taking more of the liquid with it. This results in diarrhea.

When should we contact our doctor or local hospital?

Most cases of diarrhea resolve themselves, but other cases can be very serious. You will need to contact your doctor if any red flags are present.

⏩ Diarrhea Red Flags

Your child should be seen by a doctor urgently if she has any of the following symptoms:

- **Dehydration:** This is commonly seen if your child has diarrhea and is also refusing to eat or drink. Other signs to look for include: unexplained drowsiness, dry tongue and sunken eyes/fontanelle (soft spot in babies), lack of tears, weight loss, decreased urination — this can be a tricky one to determine if your child is in diapers and is having frequent, loose stools! See Dehydration (page 150).
- **Bloody stools:** This can be either streaks of red blood; frank, bright red blood; or black stools.
- **Vomiting:** Diarrhea associated with vomiting that is bright green (bilious) can be a sign of intestinal blockage. See Vomiting (page 415).
- **Chronic diarrhea:** Diarrhea that lasts more than 2 weeks, especially with associated weight loss or poor growth, should be assessed by a doctor.

Stool Color

The color of your child's stool can offer clues to her condition.

Green

Green stool simply means that the material is passing through the intestines very rapidly.

Red

Fresh blood is red, which indicates a source of bleeding in the colon or lower part of the bowel. Causes of red blood in the stool include traveler's diarrhea and *Clostridium difficile* colitis, caused temporarily by antibiotics. Small babies may have blood in their stool if they are breastfeeding and their mother's nipples are cracked. See Breastfeeding Problems (page 93).

Other causes include an allergy to the protein in milk (see Bloody Stools, page 89) and structural bowel problems, such as intussusception (see page 20), where one piece of the bowel telescopes into the adjacent bowel, creating a blockage. If your child is constipated, it is important to check for a rectal tear or fissure (see Anal Fissures, page 90), which can also cause blood-streaked stools. One more thing to be aware of: consuming strawberry and raspberry gelatin (for example, Jell-O) can cause a red discoloration of the stool due to the dye!

> **Did You Know?**
>
> **Blood in the Stool**
>
> Many parents are very impressed by the precise shade of their children's diarrhea. This is generally not very helpful! When it comes to color, knowing about the presence or absence of blood in the stool is more important.

Black

Tar-like stools, called melena, suggest bleeding that is coming from higher up in the bowel, closer to the stomach or its outlet— the duodenum. This is less common in children but can be seen with ulcers or small tears from severe vomiting and retching.

What Causes Acute Diarrhea?

Cause	Features
Gastroenteritis (gastrointestinal tract infection) • Viral (most common): examples include rotavirus and norovirus (stomach flu). See Viral Gastroenteritis (page 209). • Bacterial: examples include salmonella, shigella, E. coli, and campylobacter. Children tend to appear more unwell with this type of gastroenteritis. Food poisoning is caused by toxin-producing bacteria, such as staphylococcus. • Parasitic: one example is giardia.	• Fever • Vomit: The color of the vomit is commonly that of recently eaten food or clear-colored. After lots of vomiting, it may be light yellow. Dark green vomitus is more concerning and might be an indication of an intestinal blockage. See Vomiting (page 415). • Stools: These are very watery, often green, foul-smelling, and may contain stringy mucus. With bacterial infections, blood may be present in the stool (this is rarely seen in viral gastroenteritis). • Duration: Symptoms usually last less than a week. In food poisoning, there is usually profuse vomiting and diarrhea that lasts only 2 to 6 hours. • Infections: With viral infections, friends, family, or schoolmates are often unwell with similar symptoms. Bacterial infections are more likely to be picked up while traveling in developing countries and by consuming foods and water that are contaminated. Parasites are sometimes ingested while drinking water from a well or when camping (beaver fever).

❷ How Is Acute Diarrhea Treated?

❶ *Intake of liquids and solids:* If there is any concern about dehydration, infants should be offered small, frequent amounts of special electrolyte solutions (oral rehydration solution), or continue breastfeeding. See Dehydration (page 150). Formula or cow's milk can be continued as well, unless it seems to be associated with worsening symptoms. Avoid giving water exclusively because it does not provide a source of much-needed sugar and salt. As for solids, let the child's appetite determine food intake. In the past, doctors recommended restricting solid food intake or very specific diets, but unless your child is vomiting nonstop or is not interested, it is better to continue offering light, tasty meals.

② *Antidiarrheal medications:* These are not recommended for children because they don't cure the problem, can lead to bad cramping, and can mask the diagnosis.

③ *Probiotics:* These can be given to shorten the duration of acute infectious viral diarrhea. It is important to know that the efficacy of probiotics is dependent on the strain and dose. The benefits seem more evident if treatment is started within the first 48 hours of illness.

④ *Antibiotics:* Some of the bacterial and parasitic causes of gastroenteritis might require treatment with antibiotics, but only after the organism has been cultured in the stool.

> **Did You Know?**
>
> **Not Hungry**
> When a child is ill with acute viral gastroeteritis, he may not want to eat. This is to be expected. Just be sure he is drinking fluids so that he does not become dehydrated.

What Causes Chronic Diarrhea?

Cause	Features
Cow's milk protein intolerance This is an allergy to the protein present in cow's milk and in many formulas. Even breastfed babies can have this disorder because these proteins can be found in their mother's breast milk. These babies may seem uncomfortable while feeding and might even vomit. Babies with cow's milk protein intolerance tend to lose microscopic amounts of protein and blood in their stools. See Bloody Stools (page 89).	• If severe, it can cause pallor from anemia, and puffiness (swelling), if the protein loss is large. • Many of the children allergic to cow's milk protein also cannot tolerate soy protein. Therefore, they may require a special hypoallergenic formula, free of both milk and soy, in order to thrive. • Fortunately, for the great majority of affected children, this intolerance seems to settle by 2 or 3 years of age.
Lactose intolerance The sugar in milk and dairy products is called lactose. In order to be absorbed, lactose must first be partially broken down by an enzyme (lactase) that is found on the microscopic tips of the intestinal wall. If the amount of lactase is reduced, the result is an inability to digest the lactose in milk products. See Lactose Intolerance (page 35).	• Abdominal cramps, bloating, and diarrhea occur after ingesting milk products because the undigested lactose passes into the large intestine and ferments. • Temporary lactose intolerance is common after a bout of viral gastroenteritis. In this case, microscopic damage to the intestinal wall reduces the amount of available lactase and results in the frequent passage of watery stools whenever milk is consumed. This problem is temporary and tends to clear up after a few weeks. • Permanent lactose intolerance is an uncommon condition in young children. It is most prevalent among children of Asian and African descent. Symptoms tend to show up when they are at least 2 to 3 years old. Teenagers and adults tend to have more symptoms.

Cause	Features
Celiac disease The small intestine is extremely sensitive to a particular protein called gluten — found in wheat, rye, barley, and often oats. Gluten damages the lining of the intestine, resulting in malabsorption (difficulty in absorbing food). Diagnosis requires an endoscopy with a biopsy to document the changes in the lining of the bowel. See Celiac Disease (page 30).	• Symptoms don't usually start until at least the end of the first year of life; children need to have had exposure to gluten in the form of infant cereal. • Most children are very irritable, have poor weight gain, diarrhea, low energy levels, and a protruding belly. • Celiac disease can sometimes be subtle in its presentation and difficult to diagnose. You may have heard of adults who only recently found out that they had celiac disease. • Celiac disease responds very well to the removal of gluten from the diet.
Cystic fibrosis (CF) This is an inherited disease where the ducts in the pancreas become blocked and are unable to pass secreted digestive enzymes into the intestines. This results in an inability to digest fat. Currently in some jurisdictions, newborn screening programs look for CF, but not every case is detected.	• Stools appear oily and tend to float on top of the water. • Children feed very well but, because of malabsorption, gain weight slowly. • Children often suffer frequent lung infections. • Parents of a young baby may notice that their baby's skin tastes salty.
Inflammatory bowel disease (Crohn's disease, ulcerative colitis) See page 32 for a full description.	• Inflammatory bowel disease often runs in families. • Children with Crohn's disease usually have diarrhea, abdominal cramping, poor growth, and weight loss. • Ulcerative colitis is characterized by diarrhea, typically bloody, and over time is associated with weight loss and poor growth.
Toddler's diarrhea This may be related to a high intake of sugary fluids, especially fruit juice. The sugar draws excess fluid into the intestines.	• Reducing sugar in the diet and increasing fiber content will improve stool frequency and consistency. • Child experiences no abdominal pain. • Child has appropriate weight gain.
Constipation Sound counterintuitive? It is true! Large stools block the rectum, and liquid stool leaks and overflows around it. See Constipation, page 124.	• Child has a history of infrequent, very hard, large-caliber stools. • Child might soil underwear. • Anal fissures may be present.

Doc Talk
An ounce of prevention is worth a pound of cure. Wash! Wash! Wash! Acute gastroenteritis is extremely contagious. Good hand hygiene is important for trying to keep other family members healthy. Rotavirus is the most common cause of gastroenteritis. Rotavirus vaccine is available for infants and taken orally. No needles! It decreases the incidence and severity of rotavirus infections. The vaccine series must be started between 6 and 15 weeks old and completed by 8 months of age.

Earache and Ear Infections
(Otitis Media, Interna, Externa)

What Can I Do?

▶ Discuss with your doctor the role of analgesics, antipyretics, and antibiotics in the management of your child's ear infection.

▶ In cases of six or more ear infections in a year, or concerns regarding hearing, consider a consultation with an otolaryngologist (ear, nose, and throat specialist).

▶ Consider otitis externa (swimmer's ear) especially in summer when your child has been doing a lot of swimming. A big clue is pain with movement of the outer ear.

❶ What Are Earache and Ear Infections?

Ear infections are one of the most common reasons for antibiotic use in young children. Experiencing at least one middle-ear infection seems to be a rite of passage for every child by the age of 1 to 3 years old. Besides middle-ear infections, the inner and the outer ear can also present problems that require medical care.

The middle ear is the small space located behind the eardrum. In young children, most commonly those between 6 months and 2 years of age, the middle ear can become infected with a bacterium or virus. The middle ear is connected to the throat by the eustachian tube. This tube helps drain the middle ear. When mucus or swelling of the tube from a cough or cold occurs, the eustachian tube can become blocked. Pressure can then build up inside the middle ear and cause pain. A blocked tube also prevents fluid from draining out of the middle ear. This fluid can become infected and cause the eardrum to bulge, resulting in more pain.

When should we contact our doctor?

Children are prone to have earaches. Some can be cared for at home with pain relievers, but a doctor is required to make the diagnosis of an ear infection. See the red flags on page 170 for further guidance.

A B C D E F G H I J K L M N O P Q R S T U V W X Y Z

▶▶ Ear Infection Red Flags

Consult your child's doctor if your child has any of the following symptoms associated with an earache:

■ You see fluid or pus draining from your child's ear.

■ Your child is still in pain or has a fever after taking antibiotics and pain medication for 48 hours.

■ You have concerns about your child's hearing.

Seek immediate medical attention at the nearest emergency department if your child has any of the following symptoms associated with an earache:

■ You see redness or swelling behind your child's ear or the ear seems like it is sticking out.

■ Your child seems excessively lethargic or irritable.

■ Your child develops a stiff or painful neck.

■ Your child's pain is not well controlled despite regular ibuprofen and acetaminophen use.

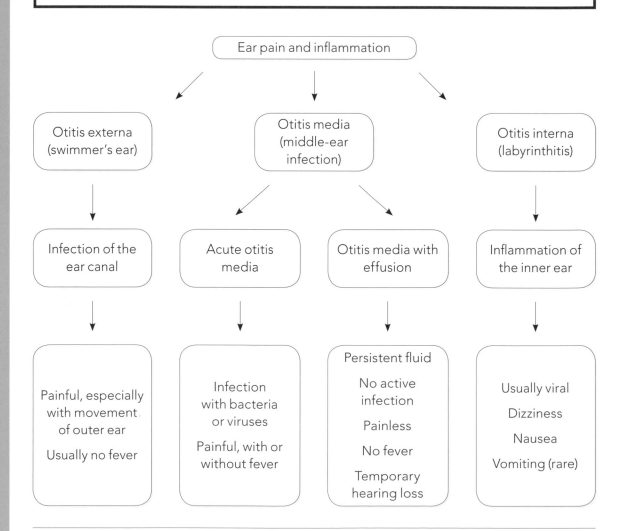

❷ What Is Acute Otitis Media?

Young children are prone to acute otitis media (middle-ear infection) because of the size and position of their eustachian tubes. The tubes of young children are small and short, allowing the tube to get blocked by a tiny amount of inflammation. Children's tubes are also more horizontal, preventing easy drainage when fluid builds up with inflammation from a cold. By the time a child is 6 years old, his tubes have grown sufficiently and they have moved into a more diagonal position, significantly reducing the chance of developing a middle-ear infection.

Signs and Symptoms of Acute Otitis Media

- Fever
- Ear pain
- Ear rubbing or pulling
- Difficulty sleeping
- Pus draining from the ear
- Decreased appetite and energy level
- Fussiness and irritability (especially in young infants)

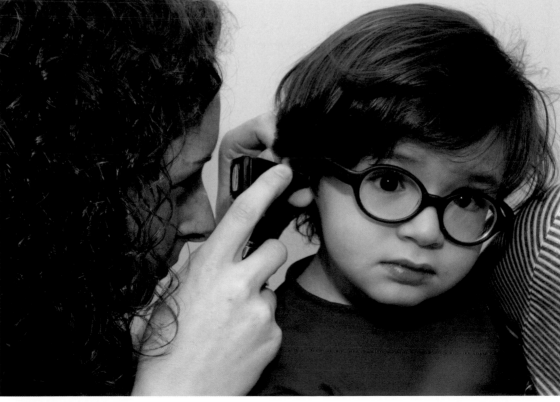

Examining for an ear infection

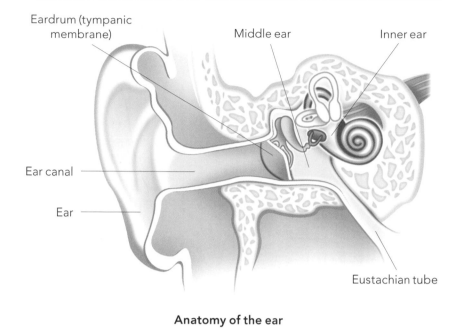

Eardrum (tympanic membrane)

Middle ear

Inner ear

Ear canal

Ear

Eustachian tube

Anatomy of the ear

Diagnosis

The diagnosis is confirmed by your doctor, who uses an otoscope to look in the ear at the eardrum. The eardrum appears red and swollen, and the middle ear behind the eardrum is filled with pus.

❸ How Is Otitis Media Treated?

How an ear infection is treated will depend on the age of the child, the duration and intensity of signs and symptoms, and whether the child has any other medical conditions predisposing him to ear infections.

Medications

Several medications are useful in reducing swelling and pain from an ear infection.

Analgesics and Antipyretics

All children with ear infections experiencing pain and fever should be treated with medications, such as ibuprofen or acetaminophen, which have analgesic and antipyretic (antifever) effects. This will make your child more comfortable until the infection clears.

Antibiotics

In older infants and children, most ear infections will get better without antibiotics. The decision tree that follows shows how your doctor considers using antibiotics.

EARACHE AND EAR INFECTIONS (OTITIS MEDIA, INTERNA, EXTERNA)

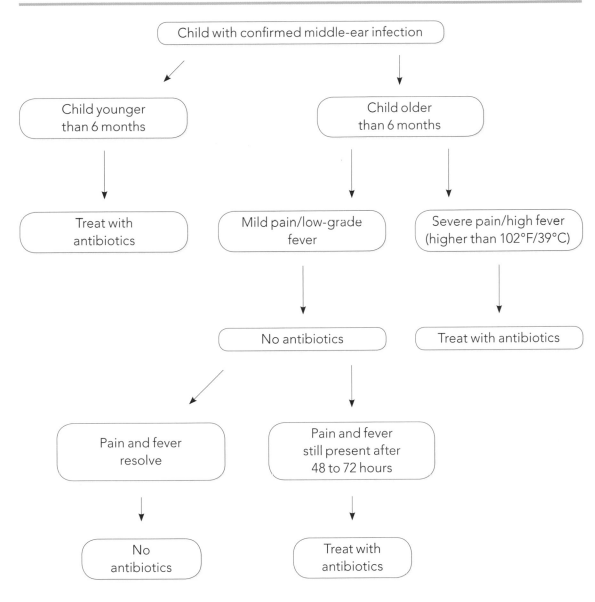

Child with confirmed middle-ear infection

Child younger than 6 months

Child older than 6 months

Treat with antibiotics

Mild pain/low-grade fever

Severe pain/high fever (higher than 102°F/39°C)

No antibiotics

Treat with antibiotics

Pain and fever resolve

Pain and fever still present after 48 to 72 hours

No antibiotics

Treat with antibiotics

FAQ

My son had an ear infection 2 weeks ago and now his doctor says there is fluid in his ear. He said not to worry about it and he'll check it again in a month or so. Should this be treated?

After acute otitis media, the pain and infection generally subside in a few days, but fluid will remain in the middle ear for some time afterward. This condition is called otitis media with effusion. It differs from acute otitis media in that there is no associated pain or fever. This stage of healing can take weeks or even months, and further antibiotic use doesn't really help.

A B C D **E** F G H I J K L M N O P Q R S T U V W X Y Z

Did You Know?

Wax Protection

Wax protects the skin of the ear canal and helps with lubrication and cleaning. Caregivers will often use cotton swabs to clean out the wax in a child's ear. This is generally not advisable because it can push the wax further down the ear canal. It can also cause accidental perforation of the eardrum. Repeated use of cotton swabs can also lead to abrasions (small scrapes) in the canal, predisposing the ear canal to infection from bacteria and fungi.

FAQs

My doctor prescribed antibiotics 3 days ago, but my daughter is feeling better now. Does she really need to finish the course?
Most infants and children feel better within the first 2 or 3 days after starting antibiotics. To cure the infection, you must complete the prescription. Failing to do so can lead to recurrence of the ear infection. It can also mean that future infections are harder to treat because the leftover bacteria become resistant to the antibiotics.

My daughter had so many ear infections this past winter. She is always getting sick and has had frequent courses of antibiotics. I've had it! When should we see an ear specialist?
Quite a few young children have such frequent ear infections, or the effusion lasts so long, that something further needs to be done. A simple surgical procedure in which tiny tubes are placed through the eardrum to better ventilate the middle ear can be performed to reduce the recurrence of otitis media. If your child has had more than three or four infections in a season, or six in a year, consider getting a referral to an ear specialist. Also, if your child has had persistent fluid for more than 4 months or his hearing is impaired, a referral is warranted.

❹ What Is Otitis Externa?

Otitis externa (swimmer's ear) refers to an infection that affects the ear canal, the passage from the outside world to the eardrum. The term "swimmer's ear" relates to the observation that these infections are more common in the summer months, especially in children who spend many hours in the water. One of the factors contributing to otitis externa is prolonged exposure to water, which softens the skin and promotes bacterial growth. Otitis externa can also be caused by trauma, such as a trauma caused by scratching or by well-meaning parents who use cotton swabs in an attempt to "clean" the ear.

Signs and Symptoms of Otitis Externa
- Itchiness of the ear canal
- Discomfort or pain in the canal
- Pain of the outer ear experienced with movement or chewing
- Ear discharge
- A feeling of blockage in the ear canal
- Temporary hearing loss from blockage of the canal with swelling and debris
- A red, scaly area around the opening of the canal
- In severe cases, the outer ear might swell or there might be fever

⑤ How Is Otitis Externa Treated?

There are a number of treatment options for otitis externa.

- Your child's doctor might prescribe different types of eardrops that can contain a combination of antiseptics, antibiotics, and steroid (anti-inflammatory) medication.
- If the pain is significant, your child should take acetaminophen or ibuprofen, as needed.
- Rarely, in more severe cases, your child might need to take oral or intravenous antibiotics.
- It is wise to keep the ear dry until the infection has healed.

> ### Doc Talk
> The approach to middle-ear infections has changed over the years. While it is still the most common cause for prescribing antibiotics in children, doctors have become much more thoughtful as to which children really need them. Many ear infections will get better with time and often some appropriate pain relief is all that may be required. Unnecessary use of antibiotics, apart from potential side effects, may also lead to more resistant germs that could be harder to treat next time around!

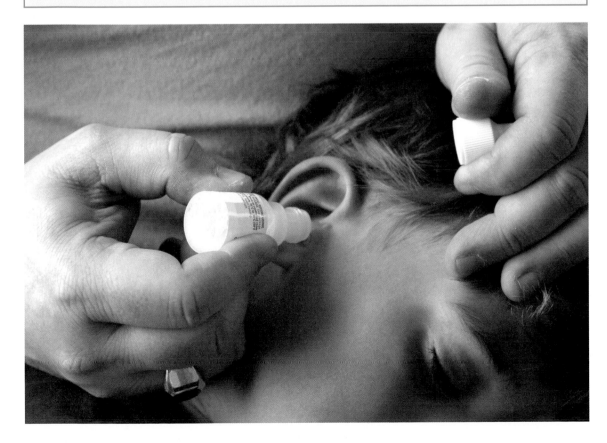

Eating Habits (Picky Eating)

What Can I Do?

▶ Limit juice to 4 ounces (125 mL) and restrict milk intake to 16 ounces (500 mL) per day after 1 year of age.

▶ Sit down for a meal as a family without any distraction (no TV) and role model healthy eating habits.

▶ As a parent, you set the mealtimes and determine what foods are offered. Let your child decide on the volume eaten.

▶ Make eating fun, not a chore.

Case Study

Emily's Appetite

Emily is 3 years old and has developed a reputation as a picky and fussy eater. Emily often refuses the food her mother prepares for the rest of the family. Her mother describes her as a "grazer," explaining that Emily has a small appetite and prefers to pick at food throughout the day. Emily's favorite foods are Cheddar cheese, fishy crackers, and yogurt. To compensate for her poor appetite, her mother gives her apple juice and is considering starting her on vitamins as well. Emily's mother is at the end of her rope. She has tried everything, including offering rewards — special desserts and special toys — if Emily improves her diet. But this never lasts. Emily is currently wearing size 3 clothing, but her mom describes her as skinny.

Emily's parents are concerned about her eating habits and behavior, and they visited their family doctor, who, after examining Emily, explained that she demonstrates a typical presentation of a picky eater. Although Emily may not seem to be eating enough, she is continuing to grow well. On her growth chart, she follows along the 25th percentile for her weight and the 50th percentile for her height. He recommended limiting her snacks, offering three meals a day, and not making a special meal for her. He also advised her parents to not use bribes or rewards to get Emily to eat.

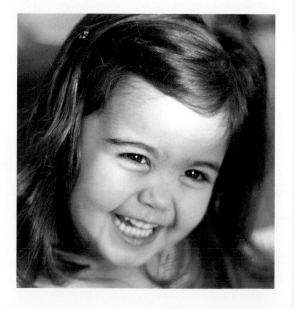

❶ What Is a Picky Eating Habit?

Perhaps the most trying eating habit your child can develop is to become a picky eater, where your child refuses to eat "perfectly good food." Most picky eaters, however, do not starve or even experience malnutrition. Research has shown that children can adequately regulate how much food they need on their own. Often a child will eat a lot at one meal, followed by a small amount at the next meal, or vice versa. It is believed that children can adjust their food intake according to the amount they have taken at the previous meal. Children might appear to eat erratically and are considered to be "picky," but they are generally adjusting their eating patterns according to their needs. About 25% to 30% of children aged 1 to 4 years are described as picky eaters.

When should we contact our doctor?

A child may be a picky eater but, in most cases, she is healthy and active. Don't be overly concerned by her skinny frame. Monitoring your child's weight and height is an important way of ensuring that her eating habits are not impacting on growth. But even this can be difficult because children with a slim or small build may just be following in your or your spouse's footprints. Recall your own childhood — were you always skinny as a child?

Did You Know?

Milk Need
Once a child is over 1 year of age, she should consume no more than 16 ounces (500 mL) of milk each day. Although milk has good nutritional value, children who drink too much milk often eat too little food. This can and does result in a condition called iron deficiency anemia. See Pallor (page 292).

⏩ Eating Red Flags

It is unlikely that there is an underlying medical problem if your child is growing along her expected growth curve. If there is absolutely no gain (or if there a loss) in weight or height, or the measurements drop considerably (from the 50th to the 5th percentile, for example), it is time for your doctor to undertake a thorough medical investigation.

FAQ

How much juice does my child need?
In short — none! Although most children love juice, it is full of sugars and they do not need it. Juice intake often results in decreased food intake. Water is a good option, and offering fruit is a much healthier option than juice.

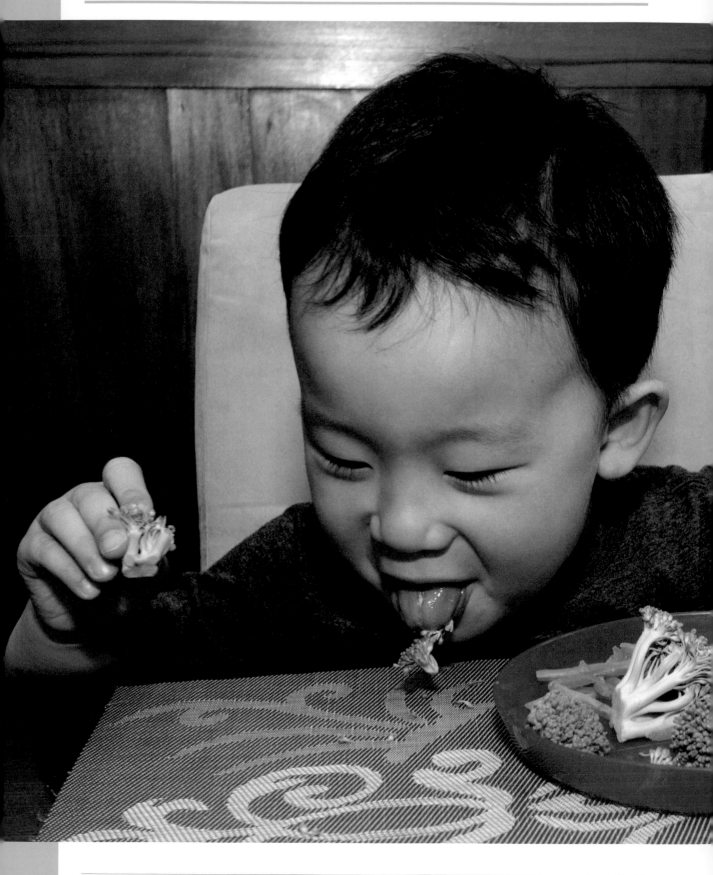

FAQ

My daughter keeps on changing her mind about foods. One day she likes tomatoes, the next day she detests them. What causes this flip-flop?

Accept the fact that children change their opinions of foods. A child who did not like a food the first time may change her mind the next time she tries it. As a parent, it is your job to offer your child healthy food choices. As a child, it is her job to determine how much she chooses to eat. Structured meal times, with little or no snacking in between meals, will enhance your child's appetite. If your child chooses not to eat a meal, this is fine. Chances are she will eat the next one.

❷ How Are Picky Eating Habits Improved?

1 Provide some structure and limit setting. As the parent, you determine the meal and the snack times, and your child will choose how much to eat at each offering. This should start as soon as your child eats solids.

2 Offer varied healthy foods from the various food groups — regardless of your own likes and dislikes.

3 Understand that some of the food you offer will be appreciated and some of it will be rejected — no matter how much effort went into preparing it!

4 Continue to offer new foods, even those that have been rejected several times in the past.

5 Do not succumb to the temptation to coerce, bribe, reward, or force-feed. Encouraging or discouraging a particular food can have the opposite effect.

6 Plan time for a family meal. Eating should be social and fun. Eating while "on the go" or in front of the TV is a setup for failure.

7 Do not let snacking replace a meal. If a child chooses not to eat a meal and is hungry, she should not be rewarded with an extra snack.

Did You Know?

Fluctuating Appetite

It is normal for a child's appetite to fluctuate from meal to meal and day to day. Toddlers demonstrate a decline in appetite as their growth velocity slows after infancy — which is normal! Pushing a child to eat when she is not hungry may backfire; she may even choose not to eat at all.

Doc Talk

If your child is not gaining weight or is losing weight, she needs to be seen by a health-care provider. On occasion, you might have to consult other health professionals, including a dietitian, an occupational therapist, or a social worker. Remember that a child's behavior around food can be directly related to their parents' behavior around food. The importance of sitting down as a family at mealtimes and role modeling good eating habits cannot be overemphasized.

Eye Problems

What Can I Do?

▶ If you suspect your child is having any problem seeing, consult with your doctor, who may refer your child for further testing. Diseases of the eye usually require an expert's opinion to diagnose.

▶ If your child has viral conjunctivitis, she should wash her hands frequently and avoid touching her eyes. This will help limit the spread to the other eye and other people.

RELATED CONDITIONS

- Blepharitis
- Cataracts
- Chalazion
- Color blindness
- Conjunctivitis (pink eye)
- Orbital cellulitis
- Periorbital cellulitis
- Refractive error (nearsightedness, farsightedness, astigmatism)
- Strabismus
- Stye
- Subconjunctival hemorrhage (bloody/red eye)
- Tearing (blocked tear ducts)

❶ What Is Conjunctivitis (Pink Eye)?

Conjunctivitis is an inflammation of the thin, transparent protective membrane that lines the eye and inner eyelids. It can occur in one or both eyes. Conjunctivitis is usually caused by a viral infection and, less frequently, by a bacterium, allergy, or chemical irritant. When caused by an infection, pink eye is contagious and spreads rapidly in household and childcare settings.

Symptoms of Conjunctivitis

- Redness of the whites of the eyes (the sclera)
- Itchiness, irritation, and a burning sensation in the eyes
- Discharge that can be watery or thick and pus-like
- Matting of the lids together, usually after sleep
- Concurrent cough, runny nose, and congestion

When should we contact our doctor or local hospital?

Fortunately, the majority of cases of viral conjunctivitis resolve on their own without treatment. However, if the symptoms are bothersome or persistent, you will need to seek medical attention.

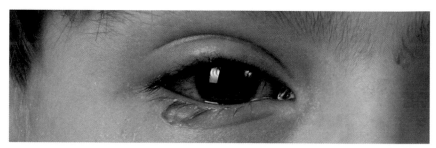

Conjunctivitis

⏩ Conjunctivitis Red Flags

Seek urgent medical attention if your child has any of the following symptoms associated with conjunctivitis:

- Eye pain
- Persistent change in vision; vision might be intermittently blurry from eye discharge but should clear with blinking or removal of the discharge
- Pain with exposure to bright lights
- Increasing eyelid swelling

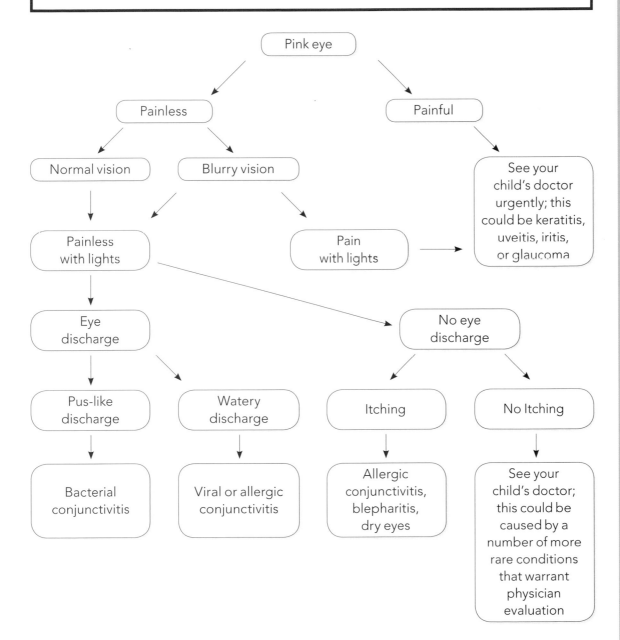

❷ What Causes Conjunctivitis?

Distinguishing between the different causes of conjunctivitis is not always easy. However, bacterial causes will usually result in a thick pus-like discharge, whereas viral infections lead to red, watery eyes. Allergic conjunctivitis is more likely when a child has been exposed to an allergen, such as pollen, and is often associated with other symptoms of hay fever (allergic rhinitis). See Allergic Rhinitis (page 38).

❸ How Is Conjunctivitis Treated?

- Wash your hands frequently to prevent the initial infection from spreading from one eye to the other.
- Do not share towels and facecloths.
- Soothe eyes with cool compresses.
- Wipe away discharge with a clean washcloth or gauze and dispose of it immediately, followed by a good hand wash.
- Use antibiotic eye drops or ointment for bacterial infections. Viral infections do not need antibiotics; these will clear up on their own in 1 to 2 weeks.
- If allergy is thought to be the cause, try oral antihistamines, such as diphenhydramine (Benadryl), loratadine (Claritin), or hydroxyzine (Atarax).
- Avoid triggers of allergic conjunctivitis.

How To: Insert Eye Drops in an Infant or Toddler

Inserting eye drops into a young child's eyes can be challenging.

1. Warm the bottle of eye drops in your hands to avoid discomfort.
2. Wrap your baby in a blanket.
3. Position your baby lying on his back.
4. Tilt your child's head backward.
5. Gently pull the lower eyelid down with your thumb, forming a pocket for the drops.
6. Place the drops on the nasal side of the corner of the eye, allowing the drops to leak into the eye.
7. If your child resists opening his eyes, drop the liquid onto the inner corner of the eye and rub gently with your fingertip. As your child opens his eyes, the medication will be absorbed.
8. Never touch the eye with the dropper.

❶ What Are Orbital and Periorbital Cellulitis (Eye Swelling)?

The term "cellulitis" refers to an infection of the skin and its underlying tissue. Periorbital cellulitis specifically refers to an infection involving the eyelids and the soft tissues in front of the eyeball itself. Orbital cellulitis is somewhat different. It is an infection of the soft tissue directly behind the eyeball. Of the two conditions, orbital cellulitis is rarer and more serious.

⏵ Orbital and Periorbital Cellulitis Red Flags

Orbital Cellulitis Symptoms

- Redness and swelling around one eye
- May have recent sinus infection or congestion
- Child may look sick and unwell
- Fever often present
- Pain with movement of eye
- May have blurry or double vision
- Eyeball may be projected forward (proptosis)

Periorbital Cellulitis Symptoms

- Redness and swelling around one eye
- May have insect bite, stye, or scratch around eye
- Generally child looks well
- Usually no fever
- Painless movement of eye
- Normal vision (unless obscured by eye swelling)

Orbital and periorbital cellulitis are always medical emergencies. See your doctor if your child shows any of the above symptoms.

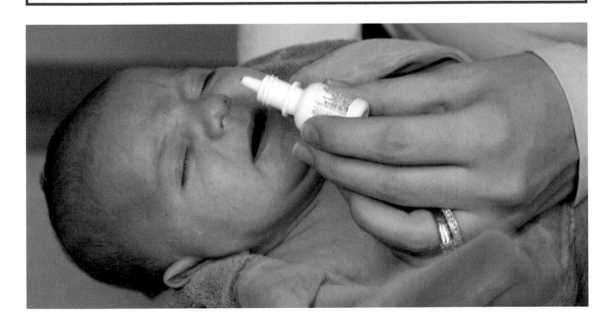

❷ What Causes Orbital and Periorbital Cellulitis?

Orbital cellulitis is most often the result of a direct extension of an infection in the sinuses. It can also be from trauma to the eye or from an infection in the skin of the eyelid.

Periorbital cellulitis is fairly common in young children. The cause is usually obvious. The cellulitis can spread from an infected scratch or insect bite, or from another infection, such as a stye. Sometimes the inflammation has spread from a sinus infection to tissue around the eye.

❸ How Are Orbital and Periorbital Cellulitis Treated?

Periorbital cellulitis is typically a bacterial infection. Milder cases can be treated with oral antibiotics. More serious cases of periorbital and all orbital cellulitis require hospitalization for intravenous therapy and close monitoring. Treatment usually involves a CT scan, and surgical drainage can sometimes be required for orbital cellulitis.

❶ What Is Tearing (Blocked Tear Ducts)?

Did You Know?

Mistaken Identity

Blocked tear ducts are often mistaken for an eye infection. If the white parts of your baby's eyes are not red and there are not copious amounts of thick pus, it is unlikely to be an infection.

Newborn babies will often cry without tears. After the first few weeks of life, you may notice your baby's tear glands starting to work, producing fluid that cleans and lubricates the eyes, creating tears when crying. Normally, tears drain through a small opening (lacrimal duct, or tear duct) in the inner, lower corner of a baby's eyelid. The tears flow through these ducts and empty into the top, inside part of the nose. It's no wonder we get runny noses with a good cry!

❷ What Causes Blocked Tear Ducts?

Nasolacrimal duct obstruction is very common, occurring in approximately 5% of healthy infants. In some infants, this drainage system is blocked or narrowed on one or both sides. The result is excessive tearing or discharge. Your baby may look like he is tearful, despite being totally happy. Sometimes there may also be a white or yellowish discharge that leads to persistent crusting in the corner of the eye. The eye may even be closed because of the sticky discharge gluing the lids together.

❸ How Are Blocked Ducts Treated?

Fortunately, in most cases, this blockage resolves spontaneously. Some experts recommend a technique called tear duct massage several times daily:

- Wipe away any obvious crusty material with a wet, clean cotton ball or gauze.
- Apply gentle pressure with the tip of your clean finger over your baby's lower eyelid, against the bridge of the nose, and "milk" downward to try to remove the tear through the duct.
- Ask your doctor to demonstrate the technique.

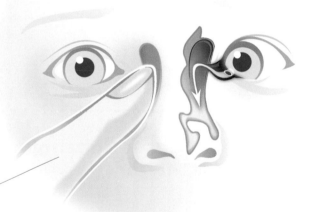

Apply gentle pressure with the tip of the finger against the nose to "milk" the tear through the tear duct.

⇥ Tearing Red Flags

Consult your child's doctor if your child has any of the following symptoms associated with tearing.

- Redness in the whites of the eyes (viral conjunctivitis)
- Thick, yellow/green discharge (bacterial conjunctivitis)
- Localized redness or swelling over the nasal portion of the lower eyelid (infection of the tear duct)
- Eye discharge beyond 1 year of age (persistent blocked tear duct potentially requiring a probe to open it)

❶ What Is Subconjunctival Hemorrhage (Bloody/Red Eye)?

A spot or patch of blood in the white part of the eye is referred to as a subconjunctival hemorrhage. The conjunctiva (thin translucent layer covering the eyeball) contains many fragile blood vessels that are easily ruptured with minimal increases in pressure. This is extremely common. It is generally harmless and painless.

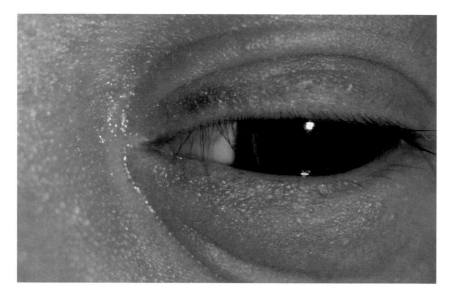

❷ What Causes Subconjunctival Hemorrhage?

- Birth (from the forceful expulsion of the baby through the birth canal)
- Coughing, sneezing
- Straining from constipation
- Head injury
- Trauma to the eye
- Vomiting

❸ How Is Subconjunctival Hemorrhage Treated?

No treatment is necessary. These generally resolve on their own within about 2 weeks. If the hemorrhage is caused by trauma to the head or eye, a child should be evaluated for other injuries.

❶ What Are Common Eyelid Problems?

Children can develop redness and swelling of the eyelids and around the eyelashes. Although these problems are usually harmless and get better without treatment, they can cause concern because they are so easily noticeable. Some of the conditions, frequently given unpronounceable names, are summarized below.

Common Eyelid Problems in Children

Stye (Hordeolum)

This is a localized bacterial infection in a gland of the eyelid.

- *Suspect if:* Your child has a red lump at the edge of the eyelid with or without yellow pus around the base of the eyelash. The lump can be painful and tender to touch and may eventually drain fluid.
- *What to do:* Styes typically disappear by themselves within 7 to 10 days. Warm compresses and antibiotic eye drops or ointment might be helpful.

Chalazion

This is an obstruction of a meibomian gland (gland that produces the oily substance making up part of a tear), which leads to a collection of fat, oil, and other tissue, called a lipogranuloma.

- *Suspect if:* Your child has a discrete, firm, non-tender bump within the eyelid.
- *What to do:* Time and warm compresses are often all that your child's doctor will recommend to treat a chalazion, although occasionally a chalazion will have to be excised surgically for cosmetic reasons or due to excess pressure on the eyeball.

Blepharitis

This is inflammation of the edges of the eyelids. It can be caused by irritation from skin conditions, such as seborrheic dermatitis, dandruff, viral or bacterial infections, or by an allergic reaction to cosmetics or ointments.

- *Suspect if:* The skin around your child's lashes appears red, itchy, or scaly. Your child might rub the eye because of burning, causing a loss of lashes.
- *What to do:* Good lid hygiene is essential. Apply warm compresses several times daily to soften lid margin debris and oil. During bath time, use a clean facecloth wet with diluted baby shampoo to gently wipe away the eyelid debris while the eyes are closed. If the problem persists, see your doctor for possible treatment with antibiotic or anti-inflammatory ointments.

❶ What Is Strabismus?

Strabismus is the medical term that describes a misalignment of the eyes, commonly called crossed eyes, squint, or lazy eye. The condition is one of the most common pediatric eye disorders; it affects about 4% of all children.

Signs and Symptoms of Strabismus

The affected eye(s) might appear turned inward (esotropia), outward (exotropia), or, less commonly, up (hypertropia) or down (hypotropia). Because the eyes aren't perfectly synchronized in these conditions, your child might experience double or blurred vision, causing him to cover or close the affected eye, hence the term "squint." He might sit in an odd position, twisting around to compensate for the misalignment and, thereby, to focus on a particular object.

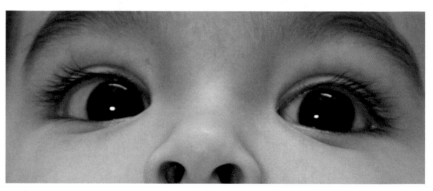

Strabismus

❷ What Causes Strabismus?

- Blurry/poor vision in one or both eyes
- Weakness in the muscles controlling eye movement
- Abnormal nerves controlling the muscles of the eye
- Cataracts (clouding of the lens of the eye)

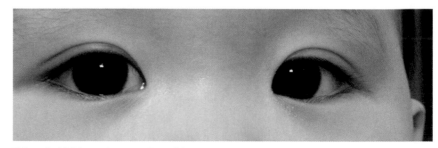

Epicanthal folds causing pseudostrabimus

When to See an Eye Specialist

Newborn infants' eyes are often out of alignment; this is normal in the first 2 to 4 months of life. Once your child is beyond 4 months of age and continues to exhibit eye misalignment, your doctor should refer him to an ophthalmologist. Any child who has constantly crossed eyes should also be referred.

❸ How Is Strabismus Treated?

The treatment for strabismus depends on the underlying cause, but there are several types of therapy that are commonly used. Children with strabismus should have their eyes assessed by an optometrist or ophthalmologist.

Treatment for Strabismus	What It Does
Wearing eyeglasses	Corrects unequal vision between the eyes or improves farsightedness or nearsightedness
Wearing a patch	Forces child to use and strengthen the weaker eye
Eye surgery	Realigns the eye muscles

❶ What Is Refractive Error?

Refractive error includes nearsightedness (myopia), farsightedness (hyperopia), and astigmatism. Normal vision is a highly complex phenomenon that requires a series of steps to occur in near perfect alignment:

- Light from an image passes through the clear cornea at the front of the eye, through the pupil, through the eye lens, through the clear fluid that fills the eye, and onto the retina, which is a thin layer of light-sensitive nerves on the back wall of the eye.
- From the retina, the signal is passed to the optic nerve, which carries it to areas of the brain that process and perceive vision.

Did You Know?

Laser Surgery
As the eye grows, the refractive error can worsen before stabilization occurs when your child has completed the growth phase of puberty. This means that laser correction therapy is not an option for children.

❷ What Causes Refractive Error?

A refractive error occurs when the image does not fall precisely onto the retina — it might fall in front or behind it, leading to blurred vision.

Types of Refractive Error

Type of Refractive Error	What Is Happening?	What Does the Child Experience?
Nearsightedness (myopia)	Image of an object is focused in front of retina	Distant objects appear blurry
Farsightedness (hyperopia)	Image of an object is focused behind retina	Close objects appear blurry
Astigmatism	Irregularities in cornea result in inability to focus on all parts of an object at the same time	Blurring of both near and distant objects

Did You Know?

Refractive Myths

Contrary to popular belief, refractive error and other visual problems are not caused by reading in dim light or sitting too close to the television; they are often inherited conditions related to the size and shape of the eyeball.

Symptoms of Refractive Errors

- Squinting
- Holding objects very close or far away in order to see them
- Eye strain
- Problems at school
- Complaints about vision

❸ How Is Refractive Error Treated?

Once a specific problem is identified, the treatment usually involves corrective lenses (eyeglasses). Teenagers sometimes prefer contact lenses, but the care requirements generally make them unsuitable for younger children.

FAQ

I thought only older people could get cataracts. Can children get them too?

Yes, although it is much rarer. A cataract is a clouding within the normally transparent lens of the eye. Depending on their size and location, cataracts can lead to visual disturbances. Normally, a child's pupils show up red when a photograph is taken using a flash. This is the same "red reflex" a doctor looks at when she looks in a child's eyes with an ophthalmoscope. If cloudy or whitish, it can suggest a cataract. Other signs of cataracts include misaligned eyes, cloudy or decreased vision, or abnormal eye movements. These signs are never normal and, if present, should be assessed promptly by your doctor.

FAQ

What is color blindness and how do I know if my child is color-blind?

Color blindness, more accurately called color vision deficiency, occurs when specialized cells in the back wall of the eye, or retina, called photoreceptors, do not function normally. There are different forms of color vision deficiency; the inability to accurately see or distinguish shades of red and green is by far the most common.

Approximately 5% to 8% of males and 1% of females have some form of color vision deficiency. In children, most instances of color vision deficiency are hereditary, meaning they are present from birth. There are various degrees of severity of color blindness and, fortunately, the condition does not worsen over time.

Your child with a deficiency of red vision will see all shades of red as dark; a child with a deficiency of green vision might not see any difference between the varying shades of green, brown, orange, and red. Color vision deficiency can usually be diagnosed by an eye doctor with specialized visual charts.

Doc Talk

During routine health examinations, your child's doctor will examine the eye and visual system in different ways, depending on the child's age. If you or your doctor have any concerns about your child's ability to see clearly, your child can undergo further specific examinations aimed at finding out how sharp his vision is and detecting any potential problems.

Failure to Thrive (Poor Growth)

What Can I Do?

▶ Ask your health-care provider to show you your child's growth chart to see where she plots for weight and height.

▶ If she plots below the 3rd percentile or has dropped off the growth curve by two or more major percentiles, she may have failure to thrive (but remember that if you and your partner were also small, then this may be genetically appropriate for her).

▶ If she has any red flag symptoms, be sure she has a detailed examination by her doctor to look for an underlying medical condition that may require treatment.

❶ What Is Failure to Thrive?

An accurate measurement of your child's weight should be obtained at birth and at each routine checkup. Remember, children come in all shapes and sizes. Just because your child is small or light does not necessarily mean there is a problem.

Growth Charts

Your health-care provider should plot your child's weight and height (as well as her head circumference in the first few years) on a standard growth chart. There is a possibility that your child has "failure to thrive" if her weight is less than the 3rd percentile for her age and sex; that is, if she weighs less than 97 out of 100 similar children. Your doctor might also suspect failure to thrive if repeat weight measurements indicate that your child's weight has fallen over two major percentiles (for example, from above the 85th percentile to below the 15th percentile) over a period of several months.

Normal Weight Gain

- Birth to 6 months: average of $\frac{2}{3}$ to 1 ounce (20 to 30 g) daily
- 6 to 12 months: average of $\frac{1}{2}$ ounce (15 g) daily
- At one year: usually three times her birth weight
- At two years: usually four times her birth weight
- To estimate weight in kilograms for children older than 2 years old: (age in years multiplied by 2) + 8 kg

Sample Growth Chart

Different growth charts are used in different parts of the world. In North America, we commonly use the World Health Organization

(WHO) charts, which allow for the fact that breastfed babies tend to gain weight a bit faster than babies fed by bottle in the first 6 months of life — although the opposite is true in the second 6 months. On this chart, you can see an example of a child who has had slow weight gain and has thus fallen over two major percentiles, which would prompt her health-care provider to investigate this issue further.

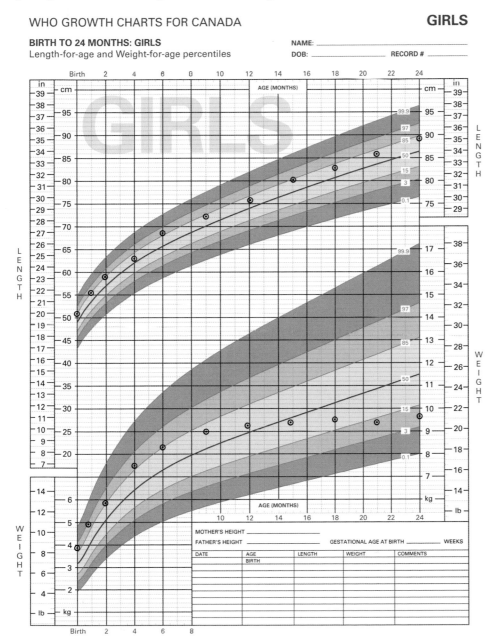

Sample growth curve demonstrating slow weight gain over time

When should we consult our doctor?

Although most children gain weight within the parameters of the growth charts, a few do not, for a variety of reasons. See the red flags below for when to consult your doctor.

➠ Failure to Thrive Red Flags

Consult your child's doctor if your child has any of the following symptoms:

- Any unexplained weight loss at any time
- Your child's weight for her age has fallen over two major percentiles (see chart, page 193)
- Persistent vomiting
- Persistent diarrhea
- Greasy, oily, loose stools
- Persistent tummy pains
- Poor energy
- Can't keep up with her peers

Specific Growth Patterns

These growth patterns affect an infant's weight and length but are somewhat less concerning:

- Some babies are born, either at term or prematurely, proportionately small for both weight and length. If these babies continue to grow well and if it seems they are "catching up," you should not be concerned — even if they are below the 3rd percentile.
- Some babies are born at an average weight and length, but by the second year of life, their weight and length are proportionately small. This often occurs if the infant's parents and extended family are small. This growth pattern should not be considered to be a problem; instead, this reflects the genetic makeup of the child.

❷ What Causes Poor Weight Gain?

Temperament

Your baby's temperament may play a role; for example, she might be a fussy or irritable infant. Another possibility is that she might not provide easy-to-read hunger cues or you may not be able to identify her cues when she is hungry. She might push away or refuse to feed.

Medical Conditions

Less commonly, there are some medical conditions that result in inadequate weight gain. In such cases, there is usually some other symptom or signal to suggest that a specific illness is present.

Vomiting

Vomiting, for example due to severe gastroesophageal reflux disease (GERD), might lead to inadequate caloric intake. See Vomiting (page 415).

Malabsorption

Your baby might be having difficulty absorbing enough calories. Malabsorption can occur as a result of certain medical conditions, such as cystic fibrosis or celiac disease.

Diarrhea

Although diarrhea usually does not last long and is due to an acute viral infection, in some cases, infants experience longer periods of diarrhea, which can lead to malabsorption. See Diarrhea (page 164).

❸ How Is Failure to Thrive Treated?

Treatment will depend on the underlying cause. In a minority of cases, an underlying medical condition may be discovered that will need to be addressed. In most cases of failure to thrive, no specific disease is present and the treatment involves a combination of strategies aimed at increasing calories and working on your child's feeding behavior. You will need input from your health-care providers as well as a dietitian.

Doc Talk	In brief, a lot of medical problems are capable of producing failure to thrive, but most of the time, no specific symptoms are present and the treatment may simply involve finding ways of increasing how many calories your child is consuming. This may involve the expert help of a dietitian.

Fainting (Syncope)

What Can I Do?

▶ If your child feels like she's going to faint, have her sit with her head between her knees or lie down with her legs elevated to increase blood flow to the brain.

▶ Call 911 if the loss of consciousness lasts more than a couple of minutes or if your child wakes up and is not back to herself.

▶ Don't panic. Reassure your child and yourself that fainting episodes, especially in teenage girls, are seldom anything serious.

Case Study

Francesca's Fainting

Francesca's mother received a call from her daughter's high school. The principal reported that Francesca had "passed out" during a pep rally in the gym and was taken to the nurse's office. She's now awake and seems back to herself. Francesca says she remembers feeling hot and light-headed, and her friend recalls that Francesca was pale before she fell to the ground. When they went to see her doctor, he did not seem overly concerned and diagnosed her as having experienced a simple faint. He reassured them both and advised Francesa's mother to observe her for any more serious symptoms.

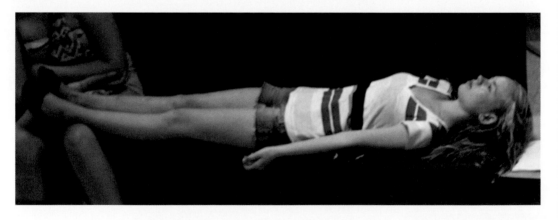

❶ What Is Fainting?

Fainting, or syncope, happens when the brain's blood supply decreases, causing the person to briefly lose consciousness, or "pass out." It usually lasts for a few seconds, or a minute at the most. Fainting is common, especially in teenage girls— about 15% of children faint at least once.

Associated Features of a Typical Faint

Before the child passes out, she will often:

- Feel light-headed
- Feel weak
- Have blurry vision
- Feel nauseous
- Look pale
- Look or feel sweaty

When the child recovers, she:

- Will not feel confused
- May feel the same sensation of being "about to faint" if she sits up or tries to stand too soon

When should we contact our doctor or local hospital?

Heart problems that lead to fainting are very rare, but are critically important to diagnose because if left untreated, sudden death can be the tragic result. See your doctor if your child has repeated episodes of fainting without an obvious cause or if there are any red flags that may suggest a cardiac cause.

RELATED CONDITIONS

- Heart problems
- Hypoglycemia
- Seizures

Did You Know?

Orthostatic Hypotension

This is similar to a simple faint, but happens when someone stands up too quickly. This is more likely to occur when the child is dehydrated or taking certain medications.

▶▶ Fainting Red Flags

Consult your child's doctor as soon as possible if your child has any of the following symptoms associated with fainting:

- Fainting with exercise
- Palpitations (feeling like the heart is beating rapidly in the chest)
- History of previous heart surgery
- Family history of sudden death, especially if family member was younger than 50 years old

If any of these symptoms are present, your child should have a detailed cardiac evaluation, including monitoring her heart rate for a prolonged period using a Holter monitor.

❷ What Are the Causes of Fainting?

In order to maintain the blood supply to the brain, you need enough blood in the blood vessels, a strong heart to pump the blood, and normal blood pressure. If a problem occurs with any of these elements, a faint may result. Sometimes the blood pressure drops suddenly in response to feelings of fear, the sight of blood, or other similar stimuli. The typical scenario is a teenager who is standing, often in hot or close quarters, for some time, which tends to "widen" the blood vessels, hence dropping the blood pressure driving the blood to the brain.

Psychological Causes

Sometimes anxiety may lead to hyperventilation, which, if severe enough, may cause a faint. Occasionally, teenagers will "fake" a dramatic fainting spell, known as a conversion reaction. This diagnosis is suggested by a history of recurrent bouts of fainting without any of the initial light-headedness, weakness, nausea, or pallor. Conversion reactions always seem to happen in front of witnesses; the teen shows little of the anxiety expected from a faint; and any fall is cushioned, so it never produces an injury.

❸ How Is Fainting Treated?

The best treatment is to lie down with the legs elevated to allow the blood to flow to the brain. The worst thing you can do is to try to get the child to stand up too quickly. Wait for her to feel better before gradually getting her on her feet again.

If the loss of consciousness lasts more than a couple of minutes or your child wakes up and doesn't seem to be acting normally, treat this as an emergency.

Other Medical Conditions Associated with Fainting

Signs or Symptoms	What This Could Mean
Child appears clammy, shaky, or weak; child is diabetic; or it has been several hours since she last ate	Low blood sugar (hypoglycemia)
Sudden onset with convulsive movements (muscle jerks), with drowsiness after the child wakes up	Seizures. See Seizures (page 332).

Doc Talk   Remember that the vast majority of all syncope is due to a simple faint. If you are concerned, take your child to your family doctor, who will ask questions, examine your child, and perhaps order some tests, such as an electrocardiogram (ECG), in order to identify any treatable cause of fainting. If the history is very suggestive of a simple faint, your doctor may well reassure you without any specific tests.

Fever

What Can I Do?

▶ Learn how to take your child's temperature accurately. Your child's exact temperature is not as important as how he looks and how he is behaving. Treat him and not the thermometer!

▶ If your child is healthy generally, looks well despite the fever, is still drinking well, and is playful and active, it is not necessary to seek medical attention in the first 48 hours unless he is younger than 3 months of age.

▶ If you feel that your child is uncomfortable as a result of the fever, you can provide fever control with antipyretics.

❶ What Is a Fever?

Fever is a sign rather than an illness. Fever means that the body's temperature is elevated, usually in response to an infection or inflammation. The fever is generated by the immune system mounting its natural response. Therefore, fever should not necessarily be seen as a bad thing, but rather as an appropriate immune reaction. Generally, finding the cause of a child's fever is the challenge, not the fever itself.

Normal Body Temperature

The body's normal temperature ranges from 97°F to 100°F (36°C to 37.8°C). There is a natural rhythm to body temperature: it is lower in the morning and increases in the early evening. A child is considered to be febrile (have a fever) if the temperature is above this range, but the exact number will vary depending on where the temperature is taken. The usual definition of fever is a temperature over 100.4°F (38°C) if taken rectally. If measured under the tongue (orally) or in the ear (tympanic), fever is a temperature over 99.5°F (37.5°C), and under the arm (axillary), it is over 99°F (37.2°C).

Did You Know?

Temperature Guide

A fever can be determined in a number of ways.

Rectally (in the anus) higher than 100.4°F (38.0°C)

Orally (under the tongue) higher than 99.5°F (37.5°C)

Tympanic (in the ear) higher than 99.5°F (37.5°C)

Axillary (under the arm) higher than 99°F (37.2°C)

❷ What Causes a Fever?

The most important question is "What is causing the fever?" — not "What can I do to stop the fever?" The most common cause of fever is some sort of infection. In children, viral illness tends to be much more common than more serious bacterial infections.

When should we contact our doctor or local hospital?

Do not assume that the higher the temperature, the more serious the illness. Children with mild viral infections can have fevers of 104°F (40°C), and those with serious bacterial infections can have a temperature of 101.3°F (38.5°C) — or, occasionally in younger infants, even subnormal temperatures. See the red flags below for when to seek medical attention.

⏩ Fever Red Flags

Seek immediate medical attention if your child has any of the following symptoms associated with fever:

- Your child is unresponsive and not interacting with you and the environment.
- Your child is listless and apathetic.
- Your child is drinking very little.
- Your child has a dry tongue and eyes.
- Your child has difficulty breathing (not just a bit congested).
- Your child has a stiff neck.
- Your child is hard to rouse or console.
- Your child has reddish or purple spots on the skin that do not blanch (disappear) when pressed.

Consult with your health-care provider if:

- Your child is younger than 6 months old.
- Your child has a known problem with his immune system.
- Your child's fever continues for more than 48 hours.
- You are not comfortable with how your child looks.

Did You Know?

Old Wives' Tale

Many people used to believe that you could use the back of your hand to touch the forehead of a child to determine if he had a fever. Unfortunately, this is not reliable and is not recommended.

❸ How Is a Fever Treated?

Start by taking an accurate reading of your child's temperature.

How To: Take Your Child's Temperature

An accurate temperature reading is very important in the first 3 months of life. A rectal temperature is the most reliable and recommended method to use. After 3 months of age, families may choose a tympanic (ear) or axillary (armpit) temperature reading until the child is about 4 years old, at which time an oral temperature becomes practical.

Rectal

Rectal temperatures are the most accurate but the least convenient. In order to use a rectal thermometer, place some petroleum jelly on the tip of the thermometer and insert the tip into the anus no farther than 1 inch (2.5 cm).

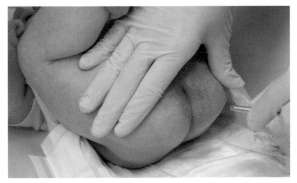

Rectal

Tympanic

Taking the temperature in the ear is easier and much quicker than other methods, but the tympanic thermometer is more expensive and not as accurate as the rectal temperature. It is sometimes difficult to fit the earpiece into a younger baby's ear, and so some authorities don't recommend its use in the first year or two of life.

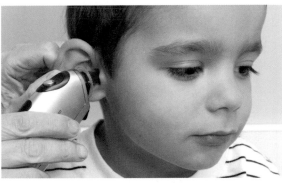

Tympanic

Axillary

Taking the temperature with an oral thermometer under the arm is the easiest method but also the least accurate. The thermometer needs to stay high in the armpit with the arm held tightly against the child's side.

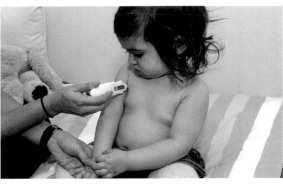

Axillary

Oral

Oral temperatures are obtained by placing the tip of the thermometer under the tongue in the mouth. This can be quite difficult in younger children due to lack of cooperation. The child needs to press his lips together without biting the thermometer until the digital thermometer beeps when it has completed recording the temperature.

Find the Cause

To determine where the fever is coming from, take a closer look at your child's symptoms. If, for example, your child has cold symptoms, the fever is likely secondary to a viral upper respiratory tract

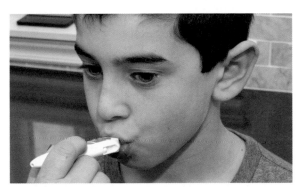

Oral

Most Common Causes of Fever By Age

Age	Cause	Symptoms	Red Flags (Seek Help)
Newborns (0 to 3 months)	• Infections are usually viral but are very difficult to distinguish from more serious bacterial infections	• Symptoms are often nonspecific (for example, poor feeding, irritability, crying)	• Always seek medical attention for fevers at this age because it is very difficult to predict which are more serious
Infants (3 to 12 months)	• Upper respiratory viral infections (colds)	• Runny nose, congestion	• Breathing difficulties (for example, fast breathing, increased breathing effort) • Fever not settling after 48 hours • Dry mouth and eyes, and decreased wet diapers • Stiff neck • Child looks unwell
	• Ear infections (especially after 6 months)	• Irritable • Pulling on ear	
	• Gastroenteritis (stomach infections)	• Vomiting, diarrhea, poor feeding	
	Note: teething does not cause fever		
Toddlers, preschoolers (1 to 6 years)	• Upper respiratory viral infections (colds)	• Runny nose, congestion	• Breathing difficulties (for example, fast breathing, increased breathing effort) • Fever not settling after 48 hours • Dry mouth and eyes, and decreased wet diapers • Stiff neck • Child looks unwell
	• Ear infections	• Irritable • Pulling on ear	
	• Sore throat, tonsillitis	• Sore, red throat with pus on tonsils	
	• Gastroenteritis (stomach infections)	• Vomiting, diarrhea, poor eating	
	• Respiratory infections (pneumonia, bronchitis)	• Cough, breathing difficulties	
Schoolchildren (6 years and older)	• Respiratory infections (pneumonia, bronchitis)	• Cough, breathing difficulty	• Breathing difficulties (for example, fast breathing, increased breathing effort) • Fever not settling after 48 hours • Dry mouth and eyes, and decreased urination • Stiff neck • Child looks unwell
	• Sore throat, tonsillitis	• Sore, red throat with pus on tonsils	
	• Urinary tract infections (especially in girls)	• Pain with urination, foul-smelling urine	
	• Gastroenteritis (stomach infections)	• Vomiting, diarrhea, poor eating	

infection. If he is vomiting and has diarrhea, the fever is likely caused by a viral stomach flu. This may not always be straightforward: your child may have fever with absolutely no other symptoms, or he may have a wide range of symptoms fitting with more than one cause. In both of these scenarios, the underlying cause is still usually a viral infection, which can cause fever and nothing else, or can cause fever with cough, cold, tummy, and ear symptoms!

FAQs

Can the fever do any harm?

Fever on its own is not dangerous to the child unless it reaches extremely high levels (over 104.9°F/40.5°C), which is very unusual. Children between the ages of 6 months and 6 years can occasionally have a convulsion with the fever, called a febrile convulsion. See Seizures (page 332). This occurs in about 4% of all children. Although it is an extremely frightening and distressing experience for the parents, febrile convulsions are not dangerous and do not lead to any brain damage. Studies have shown that 97% of these children tend to grow out of the seizures by the age of 6 years and will function normally at school and university. There is no evidence to suggest that lowering the fever with acetaminophen will decrease the likelihood of the child having a febrile convulsion. That said, most physicians and parents do treat fevers more readily with acetaminophen in children with a past history of febrile convulsions.

Which should I use: a digital or a mercury thermometer?

Digital thermometers have now replaced the older glass mercury thermometers. Most pediatric authorities do not recommend using mercury thermometers because the glass can break, leading to an accidental exposure to mercury and environmental contamination. The newer plastic digital thermometers are inexpensive, easy to use, and give a much quicker reading. Both types provide comparable accuracy for assessing your child's temperature.

Medication

Since most fevers are viral in origin, no specific treatment is available to treat the infection. Antibiotics do not work against viruses, so they should not be used for children with colds, flu, or sore throats that are not caused by strep. If the fever has a bacterial cause, such as a urinary tract infection, strep throat, or one of a few kinds of ear infection, then it is likely that your child will require antibiotics.

Did You Know?

Behavior
Some children with fever may initially look quite well but then start to get "sicker." For example, if the fever remains high and your child progresses from having cold symptoms (runny nose, cough, congestion) to having increased difficulty breathing, then he may have developed a more serious problem, such as a chest infection (pneumonia). To tell the difference between a mild viral infection and a more serious bacterial infection, you need to look not so much at the fever but more at your child's behavior in general.

Antipyretic medication is only necessary if your child appears to be uncomfortable or irritable as a result of the fever. The evidence from studies suggests that antipyretic medication will not alter the course of the illness.

Medication	Dose	Frequency
Acetaminophen (Tylenol, Tempra)	10 to 15 mg per kg	Every 4 to 6 hours, if necessary
Ibuprofen (Advil, Motrin)	5 to 10 mg per kg	Every 6 to 8 hours, if necessary

FAQ

Should I give my child acetaminophen or ibuprofen?

The answer is not black or white. The most commonly used antipyretic drug is acetaminophen, which is available in drops, syrup, chewable tablets, capsules, and suppositories (good for use in children who are vomiting or refuse to take medication by mouth). The dosage will depend on the weight of the child (10 to 15 mg/kg given every 4 to 6 hours, if necessary). Another very commonly used option is ibuprofen, which studies have shown to be equally effective and as safe as acetaminophen. It is only required every 6 to 8 hours at a dose of 5 to 10 mg/kg.

Some parents have started to use acetaminophen and ibuprofen on an alternating basis for particularly high fevers that seem to be causing the child discomfort. If dosed correctly (do not exceed the maximum for either of the two medications), this appears to be reasonably safe and may result in less fever. Remember that this will not change the course or outcome of the particular infection!

Increase Comfort

We generally recommend dressing your feverish child lightly (rather than bundling him up) because bundling can prevent the escape of the body's excess heat. If your child is feeling cold and is shivering, it is acceptable to cover him with a light blanket until the shivering stops. It is also important that children stay well hydrated when they are feverish; offer your child plenty of liquids.

Tepid water sponging when combined with antipyretics has shown a slight advantage in trials over medication alone in bringing the fever down in the first 30 minutes after treatment. Avoid using water so cold that it makes your child shiver and generate more body heat. Sponging with rubbing alcohol is definitely not recommended.

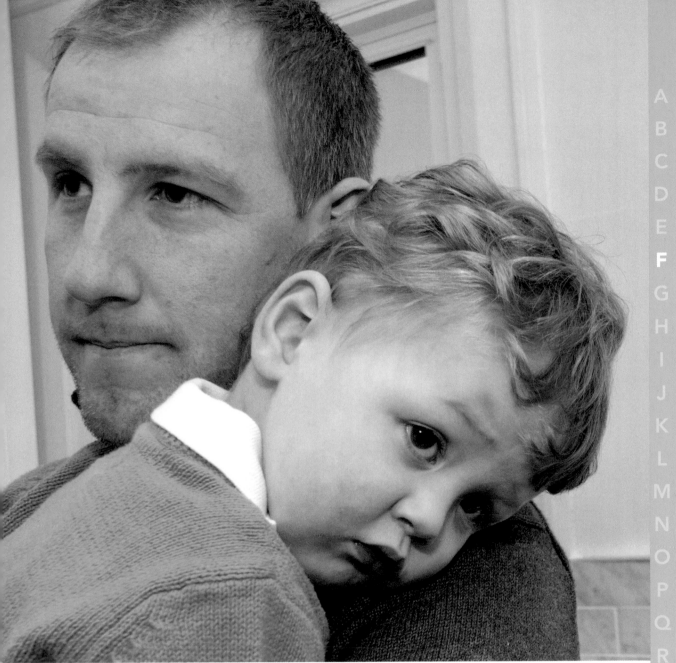

Doc Talk Most children with a fever will typically perk up as the fever breaks. Still, there are certain scenarios where a fever needs to be immediately attended to by a health-care practitioner. In the case of a child whose immune system is compromised — for example, a child with cancer or sickle cell disease — a fever may be the first sign of a life-threatening infection. His body may be unable to fight off the infection without medication. A more common problem would be the infant who develops a fever in the first 3 months of life. In this case, the immune system is still developing: the signs and symptoms of a very serious infection, such as meningitis, can be very nonspecific. Fever might be the only clue that something serious is brewing.

Flat Feet

When should we contact our doctor?

In most cases, flat feet are normal and require no special treatment.

❶ What Is a Flat Foot?

If your child has a flat foot, the entire sole of the foot touches the ground while she is standing. The arch, usually seen under the foot, is not present.

❷ What Causes Flat Feet?

In young children, flat feet are caused by a looseness of the tendons that hold the foot bones together. This is normal. The arch may only become apparent between 5 and 10 years of age. Very rarely, flat feet are caused by bone, joint, or neuromuscular problems.

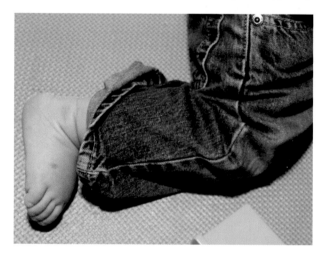

❸ How Is a Flat Foot Treated?

Sometimes special shoes, orthotics, or inserts are recommended, but these are not usually necessary. Most children with flat feet should wear regular shoes; they may also go barefoot without causing problems. Special inserts or arches in childhood will not prevent or reduce the degree of flat feet as the child ages.

Doc Talk

Flat feet are normal in babies because of the fat pad at the bottom of their feet, which hides their arch. Virtually all children under 18 months of age have flat feet. As they grow, the arch of the sole of the foot will start to form. Contrary to popular belief, people with flat feet do not have more foot pain or foot issues than people with arched feet. In fact, some studies suggest that people with flat feet have fewer problems.

Flu (Influenza, Gastroenteritis, and Epstein-Barr Virus)

What Can I Do?

▶ Distinguish between "true" influenza and the "flu" caused by the common cold, "stomach" flu (gastroenteritis), or infectious mononucleosis ("mono").

▶ Look for the red flags that signify dehydration in stomach flu that will require medical attention.

▶ Treat the flu with acetaminophen or ibuprofen, lots of fluids, and rest.

▶ Consider having your child vaccinated annually against the influenza virus.

❶ What Is the Flu?

Many of us will use the term "flu" to describe a feeling of generally being unwell. In medical terms, flu refers specifically to respiratory infections caused by influenza viruses in the fall and winter months. Much of what lay people refer to as the flu is actually a bad cold as a result of a common cold virus. See Common Cold (page 120). What is usually referred to as the "stomach flu" is actually viral gastroenteritis.

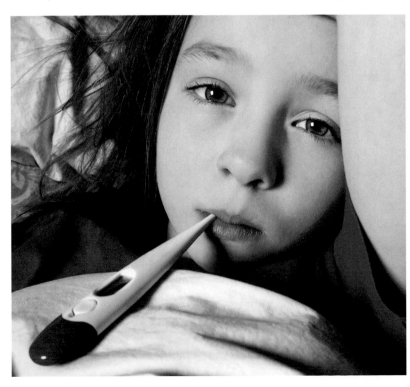

RELATED CONDITIONS

- Epstein-Barr virus
- Gastroenteritis
- Influenza

Did You Know?

Very Catchy

Influenza is transmitted from person to person by droplets of secretions containing the virus. The droplets are spread by coughing or sneezing, or by direct contact with articles, such as toys, recently contaminated by an infected child's coughing or sneezing. Influenza is most infectious during the 24 hours before the onset of the symptoms. This means it may be spread before you even know you have it!

See Viral Gastroenteritis (page 209). Flu can also occasionally be confused with the Epstein-Barr virus (the mononucleosis virus or "mono").

The Common Cold Versus the (True) Flu

Symptom	Common Cold	Flu (Influenza Virus)
Fever	Occasionally; if present fever is typically low grade (lower than 102°F/39°C)	Usually; onset is sudden, fever is high (higher than 102°F/39°C)
Headache	Rare; if present, usually mild	Usually
Muscle aches and pains	Sometimes; often mild	Usually; often severe
Runny nose, congestion	Common	Common
General discomfort; feeling "out of sorts"	Sometimes; when present, mild	Common; often severe
Sore throat	Common	Common
Sneezing	Common	Occasionally
Complications	Can get ear or sinus infection	Can get pneumonia, with severe respiratory symptoms
Prevention	Frequent hand washing	Frequent hand washing and annual immunization

When should we contact our doctor or local hospital?

One in 100 children with influenza will be hospitalized for complications related to their infection. In young infants, influenza can look like a very serious illness and be mistaken for meningitis. Other complications of influenza include pneumonia and encephalitis (infection of the brain). If any red flags are present, seek medical attention.

▶▶ Flu Red Flags

- Rapid breathing
- Refusal to drink
- Recurrent vomiting
- Drowsiness

- Lips look blue
- Severe headache
- Stiff neck

❷ How Is the Flu Treated?

Comfort and hydration are key to getting through a bout of the flu.

How To: Treat the Flu

- Control the fever and muscle aches with acetaminophen or ibuprofen. These are useful and should be used liberally.
- Encourage your child to drink fluids. Your child may not feel like eating — this is expected and fine — so ensure that he continues to drink lots of fluids.
- Give antiviral medications as prescribed by your doctor, depending on the age and underlying medical conditions of your child.

❶ What Is Viral Gastroenteritis ("Stomach Flu")?

When a child has vomiting, diarrhea, and painful abdominal cramps, we will often say a child has the stomach flu. This type of viral illness, which leads to inflammation of the stomach and intestines, is caused by any one of a number of common stomach bugs, including norovirus (Norwalk), rotavirus, and adenovirus. Other family members or friends at daycare may also have an upset stomach. Infected toddlers may also have a low-grade fever, have decreased energy and appetite, and feel generally under the weather.

Did You Know?

Aspirin Caution
Children with influenza should not take salicylates, such as aspirin (ASA). This combination results in an increased risk of developing a condition known as Reye's syndrome, a very serious condition, often fatal, which produces headache, vomiting, liver inflammation, and low blood sugar.

⯈ Viral Gastroenteritis Red Flags

Consult your child's doctor if your child has any of the following symptoms associated with viral gastroenteritis:

- Sunken eyes
- Decreased urine output
- Sticky mouth
- Dizziness
- No tears with crying
- Lethargy (difficult to rouse)
- Inability to keep fluids down because of recurrent vomiting

Annual Vaccination

Annually, a new influenza vaccine is available to protect us against the flu virus. A new vaccine is required each year because there are minor changes in the strain of virus most prevalent every season. This means that the immune system doesn't recognize the virus from year to year and needs to be reminded with the latest version of the flu vaccine.

❷ How Is Viral Gastroenteritis Treated?

Like most viral infections, the mainstay of treatment is comfort and hydration. Pain relief can be achieved with acetaminophen or ibuprofen. Staying well hydrated is often the more challenging part, especially with increased fluid losses from vomiting and diarrhea. Giving your child frequent, small amounts of fluid is key to maintaining hydration (see Dehydration, page 150).

❶ What Is Epstein-Barr Virus (Infectious Mononucleosis)?

Infectious mononucleosis is a well-known infection caused by the Epstein-Barr virus (EBV). EBV is transmitted primarily in the saliva, hence the term "kissing disease." EBV infection is common, and in some developing countries, 80% to 100% of children are infected by the age of 3 to 6 years. In more developed countries, infection tends to occur mainly in adolescents or young adults.

Symptoms of EBV Infection

In young children (usually milder):

- Cough, congestion, runny nose
- Sore throat
- Low-grade fever
- Enlarged spleen or liver

In older children:

- Initially feel generally unwell
- Decreased appetite
- Chills
- Fever that can last 1 to 2 weeks
- Sore throat that appears red and inflamed, often with a whitish coating
- Swollen glands (lymph nodes)
- Some older children may have fatigue for weeks or even months
- Enlarged spleen or liver
- Swelling around the eyes

Diagnosis

If your child presents with a number of EBV features, your doctor may do a complete blood count, which often gives clues that the infection is from EBV. Infectious mono can be confirmed by a blood test that detects antibodies produced by the body against the virus. Your doctor may also do a throat swab to exclude the possibility of strep throat, which has some similar features. See Sore Throat (page 371).

❷ How Is Epstein-Barr Virus Treated?

Unfortunately, like the influenza virus and many other viruses, there is no specific treatment for an EBV infection. Acetaminophen or ibuprofen can be used to control fever and pain from muscle aches. The virus will eventually run its course. Antibiotics are not useful (because it is caused by a virus, not a bacteria) and often actually make things worse by producing a rash. Children who have an enlarged spleen should avoid contact sports until the infection has passed to prevent the rare chance of an injury to the spleen.

| Doc Talk | "Flu shots" remain an issue, with most authorities recommending vaccination, while other parties are worried about possible side |

effects. The American Academy of Pediatrics recommends an annual influenza vaccine for all children and adolescents aged 6 months and older. Special efforts should be made to vaccinate specific children and adults:

- All children born preterm who are older than 6 months of age
- Children who have chronic medical conditions (such as asthma, diabetes, heart or lung diseases, or any form of immunosuppression); these conditions increase the risk of serious disease from influenza
- All household contacts and care providers of the children described above and those with children younger than 6 months of age (because they cannot get the vaccine themselves)
- All pregnant or breastfeeding women, or women considering pregnancy

Frostbite

What Can I Do?

▶ Prevent frostbite by dressing your child appropriately, ideally in waterproof layers.

▶ Warm your child slowly if you suspect he has frostbite. Encourage him to sip on warm drinks. Use acetaminophen or ibuprofen if your child feels pain.

▶ Don't use direct heat, such as a stove, radiator, heat lamp, fireplace, heating pad, or hairdryer because they can cause burns before your child can feel them on numb skin.

Case Study

Michael's Frostbite

Michael is a 10-year-old boy who was playing hockey with his friends at a nearby outdoor ice rink. He was having so much fun that he played for a few hours without noticing the cold. When he was done, his hands were numb and he had difficulty taking off his skates. When he got home, he found that his socks were wet and his feet were also numb.

Michael stayed outdoors in the cold for several hours. His hands were exposed to the cold for quite a while and his feet were constricted in tight skates. This put him at risk for frostbite. Michael's mom removed his wet socks and wrapped him in a warm blanket. She soaked his feet and hands in a bucket of lukewarm water for half an hour, until sensation returned. Michael started complaining of pain in his hands and feet. His mom gave him some acetaminophen for the pain. She called their family doctor, who instructed her to bring Michael in right away so that she could assess Michael further for possible frostbite.

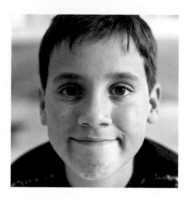

❶ What Is Frostbite?

Frostbite is damage to the skin from freezing due to exposure to cold temperatures. Ice crystals form in the skin or deeper tissue. The nose, cheeks, ears, fingers, and toes are most commonly affected. The severity of frostbite depends on several factors, including temperature, length of exposure, wind-chill factor, dampness, and type of clothing worn. Kids are more prone to frostbite than adults because they lose heat from their skin more rapidly. They also have a tendency to ignore the cold when having fun playing outdoors.

Factors That Increase Frostbite Risk

- Very young age
- Hunger or dehydration
- Prolonged outdoor play
- Previous frostbite
- Skin damage
- Tight clothing or footwear
- Windy or wet weather

When should we contact our doctor or local hospital?

The symptoms of frostbite range from mild pins and needles that can be treated at home to severe pain on warming and gangrene. Consider contacting your doctor if the mild red flags don't settle quickly. Severe red flags require urgent medical attention.

⏩ Frostbite Red Flags

Mild Red Flags	Severe Red Flags
■ Aching or throbbing	■ Blackened skin (gangrene)
■ Burning	■ Blisters
■ Itching	■ Blue or purple skin on rewarming
■ Numbness	■ Hard skin
■ Pins and needles	■ Severe pain on rewarming
■ Redness and pain on rewarming	■ Swelling
■ Tingling	■ White, yellow, or waxy skin

❷ How Is Frostbite Treated?

The best treatment is prevention, but if your child has frostbite, there are a few procedures you should follow to avoid further tissue damage and pain.

- **Protect skin from further exposure.** If you're outside, warm frostbitten hands by tucking them into your armpits or against your belly. Protect a frostbitten face, nose, or ears by covering the area with dry, gloved hands. Don't rub the affected area and never rub snow on frostbitten skin.

- **Get out of the cold.** Once you're indoors, remove wet clothes or any constricting clothes or jewelry. Put on dry clothes or wrap your child in warm blankets.
- **Assess your child for hypothermia (lowered body temperature).** Signs of hypothermia are uncontrollable shivering, rapid or slow breathing and heart rate, weakness, agitation, confusion, and drowsiness. If there are signs of hypothermia, call 911.
- **Give plenty of fluids and warm drinks.** This will replace lost fluids and warm his core body temperature.
- **Gradually warm frostbitten areas.** Put frostbitten hands or feet in lukewarm (not hot!) water at about 100°F (38°C). Place a warm, wet cloth on other frostbitten areas, such as nose, cheeks, and ears; keep replacing with a new warm, wet cloth as it cools. There may be pain as the numbness goes away; acetaminophen or ibuprofen may be used.
- **Don't walk on frostbitten feet or toes.** This further damages the tissue. Carry your child, if possible. Move any frostbitten areas as little as possible and try to keep them elevated to prevent swelling.

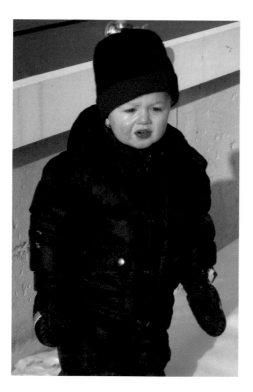

Prevention

- Dress your child in layers. The outer layer should be waterproof.
- Avoid tight-fitting clothes and footwear.
- Put mittens or gloves on his hands. Mittens are warmer, but kids may keep gloves on longer.
- Ensure he wears a hat or balaclava that covers the ears.
- Change wet clothing immediately, especially socks and mittens.
- Make sure he comes inside often to warm up. If your child is shivering, it's time for a break.
- Drink plenty of fluids and eat plenty of food during lengthy outings.
- Know the early signs (numbness or tingling).
- In older children and teens, use a buddy system to monitor each other for early signs of frostbite.
- Stay updated on weather forecasts and make plans accordingly.

Doc Talk Go gradually. All rewarming methods for frostbite should be done gradually. Slow rewarming optimizes tissue healing.

Hair Loss (Alopecia)

What Can I Do?

▶ Don't worry if your baby loses her hair within a few weeks of birth. This is normal.

▶ Discourage tight hairstyling and chronic hair-pulling or twisting.

▶ If the cause of the hair loss is not obvious, arrange for your child to be examined by a health-care provider to help diagnose the cause and to begin appropriate treatment.

Case Study

Samantha's Hair Loss

Samantha is a healthy 3-year-old with a beautiful head of thick, curly hair. She prefers to wear it in a tight ponytail, in braids, and sometimes with a hair barrette. Samantha's mother noticed that she has some thinning of her hair along her hairline and wondered if it could be an infection. She made an appointment with their family doctor to have Samantha's scalp and hair examined. Samantha did have some thinning of her hair at her hairline, which matched the area under the tightest traction from her braids and ponytails. Her doctor recommended wearing her hair down or in a loose ponytail to release the pressure on the hair and give it a chance to regrow.

❶ What Is Alopecia (Hair Loss)?

The term "alopecia" simply means hair loss. The hair loss can be restricted to the scalp or it can include body hair too. In children, hair loss has five main causes: trichotillomania, alopecia areata, traction alopecia, tinea capitis, and telogen effluvium.

RELATED CONDITIONS

- Alopecia areata
- Telogen effluvium
- Tinea capitis
- Traction alopecia
- Trichotillomania

Trichotillomania

- *Symptoms:* Patchy hair loss anywhere on the scalp or face (eyebrows and eyelashes)
- *Causes:* Children develop a compulsive urge to pull out their hair. It is most common in girls 9 to 13 and can be triggered by anxiety, stress, or depression.
- *Treatment:* In young children (5 years and under), the condition usually resolves without intervention. Older children (6 years and over) should be evaluated for underlying mental health problems, such as anxiety.

When should we contact our doctor?

Alopecia is not an emergency, though it can certainly be alarming for a parent or child. Unless aggressive hairstyling is the obvious cause, hair loss should always be evaluated by your health-care provider.

Alopecia Areata

- *Symptoms:* This is a type of patchy hair loss seen in children. You may notice your child's hair falling out in clumps or patches, or more hair on her pillow. This will leave single or multiple round patches of bald scalp. Hair loss can be isolated to the scalp or include hair loss over the entire body.
- *Causes:* Alopecia areata is presumed to be the result of the immune system attacking the hair follicles, leading to hair loss. Sometimes the immune system can attack other organs, such as the thyroid or adrenal glands. Your doctor may do blood tests to look for these problems.
- *Treatment:* Children who have alopecia areata can occasionally recover spontaneously; however, most cases require treatment with topical medications that prevent the immune system from attacking hair follicles.

Traction Alopecia

- *Symptoms:* Typically, hair loss is most noticeable along the hairline.
- *Causes:* This hair loss is a result of tight braiding or the child pulling on or twisting her hair.
- *Treatment:* Once the child wears her hair loosely on a regular basis, the hair will grow back normally.

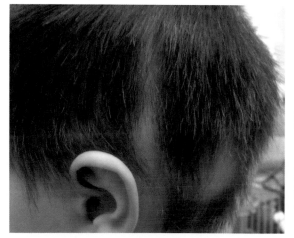

Alopecia areata

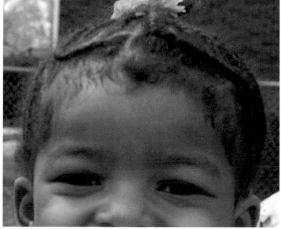

Traction alopecia

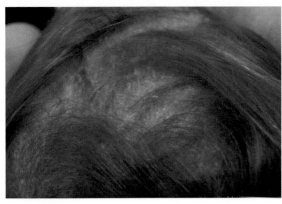
Tinea capitis

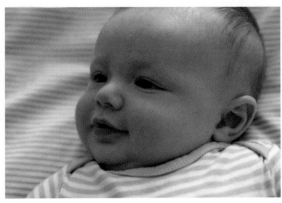
Normal hair loss in infants

Tinea Capitis

- *Symptoms:* Typically, children complain of a round, scaly, itchy patch on their scalp and present with hair loss. The patch might be tender, and you may notice enlarged bumps (lymph glands) at the base of the scalp or around the neck.
- *Causes:* This is a fungal infection of the scalp that can cause hair loss.
- *Treatment:* Oral antifungal medication prescribed by your doctor can treat this condition.

Telogen Effluvium

- *Symptoms:* Hair loss or thinning occurs as hairs enter their "dormant" phase.
- *Causes:* This typically happens a few months after a period of illness, infection, or stress.
- *Treatment:* Hair growth usually resumes several months after the initiating event has resolved.

Other Causes

Other causes of diffuse alopecia include aggressive hairstyling, straightening, and perming of the hair. Certain medical conditions are associated with hair loss, such as thyroid disease and lupus. However, hair loss alone is usually not the only symptom that children experience with these conditions.

Did You Know?

Bald Baby

It is entirely normal for babies to lose their hair within a few weeks of birth, and it can sometimes take months before it grows back. Infants often have bald patches over the back of their head; this is because babies are often lying down, and the friction of the bed or carpet on their scalp causes the hair to fall out. Hair in that spot grows back as the child becomes mobile.

Doc Talk Hair loss is caused by a variety of conditions. Unless tight hairstyling or chronic hair-pulling or twisting is the obvious cause of hair loss, an examination by a health-care provider is recommended to help diagnose the cause and to begin the appropriate treatment.

Head Injuries

What Can I Do?

▶ Prevent head injuries by using appropriate safety headgear for all sporting activities where a child might sustain a blow to the head.

▶ Ensure child safety gates are installed and CLOSED to prevent children from tumbling down the stairs.

▶ Never leave infants and young toddlers alone on a bed or a change table — even for a second!

▶ If you suspect a concussion, ensure that your child does not continue to play.

RELATED CONDITIONS

• Brain trauma
• Concussions

Did You Know?

Mild Headache
It is normal after a bump to the head to have a mild headache with some tenderness, swelling or bruising of the scalp.
If your child's headache is more severe or worsens significantly over time, seek medical attention.

❶ What Is a Head Injury?

Unfortunately, young children often bump their heads. Fortunately, most of these bumps are minor and should not be a cause for concern. The big questions for most parents relate to when to worry, and what to do to make sure that everything is okay. The mechanism of injury (for example, falling down the stairs), the type of injury (for example, a large cut with bleeding), and the age of the child are three important factors in deciding what to do. In the majority of cases, if your child is behaving appropriately and does not show any of the worrisome features, then it will usually be adequate to observe her at home, checking in on her from time to time over the next 24 hours to make sure that she hasn't developed any new symptoms.

Causes and Consequences

A head injury may occur from:

• A fall from a height
• A blow to the head

A head injury may result in:

• A cut to the scalp or face
• A bump, or "goose egg," over the scalp or forehead
• A "shake" to the brain that results in a brief loss of consciousness or affects the ability to think clearly for a brief period (concussion)
• A skull fracture (a crack in one of the skull bones)
• A bleed underneath the skull or even inside the brain (uncommon)

When should we contact our doctor or local hospital?

Minor blows to the head are common and tend to resolve by themselves, If your child appears well and is not complaining of pain, and the injury was mild, you can stay home and monitor your child for worsening of symptoms. If symptoms progress or any red flags are present, seek medical attention.

➤➤ Head Injury Red Flags

Consult your child's doctor if your child has any of the following symptoms associated with a head injury:

- A blow to the head from a fall greater than 3 feet (1 meter)
- Any head injury in the first 12 months of life
- Any loss of consciousness at the time of the injury
- Any cut to the head that does not stop bleeding after holding pressure on it for 5 to 10 minutes
- Any cut that is gaping open or deep and might need sutures, glue, or staples to close it
- A bad headache that is getting worse or just does not go away
- Repeated vomiting after the head injury
- Any decrease in the level of her alertness
- Appears confused or disorientated
- Difficulty with seeing, moving, or speaking
- Complains of neck stiffness

Bleeding

The scalp and face have an abundance of blood vessels. Consequently, if your child cuts herself in one of these areas, she will likely bleed a lot. This can be scary, but it is quite normal. This rich blood supply also means that cuts tend to heal nicely and quickly.

How To: Stop the Bleeding

- Apply firm pressure for 5 to 10 minutes with a clean cloth.
- Keep the head positioned above the body (with the child sitting or propped up).
- See your health-care provider if the bleeding continues after holding firm pressure or if the cut is more than a superficial scrape. Also see Cuts (page 144).

Did You Know?

Serious Signs

In young babies, signs of moderate to severe head injury may be less specific than in a toddler or child. Signs and symptoms that suggest a more serious injury in babies include irritability, difficulty to console her crying, lethargy or inappropriate sleepiness, poor feeding, or repeated vomiting.

Swelling

A "goose egg" often appears after a blow to the head from an object or person or when a child falls and hits her head on a hard surface. The blood vessels between the skull and just under the skin get compressed and break with the injury, leading to bleeding under the skin and swelling. The ensuing bump can occur rapidly and be quite impressive. A goose egg does not mean that the bone is broken or that any bleeding has occurred underneath the skull.

How To: Reduce the Swelling

- Wrap some ice in a cloth (or improvise with a pack of frozen vegetables) and place it over the swollen area for at least 15 to 20 minutes, as soon as possible after the injury.
- Ice the bump on and off for as much time as your child will tolerate over the next few hours.
- If she is complaining of pain (which is likely!), then go ahead and give her something to relieve the pain, either a dose of acetaminophen or ibuprofen.

FAQ

Should I be checking and waking my child at night after a head injury?
This is a controversial area. Here's a three-part answer.

- Some authorities recommend letting the child sleep through the night if it is close to her regular bedtime; others tell parents to wake their children once or twice through the night to ensure that they are looking okay. The difficulty with this is that most children (and adults) woken in the middle of the night tend to be drowsy, a bit confused, and often quite cranky, even if they didn't bump their head!
- The safest course is to be guided by your and your health-care provider's degree of worry. If you are not particularly worried, for example, and the mechanism of injury was pretty minor — and your child seemed pretty well afterward, apart from a mild brief period of discomfort — then letting her sleep through the night is appropriate. On the other hand, if it was a more severe blow to the head and your child had some symptoms, with headache and drowsiness, then it is likely that you will be advised to check in on her. This is done by waking her midway through the night to assess if she seems to be her normal self (for someone being woken in the middle of the night) or by at least checking that she is sleeping comfortably and that her color and breathing seem regular and normal.
- If you are worried, the safest thing would be to have her assessed after the head injury, and then go with the advice of the health-care provider. She will have done a complete assessment and should be well positioned to advise you as to how closely you need to observe your child.

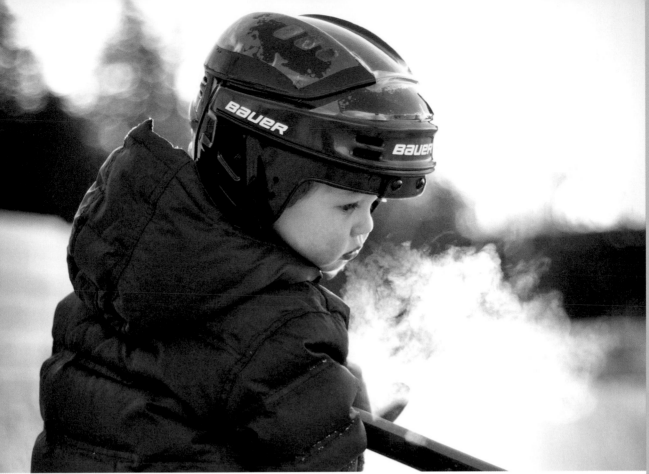

❶ What Are Brain Injuries?

More serious brain injuries are rare, but they do happen.

- *Skull fracture:* The skull bone is cracked from a blow or fall, leaving some bruising on the outside of the brain. Most skull fractures will heal very well without problems, but if the bone is dented inward and is putting pressure on the brain, this may require specialized treatment.
- *Epidural hematoma:* This is a bleed between the skull and the outer lining of the brain. It usually occurs if the skull fracture tears through a blood vessel just under the skull and the blood forms into a bruise/hematoma, which then puts pressure on the underlying brain.
- *Subdural hematoma:* This is a slightly deeper bleed between the outer and inner linings of the brain. It is also caused by the tearing of a blood vessel. These veins tend to bleed more slowly than those in the epidural space, so the child's symptoms can get gradually worse over the course of a few days.
- *Intraparenchymal hematoma:* This refers to bleeding inside the brain tissue itself.

A B C D E F G H I J K L M N O P Q R S T U V W X Y Z

❶ What Is a Concussion?

Concussion refers to a traumatic injury to the brain that temporarily affects the way you think and remember things. Any blow to the head, face, or neck, or somewhere else on the body that causes a sudden jarring of the head, may cause a concussion. Some examples of this kind of injury are being hit in the head with a ball or being checked into the boards in hockey.

Signs and Symptoms of a Concussion

A child does not need to be knocked out (lose consciousness or pass out) to have had a concussion. Signs and symptoms might include:

- Headache
- Nausea or vomiting
- Dizziness, balance problems, or poor coordination
- Decreased playing ability
- Changes in behavior (for example, anxiety or sadness)
- Confusion or feeling "dazed"
- Slowed thinking
- Difficulty concentrating
- Difficulty remembering
- Difficulty with sleeping (too much or too little)
- Ringing in the ears
- Sensitivity to loud noises or bright lights

In younger children, the signs and symptoms may be very general:

- Tummy pains
- Irritability
- Behavioral changes

▶▶ Concussion Red Flags

If you suspect that your child has a concussion, she should be evaluated by your health-care provider. Consult your child's doctor immediately if your child has any of the following symptoms:

- The headache is getting worse
- There is ongoing vomiting
- There is a decreased level of alertness/wakefulness
- There is difficulty walking

❷ How Is a Concussion Treated?

Rest

The most important part of treatment is rest. Initially, this means no exercising or even "energetic" playing. If a child is in the middle of playing a game, she should stop immediately.

It is also important to refrain from playing on the computer or video games. If the concussion symptoms seem to be worse with minimal activity (for example, concentrating at school), your child may need to rest at home until the symptoms are better and she has been assessed by her health-care provider. Certainly there should be no return to physical activity until all the signs and symptoms have entirely resolved. This could take days or weeks. When she is symptom-free, she can start a very gradual reintroduction of activity, starting with very light exercise and slowly increasing the level of intensity over days.

> **Did You Know?**
>
> **Repeat Concussion**
> When an athlete has a concussion, there is a significant chance that a second and more damaging concussion will follow that same season.

Principles of Concussion Management in Sports

Sports concussions have come to the forefront as more and more athletes suffer head injuries. Here are some guidelines to play by:

- Remove the injured player from play immediately.
- Do not allow the child to return to play in that game.
- Watch closely for symptoms (described on page 222).
- Have a health-care provider evaluate your child.
- Rest from exercise and school until symptoms have resolved.
- Once symptom-free for several days, begin a medically supervised stepwise return-to-play protocol.
- Return to sports should be cautious and individualized.

A responsible adult who understands the classification and management of concussion should be on the sidelines for all contact sports.

Doc Talk Sports concussions have been front and center in the press recently as hockey and football players have stepped up to the podium to discuss the effect of concussions on their game and life. Everybody should follow safe preventive practices. This includes wearing appropriate, well-fitting equipment when needed for sports or other physical exercise. Helmets are an absolute must for biking, hockey, and inline skating. Diving into unknown water is also an invitation for disaster.

Headache

What Can I Do?

▶ Avoid known triggers. Provide fluids if headache is thought to be related to a long day of sports in the hot sun.

▶ Provide comfort measures. Rest in a quiet and darkened room. Administer over-the-counter pain medicine (ibuprofen or acetaminophen). Ensure your child is well hydrated.

▶ For migraine sufferers, the sooner these medications are offered (ideally within 30 minutes of onset), the better the effect. It is important to recognize the first signs of your child's migraine episodes.

Case Study

Hayden's Headache

Hayden is a 9-year-old boy who has been experiencing headaches once every couple of weeks for the past 5 months. They are usually on one side of his head and he complains of intense throbbing and pounding. The headaches have been interfering with his activities, and he has occasionally had to miss school or a hockey game because of his pain. When he has a headache, he complains of nausea and occasionally will vomit. He prefers lying in a dark, quiet room and likes to "sleep off" the headache. When his parents took him to see the family's doctor, he indicated that Hayden was experiencing migraine headaches. He advised Hayden to drink lots of fluid, and at the onset of a headache, take a dose of acetaminophen or ibuprofen. He also encouraged Hayden to keep a headache diary to review possible triggers for his migraines.

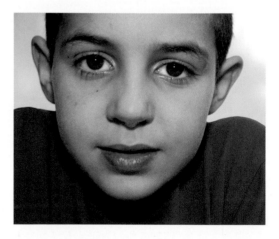

❶ What Is a Headache?

Virtually all adults have experienced a headache at one time or another and can recall the pain, pressure, throbbing, tightening, or other uncomfortable sensation in their scalp, forehead, "behind their eyes," or vaguely within their head. Children, especially after they enter school, also commonly experience headache. Most childhood headaches go away on their own without any long-term consequences. However, some types of headache in children can be very bothersome and disruptive to day-to-day activities. Although parents naturally worry that their child's headache indicates a significant underlying disease (such as a tumor or meningitis), these situations are very rare and almost always occur with many other symptoms (red flags) apart from the headache itself.

Migraines

Migraines are relatively uncommon in young children, but up to 15% of children aged 14 years have experienced migraines. Why some people but not others get migraines remains an incompletely answered question for researchers. In some children, triggers such as specific foods or sleep deprivation may become recognizable over time.

When should we contact our doctor or local hospital?

It is generally a good idea to seek a physician's assessment when you are unsure of the cause of your child's headache, or the intensity or pattern of the headache is out of keeping with what you have managed in the past.

▶ Headache Red Flags

Several red flags are rare but important signals that you should be seeking urgent medical evaluation:

- You think your child looks very sick
- Excessive sleepiness or irritability that does not resolve with comfort measures
- Fever or stiff neck (difficulty touching chin to chest)
- Fainting ("passed out") or collapse
- Abnormal movements (such as seizures), altered speech, blurred vision, weakness or loss of use of a limb, or unexplained behavioral changes
- Increase in headache severity over time
- Night wakening or early morning vomiting
- Weight loss
- Young children in the preschool age (when headaches are uncommon and the cause is difficult to determine)
- A nurse or doctor has previously detected a neurological abnormality, high blood pressure, or a slowing of the child's growth in height

❷ What Causes Acute Headaches?

"Acute" means that an episode starts abruptly, as if a headache switch was turned on. Most acute headaches in children are short-lived episodes caused by one or more typical stressors.

Features of Acute Headaches

Onset	• Abrupt, like a light switch has been turned on
Duration	• Several minutes to a few hours
Typical triggers	• Hunger • Dehydration • Physical exertion • Prolonged period of time in heat or sun • Recurrent coughing
Severity	• Mild with minimal interference to severe
Long-term consequences	• None
Treatment	• Elimination of the trigger (eating, drinking fluids, moving to the shade, etc.) • Comfort measures to directly address the pain

Causes of Acute Headaches

Viral illnesses	• Quite commonly, viral illnesses, such as influenza or the common cold, are accompanied by headaches, which can last 2 to 3 days.
Streptococcal bacteria	• Sore throat caused by an infection ("strep throat") can also cause headache.
Meningitis	• It is a very rare cause of acute headache, but is almost always accompanied by other signs of severe illness, such as fever, excessive sleepiness, or irritability.
Sinusitis	• Occasionally, frontal sinusitis (a bacterial infection of the sinuses above the eyebrows) can cause forehead pain; this is uncommon in children under age 10 because the sinuses are not fully formed. Other types of sinusitis cause facial pain rather than headache.
Head injury	• A blow to the head or fall from a height can result in headache.

Other severe causes of acute headache, including spontaneous bleeding from blood vessels in the brain, are exceedingly rare in healthy children. However, a very sudden-onset and severe headache (beyond the level of any other headache experienced by the child before), head injury, or other signs of severe illness (for example, very sleepy or unresponsive child) should prompt you to seek an immediate medical evaluation of your child.

❸ What Are the Causes of Acute Recurrent Headaches?

"Recurrent" means that the on/off headache switch is repeatedly turned on, but is completely turned off between episodes. There are essentially two types of acute recurrent headaches in children — migraine headaches and tension-type headaches.

Features of Migraine Headaches

Onset	• Over several minutes
Duration	• A few hours to a few days
Frequency	• A couple of times per week to once every several months. Child is well between headaches.
Location	• Often one-sided throbbing or pounding, but can be both sides
Common triggers	• Sleep deprivation • Certain foods (tannins, MSG)
Severity	• Commonly debilitating (child cannot engage in regular activities during this period)
Associated features	• Nausea/vomiting • Photophobia (bothered by bright light) • Phonophobia (bothered by loud noise) • Worse with physical activity • Pallor • Auras (vision changes, flashing lights) • History of migraines in the family
Long-term consequences	• May have school/activity absenteeism
Treatment	• Rest in a dark, quiet room • Give acetaminophen or ibuprofen as soon as possible after the headache begins • Ensure child is well hydrated by giving lots of fluids

❶ What Are Tension-Type Headaches?

Older children and adolescents may experience recurrent headaches that are described as an aching or pressure sensation in a "hat-band" distribution. This type of headache is due to unconscious contractions of the muscles in the neck, jaw, and face.

Features of Tension-Type Headaches

Onset	• Slow and steady over several minutes to hours
Duration	• A few hours
Frequency	• Daily
Location	• Hat-band distribution
Common triggers	• Stress: upcoming tests or examinations, scholastic difficulty, peer group conflict, family discord
Severity	• Low intensity
Long-term consequences	• School/activity absenteeism
Treatment	• Relief of the underlying stressor • Ensure child is well hydrated by giving lots of fluids

❶ What Is Chronic Progressive Headache?

In chronic headaches, the on/off switch stays in the on position for a prolonged period of time, or never completely switches off. "Progressive" means that the headache is worsening over time. Chronic and/or progressive headaches may be caused by increased pressure on the brain due to excessive fluid or an abnormal growth of tissue (tumor). These types of headaches are very rare, but should prompt immediate medical attention.

❷ How Are Headaches Treated?

The first step is to identify and address any obvious injuries or underlying illnesses. For example, if your child hit his head during a sporting event, and subsequently experiences headache, a physician assessment to consider concussion is warranted. Or if your child has a viral infection, your efforts should be directed at the whole illness. However, most uncomplicated acute headaches can be treated at home with acetaminophen or ibuprofen.

Keeping Track

A headache "diary" may aid a physician's assessment of your child's headache. This journal should track the timing of each headache episode's onset, duration, and resolution, and include details about possible triggers (for example, activities, sleep patterns, and foods eaten prior to the headache) and relieving factors (such as medications). Also be sure to make note of any specific accompanying features, such as dizziness or blurry vision.

Doc Talk Young children are typically unable to pinpoint the specific location or nature of their discomfort. This can be frustrating to parents, who want to understand their child's experience so that they can help relieve any suffering. If you are not sure whether your child's ongoing discomfort is due to a headache, you should consult a physician.

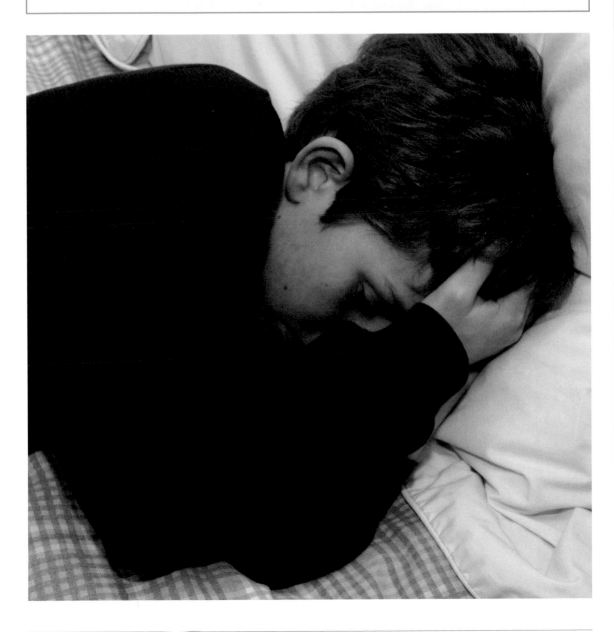

Hearing Loss

❶ What Is Hearing Loss?

Hearing loss is defined based on its severity (from mild through to profound) as well as by its cause. Conductive hearing loss results from problems with the outer and middle ear, resulting in sound waves that are blocked from entering the inner ear. Sensorineural hearing loss occurs when there is a problem with the inner ear or the pathways

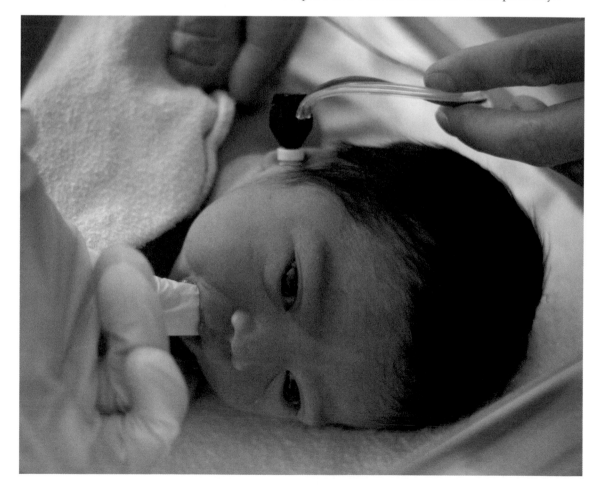

that transmit information from the ear to the brain, resulting in an abnormal response to the sound waves.

❷ What Causes Hearing Loss?

Hearing loss in children has many causes, some of which are present at birth (congenital); others are acquired during infancy or childhood. In general, many types of conductive hearing loss are temporary and sensorineural hearing loss is often permanent.

When should we contact our doctor?

Hearing loss is not an "emergency," but hearing loss in the first years of life can lead to delays in speech, language, and cognitive development. You are usually the best judge of your child's ability to hear, and studies have shown that a parent's concern about their child's hearing indeed predicts a hearing problem.

Even with a normal newborn hearing screening test, a number of children will have a delayed onset of hearing loss or will develop conditions later in life that will lead to impaired hearing.

Newborn Screening

Congenital hearing loss is relatively common, occurring in 1 to 3 of every 1,000 newborn babies. Although we know that several conditions put babies at risk of hearing loss (inherited diseases or serious infections during pregnancy, for example), 50% of babies born with hearing loss do not in fact have any risk factors.

Both the Canadian Paediatric Society and the American Academy of Pediatrics recommend a newborn hearing screen for every baby. Newborn hearing screening programs are now well established in most communities and hospitals across North America. We know that diagnosing and treating hearing problems promptly results in better outcomes in hearing-impaired children. These hearing tests are fast, do not hurt the baby, and can be performed at the bedside in full-term and premature infants.

Developmental Milestones

If you suspect your child has a hearing problem, talk to your child's doctor about arranging a proper hearing assessment. If your child does not meet any of the standard development milestones listed here, she should have a hearing evaluation.

Did You Know?

Screening Facts

Without newborn screening, hearing loss is diagnosed at approximately 24 months of age, with mild and moderate hearing loss often not detected until the child starts school. With newborn screening in place, hearing loss is diagnosed at an average age of 3 months, with treatment starting by 6 months of age. What a difference!

By 3 months, a child should:

- Startle to loud sounds
- Smile in response to soothing sounds
- Make certain sounds (for example, "ooo" and "aah")

By 6 months, a child should:

- Turn toward a sound
- Make several different sounds (often in reaction to a parent's sound)

By 9 months, a child should:

- Respond to her name
- Babble, often with a speech-like quality (for example, "gaga" or "baba")
- Understand "no"

By 12 months, a child should:

- Understand some words and simple phrases
- Communicate by using a combination of sounds and gestures

❸ How Is Hearing Loss Treated?

Because the ability to hear is critical for normal language development, early identification of hearing impairment is essential to allow for timely intervention. If hearing impairment is detected on a newborn screening or testing in early childhood, your child will be referred to a team that may include an audiologist, an ear, nose, and throat specialist (otolaryngologist), and a speech pathologist.

The specific treatment will depend on the underlying cause of the hearing loss. For example, if the doctor finds persistent fluid in the middle ear (otitis media with effusion), she may recommend that ear tubes be inserted. See Earache and Ear Infections (page 169).

Did You Know?

Implants

If profound hearing loss is determined in infancy, it may be treated with electronic devices surgically implanted in the inner ear, which allows for age-appropriate language development.

Doc Talk Regardless of the cause and treatment, parental or caregiver involvement is a vital part of a hearing-impaired child's language development. Be sure to reach out for support, and ask your health-care team how you can help.

Hiccups

What Can I Do?

▶ While most cases of hiccups resolve on their own, you may be able to help by asking your child to hold her breath, sip on water, gargle cold water, or bear down as if having a bowel movement.

▶ If hiccups do not resolve after 48 hours, you should visit your doctor.

❶ What Are Hiccups?

Hiccups are common, involuntary, intermittent, brief contractions of the diaphragm (the muscle that separates your lungs from your belly). As the contraction of the muscles ends, the vocal cords abruptly close, leading to the distinctive "hic" sound. The medical word for hiccups is singultus, meaning "a gasp" or "a sob."

When should we see our doctor?

There is little evidence for any effective treatment for hiccups, but you should take your child to his doctor for assessment if his hiccups persist for 48 hours.

❷ What Causes Hiccups?

Scientists have not been able to decisively determine what causes hiccups. It is thought that a distension or fullness of the stomach from overeating, carbonated beverages, or swallowing air (for example, from chewing gum) may precipitate hiccups. They may also be provoked by sudden excitement or emotional stress. Medical causes of persistent hiccups are very rare and are usually caused by something that irritates the nerve that stimulates the diaphragm.

❸ How Are Hiccups Treated?

Most bouts of hiccups are self-resolving, but your child can try:

- Holding his breath for several seconds
- Bearing down as if he is trying to have a bowel movement (Valsalva maneuver)
- Sipping or gargling cold water
- Pulling his knees to his chest and leaning forward to compress the chest

Doc Talk Unfortunately for the hiccupping child, there is little evidence for any effective treatment for hiccups. Fortunately, most cases of hiccups go away on their own in a short period of time, but if they persist, you should have your child's doctor assess his symptoms. Attempts to scare him to stop his hiccups have not proven to be effective and can be mildly traumatic.

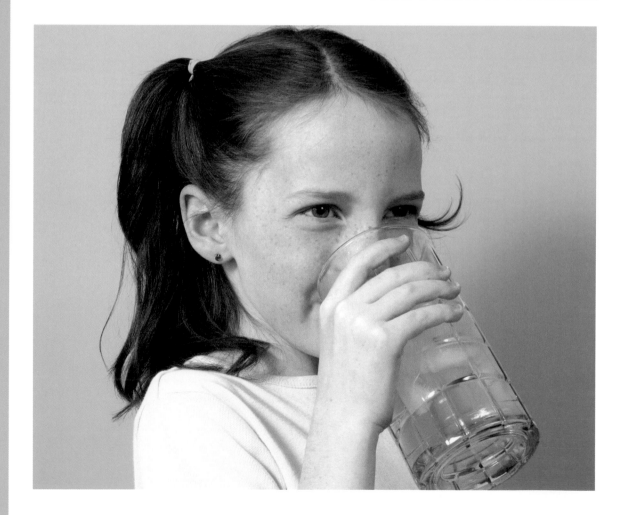

Ingrown Toenails

What Can I Do?

▶ Be sure your child's shoes are not too tight, especially surrounding the big toe.

▶ Do not cut your child's toenails too short.

▶ Try soaking the toe in warm water for 15 to 20 minutes, two to three times daily, to relieve pain and swelling.

▶ If the toe area becomes infected, your child may require topical or even oral antibiotic treatment.

Case Study

Angela's Big Toe

Angela was not a happy camper! She was at her first summer camp and had been enjoying all of her activities, but in the last few days had felt a huge pain over her big toe every time something touched it. She never realized just how often things banged against her toe until now! She didn't remember hurting it. Nothing had dropped on it and she hadn't even stubbed it hard.

The nurse at the camp took a look at Angela's big toe. The top corner of her toe, where the skin met the nail, looked red, swollen, and angry. There was a little bit of yellowish fluid leaking out, forming a brown crust. It was too tender to even touch. The nurse was quite sure that Angela had an ingrown toenail and advised her parents that she would need to soak the big toe in warm water for 20 minutes three times daily. She should then pat it dry and apply some topical antibiotic ointment. If it didn't look like it was improving within a few days, she advised them to take Angela in to see her regular family doctor for further treatment.

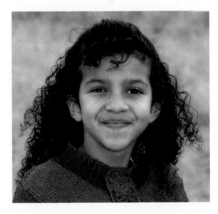

❶ What Is an Ingrown Toenail?

An ingrown toenail is a nail that grows into the skin at the corners of the nail. The big toe is most commonly affected. The skin around the corner of the toenail looks red and swollen. It is often quite painful, especially when pressure is applied. If the area is infected, it can

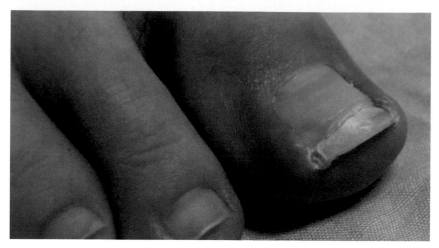

Ingrown toenail

Did You Know?

Surgery for an Ingrown Toenail

If an ingrown toenail is a recurring problem or if a lot of scar tissue forms around the affected area, the part of the nail that is embedded in the skin may have to be removed. This procedure is usually done by a surgeon or podiatrist, using local freezing.

become very red and swollen, and pus may appear next to or under the nail. After a while, granulation tissue may develop, which looks like a dark red piece of fleshy tissue with a moist, crusted surface.

❷ What Causes an Ingrown Toenail?

Some people just seem to be prone to ingrown toenails. They can also be caused when toenails are cut too short, because the nails can grow back into the surrounding skin. Tight shoes can make the nails grow into the skin, by pushing the skin up over the corners of the nails. Sometimes a toe injury that affects the nail will cause an ingrown toenail.

❸ How Is an Ingrown Toenail Treated?

If the area is not very swollen and painful, soaking the toe in warm water for 15 to 20 minutes, two to three times daily, may relieve pain and swelling. An antibiotic ointment over the painful area two to three times daily may also be helpful. If the area is very red, swollen, and painful, you should see your doctor; an oral antibiotic may be necessary. If there is a lot of pus in the area, it may have to be drained.

Doc Talk Don't cut your child's toenails too short! Nails should be allowed to grow to the end of the toe so that they can't grow into the skin. Cut the nails straight across. Make sure that your child's shoes do not fit too tightly across the toes, and encourage him to wear sandals or open shoes when possible.

Insect Bites

What Can I Do?

▶ Prevention remains the best treatment. Reduce your child's exposure to biting insects by wearing long sleeves and pants, avoiding standing water, and wearing bug spray when outdoors.

▶ If your child shows signs of anaphylaxis when bitten by any insect, call 911 and seek emergency treatment at your local hospital.

▶ Try the helpful tips outlined on page 239 to treat the itching, pain, and swelling that often accompany the bite. Ice, soothing lotions, and antihistamines are often helpful remedies.

❶ What Is an Insect Bite?

The most common insect bite your child will suffer from is a mosquito. Other biting insects include black flies, bed bugs, and scabies, as well as tics, fire ants, and spiders. Most insect bites present no danger to your child's health, although some bites, like bee stings (which are not true "bites"), can have serious consequences, such as anaphylaxis. See Bee and Wasp Stings (page 75).

RELATED CONDITIONS

- Bed bug bites
- Black fly bites
- Mosquito bites
- Scabies
- West Nile virus

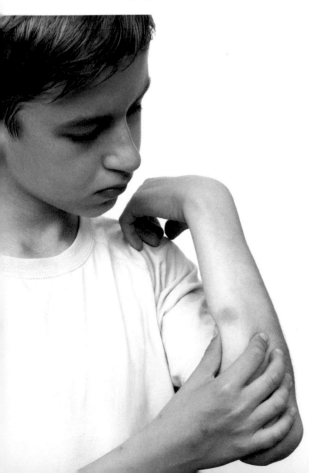

⏩ Insect Bite Red Flags

Generally, it is not necessary to call the doctor when insect bites occur. However, seek medical attention if there are any of these signs:

■ Lip or tongue swelling, or difficulty breathing

■ Spreading redness at the site of a bite, especially after the first 24 hours

■ Fever

■ Muscle pain

■ Cramping

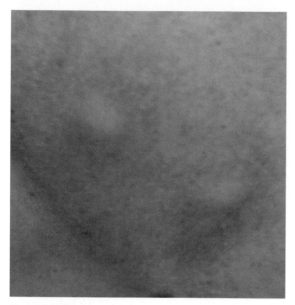

Mosquito bites

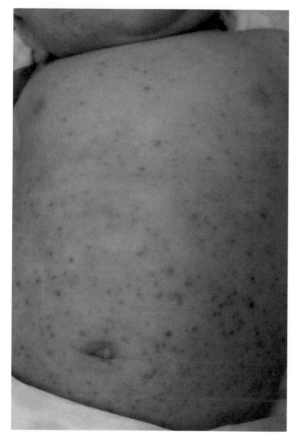

Scabies

Signs and Symptoms of Insect Bites

The characteristics of bites will vary depending on what type of insect caused the bite. Most commonly, you will see a small, round, swollen area with redness, pimples, or blisters. Shortly thereafter, your child may experience intense itching at the site, lasting several hours to a couple of days.

Mosquito

Bites from mosquitos can occur anywhere on exposed surfaces of the body. They tend to be small: less than a $\frac{1}{2}$-inch (1 cm) raised red bump that disappears in a couple of days.

Black Fly

A black fly tends to leave a red bump that is slightly larger ($\frac{1}{2}$ to $1\frac{1}{4}$ inch/1 to 3 cm) than a mosquito. These bites can be intensely itchy and painful. There will often be a central area with a small bite mark.

Bed Bugs

Bed bug bites often show up in groups of three: "breakfast, lunch, and dinner." Red and itchy flat lesions are often seen, but small, raised, red swollen bites are also common. Bites can occur anywhere on the body. Bed bugs usually live in and around beds, but they are also known to hide in couches, soft chairs, books, pillows, and stuffed animals.

Scabies

Scabies bites are caused by tiny mites that burrow under the child's skin, causing intense itching. Bites are most commonly seen on the hands, feet, buttocks, external genitalia, back, and elbows. Except in infants, bites are not usually seen on the face or scalp. Linear tracks are commonly seen with rows of small pimples.

❷ How Are Insect Bites Treated?

Try these remedies for insect bites before seeking medical advice.

For Itching
- Apply soothing lotions, such as calamine, or anti-itch creams, such as 0.5% or 1% hydrocortisone.
- Apply baking soda mixed with water as a paste to the affected area.
- Give an antihistamine if your child is unable to sleep because the itching is keeping him awake.

For Swelling
- Apply ice or a cool compress to the area.

For Pain
- Give a dose of ibuprofen or acetaminophen, as needed.

Prevention

Prevention remains the best treatment. Look for ways to reduce your child's exposure to biting insects.

- Reduce the amount of time spent outside during the dawn or dusk hours.
- Use barriers, like mosquito nets or screens, on baby strollers.
- Make sure windows and doors are properly screened, and that screens are in good repair.
- Wear protective clothing when possible: light-colored clothing with long sleeves and cuffs, long pants tucked into socks or shoes, and hats.
- When outdoors in parks or rural settings, apply insect repellents containing DEET.
- Citronella (5% to 15%) is a natural repellent, but its effectiveness is short-lived, only about 20 minutes. Its value is therefore limited.

Insect Repellent Precautions
Do not use insect repellent without taking these precautions:

- Apply insect repellent to your hands and then put it on the child's skin, avoiding his eyes, mouth, and palms. Using a spray can lead to inadvertent administration of the repellent into a child's eye or airway.
- Do not allow young children to apply DEET products themselves.
- Avoid repellent on cuts or irritated skin.

Did You Know?

Preventing Infection
Infection is always a possibility following an insect bite. To prevent infection, keep the area covered by a long-sleeved shirt or pants to prevent your child from scratching the area. Cut your child's fingernails so that he is less likely to break the skin; breaking the skin creates an opening for infection to enter the body.

Did You Know?

DEET Caution
Insect repellents that are used on children should have a small concentration of DEET, depending on the age of the child. These products should not be used on children younger than 6 months old.

- Reapply after swimming.
- Wash treated skin and clothing with soap and water after returning indoors.
- Store DEET out of reach of children.

❸ What Is West Nile Virus (WNV)?

Although malaria is the most worrisome disease transmitted by mosquitoes in tropical parts of the world, West Nile virus (WNV) seems to be increasing in North America. Nevertheless, the chance of your child getting this virus and being sick with it is very tiny.

WNV was first discovered in Uganda in 1937 and only recently has become a problem in North America. WNV is transmitted by mosquitoes. Not every mosquito carries WNV and not every person bitten by a mosquito will get infected with WNV. In North America, the virus is active from May until the end of October, with a peak in late August to early September.

Signs and Symptoms of West Nile Virus

Only 1 in 5 individuals infected with WNV will actually develop any symptoms. If symptoms do appear, they usually show up between 3 and 14 days after an infected mosquito has bitten the person. They are often flu-like and can include fever, aches and fatigue, weakness, headache, and a rash.

❹ How Is WNV Treated?

Currently, there is no treatment or vaccine to prevent the disease. The best protection against West Nile virus is to avoid mosquito bites and reduce mosquito breeding spots. Insect repellents containing DEET are most effective at preventing mosquito bites and are safe if used appropriately.

Doc Talk

Mankind does not occupy the planet alone. We share it with billions of insects. Insect bites are an inevitable part of your child's life. In some parts of the world, insect bites have immense consequences: malaria, for example, transmitted by a mosquito bite, kills thousands of children annually in tropical areas. In North America, although serious problems can sometimes occur, the great majority of insect bites merely result in an irritating annoyance.

In-Toeing (Pigeon Toe) and Out-Toeing

What Can I Do?

▶ Don't worry. Most cases of in-toeing and out-toeing resolve with age.

▶ Discourage your child from sitting with his legs in a "W" shape.

▶ If your child has any of the red flag symptoms, then seek medical advice.

❶ What Are In-Toeing and Out-Toeing?

Some children's toes point inward when they stand or walk. This is known as in-toeing or "pigeon toe." In-toeing is a common condition, most often noticed in toddlers, which typically improves as a child grows. The reverse of in-toeing is out-toeing.

Causes of In-Toeing

- Metatarsus adductus: when the big toe turns inward.
- Tibial torsion: when the shinbone twists inward.
- Femoral anteversion: when the thighbone turns inward.

When should we contact our doctor?

Neither in-toeing nor out-toeing are medical emergencies, but some symptoms associated with in-toeing and out-toeing require medical attention. These include knee, hip, and foot pain or difficulty walking.

Did You Know?

No Long-Term Problems

In-toeing and out-toeing do not usually cause problems. Occasionally, children with in-toeing trip more than other children their age, but this usually improves as they get older.

➤➤ In-Toeing and Out-Toeing Red Flags

Consult your child's doctor if your child has any of the following symptoms associated with out-toeing:

- Your child complains of leg or hip pain.
- The deformity worsens with age (it should be getting better).
- Your child seems to trip and fall much more than her peers.

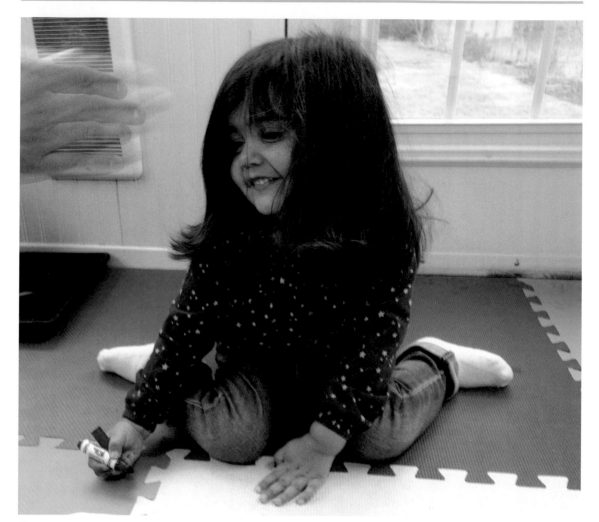

W-sit

❷ How Are In-Toeing and Out-Toeing Treated?

Since in-toeing usually improves on its own and does not cause long-term problems, no treatment is indicated for most children. Special shoes and braces are not helpful. Children with femoral anteversion often sit with their legs in a "W" shape; this should be discouraged. Rarely, if the deformity is rigid, children with metatarsus adductus require surgery or casting.

Doc Talk Like children with in-toeing, children with out-toeing tend to improve as they get older. The usual cause is a twisting outward of the lower leg, called external tibial torsion. This is a normal healthy variant. Only very rarely is out-toeing related to an orthopedic problem.

Itch (Skin and Scalp)

What Can I Do?

▶ Prevent itch. Avoid known allergens and irritants. Wear sunscreen before going out in the sun, and use bug spray to prevent bug bites.

▶ Keep your child's skin moisturized and ensure he drinks plenty of water.

▶ Give your child an oral antihistamine to reduce the itch and help with sleep.

Case Study

Maya's Eczema

Maya is a 3-year-old girl who has had dry skin since she was a few months of age. She sometimes breaks out in a red, bumpy rash. The rash used to affect only her face but is now on the inside of her elbows and knees. When the rash erupts, she is very itchy, scratches all the time, and has difficulty sleeping. Maya's mom uses lotions on the rash when it appears, but nothing seems to help. When Maya's doctor examines her, she finds a healthy girl with dry skin. The insides of her elbows have red bumps and lots of scratch marks.

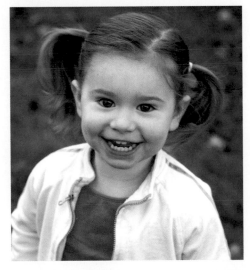

Maya's doctor diagnosed these symptoms as atopic dermatitis, better known as eczema. Her doctor recommended that Maya's mom bathe her in warm (not hot) water with a few drops of Aveeno or Alpha Keri oil at least once daily. She prescribed a steroid ointment to apply to the rash immediately after coming out of the bath, and then two more times during the day. She instructed Maya's mother to apply petroleum jelly liberally to her skin three times daily.

❶ What Is an Itch?

An itch is a subjective sensation of the skin or the scalp caused by inflammation or irritation. Itchiness is a very common reaction to a variety of conditions. It can be localized (in one area) or generalized (all over the body). An itch may or may not be accompanied by lesions on the skin, such as bumps, blisters, redness, or flakiness.

When should we contact our doctor or local hospital?

Itch can be so aggravating that you want to find relief for your child immediately. If you are not able to provide relief with home treatments, see your doctor. Itch can also be associated with symptoms of anaphylaxis. If you think your child may be having a severe allergic reaction, contact your local hospital.

➤➤ Itch Red Flags

Call 911 if your child has any of the following symptoms associated with itch:

- Difficulty breathing
- Swelling of the tongue, throat, or mouth area

Consult your child's doctor if your child has any of the following symptoms associated with itch:

- Itching is severe
- Home treatment isn't helping
- Itching persists or worsens with time
- Scratching is damaging the skin
- The itch is disturbing sleep
- The itch occurs with other unexplained symptoms

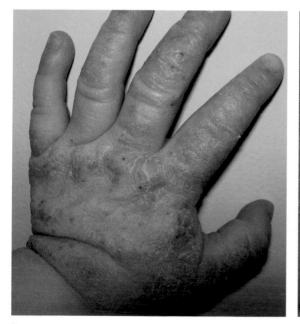

Eczema

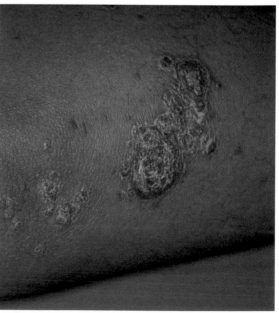

Psoriasis

❷ What Are the Causes of Itchy Skin?

There are a number of causes of itchy skin. Look through this list to see if you can find the cause of your child's itch.

Allergic reactions	Can be all over or localized (hives)
Contact irritants	Metals, soaps, chemicals, wool, poison ivy, or poison oak cause an itchy rash where they contact the skin.
Dry skin	Flaky, rough skin (e.g., eczema)
Hives	Allergic reactions or viral illnesses (see Rashes in Children, page 315)
Insect bites or stings	Mosquitos, bees, bed bugs, scabies, lice (see Insect Bites, page 237)
Chronic skin diseases	May wax and wane (for example, atopic dermatitis (eczema), psoriasis
Sunburn	In sun-exposed areas; may be painful
Medications	Some antibiotics
Skin infections	Ringworm, chicken pox

How To: Treat Itchy Skin

- Avoid scratching or rubbing. Keep fingernails short and keep itchy areas covered with long sleeves or pants.
- Have your child wear cool, light, loose clothing. Avoid rough clothing, particularly wool, over an itchy area.
- Cool the itchy area. Cold water, ice packs, or a cold, clean washcloth over the affected area can be soothing.
- Avoid heat. Lengthy exposure to too much heat and humidity can make an itch worse.
- Take brief lukewarm baths (5 to 10 minutes) using just a little soap, and rinse thoroughly. Try adding oatmeal (1 to 2 cups/125 to 250 mL, ground into a powder), or cornstarch ($\frac{1}{2}$ cup/125 mL), or a few drops of emulsifying oil (such as Oilatum, Aveeno oil or Keri oil) to the water. This can help retain skin moisture.
- Apply unscented, hypoallergenic cream after bathing. This will soften and cool the skin.
- Use moisturizer on the skin regularly, particularly in the dry winter months. Dry skin is a common cause of itching and can make any type of itching worse. Creams work better than lotions at holding in the moisture.
- Apply over-the-counter anti-itch creams and lotions, which can help numb the skin and reduce the feeling of itchiness.

❸ What Are the Causes of Itchy Scalp?

Itchy scalp shares with itchy skin the "itch," but the causes and treatments differ. In addition, not all itchy scalp in children should be blamed on lice (see page 270) or on tinea capitis (see page 217). In fact, there are many common conditions that can cause an itchy scalp.

Cause	Treatment
Seborrheic dermatitis	• Mild forms can be treated regularly with over-the-counter (non-prescription) antidandruff shampoos containing selenium sulfide, tar, or zinc pyrithione. • Antifungal shampoos containing ketoconazole or ciclopirox also yield good results.
Atopic dermatitis (eczema)	• Topical corticosteroids (creams) can be effective. • Antihistamines can be given orally if itchiness is distressing or preventing sleep. • Extensive eczema of the scalp is best treated with corticosteroid lotions or foams.
Dry scalp or dandruff	• Over-the-counter antidandruff shampoos work best.
Psoriasis	• Mild to moderate severity is often treated with topical corticosteroids and tar shampoos.

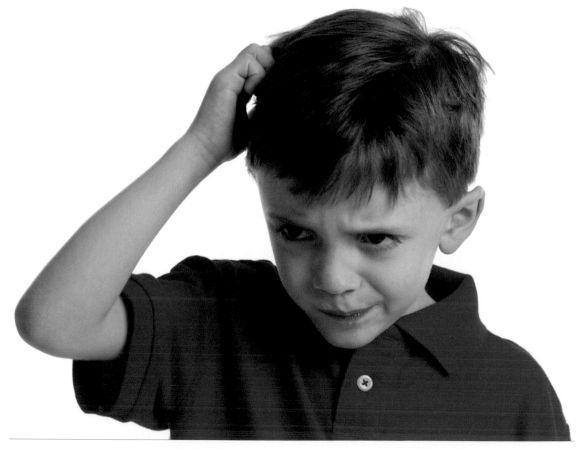

Seborrheic Dermatitis

Also known as cradle cap in infants, seborrheic dermatitis is a red, scaly, and sometimes itchy eruption that develops in areas rich in oil glands, such as the scalp. It can occur in infants, children, and even adults. It is believed that seborrheic dermatitis is caused by an interaction between the scalp and a type of yeast called malassezia.

Atopic Dermatitis (Eczema)

Children prone to asthma and allergies or who have had eczema on other parts of their body can develop patches of flaky, itchy eczema on the scalp. The most common location on the scalp is on the back of their head.

Dry Scalp or Dandruff

Dandruff is considered to be a mild form of seborrheic dermatitis but usually presents with very little inflammation or redness. Children can, however, still have dry, itchy, and flaky scalps.

Psoriasis

Psoriasis is a chronic skin condition that is more common in adults but can occur more rarely in children. There is often a family history of psoriasis. Psoriasis is often seen on the elbows and knees but can also be seen along the hairline and scalp. The causes of psoriasis are not known, but it is believed to be a condition where unknown triggers lead to overstimulation of the immune system. This overstimulation leads to flaky, silvery plaques on the skin and scalp, with redness and inflammation. They may or may not be itchy.

❹ How Is Scalp Itch Treated?

At-Home Treatment First

There are several causes of itchiness and flakiness of the scalp. It is fair to first try an over-the-counter (non-prescription) antidandruff shampoo at home. However, if the symptoms do not improve, then a visit to your child's health-care provider will help you to diagnose and best treat the problem.

> **Doc Talk** Treating skin and scalp itch can be frustrating because completely eliminating symptoms is not always easy. Try giving diphenhydramine (Benadryl) at 1 mg/kg every 6 hours. Alternatively, if this is not enough, consider getting a prescription from your doctor for hydroxyzine (Atarax) which may also alleviate symptoms.

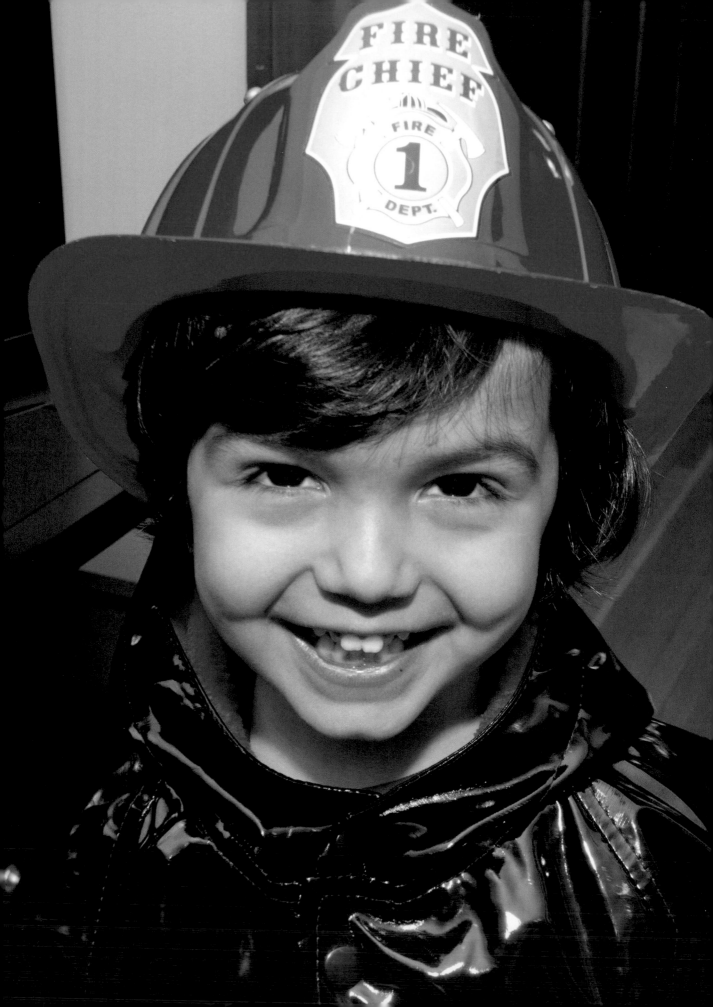

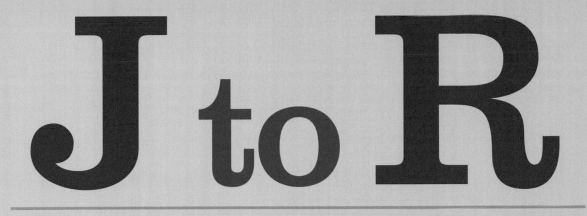

J to R

Jaundice

❶ What Is Jaundice?

Jaundice is a medical term familiar to many parents. It refers to the yellow pigment of the skin or in the whites of many newborn eyes. Jaundice is caused by excess bilirubin, a product of the natural breakdown of red blood cells. Normally, bilirubin is processed through the liver and excreted primarily in the stool. In newborn babies, several aspects of bilirubin metabolism are not yet fully developed, resulting in the appearance of jaundice as part of a physiologic, or normal, process.

Did You Know?

Early Discharge Caution

Many infants are discharged from hospital by 24 hours of age. Babies who are home within this short period of time should be evaluated for jaundice within 1 to 2 days of discharge by a health-care professional.

Signs and Symptoms of Jaundice

Jaundice first affects the whites of a baby's eyes: as the bilirubin level increases, the yellow appears to spread downward, from head to toe. Although jaundice is easiest to see in Caucasian babies, it is evident in darker-skinned babies by looking at their eyes as well as the palms of their hands and soles of their feet. Some clinicians try to predict the bilirubin level based on the extent of jaundice affecting the baby's body, but this estimation is not reliable!

Newborn Jaundice

Jaundice typically begins in a full-term infant after the first 24 hours of life. The bilirubin level, or degree of jaundice, peaks at 3 to 5 days, and then gradually decreases over approximately 2 weeks. If your baby is healthy, and the bilirubin level is not too high, the jaundice is harmless and will resolve naturally.

Although approximately 60% of newborns develop jaundice that is harmless, about 2% will have very high bilirubin levels that can be dangerous. In these cases, the bilirubin is toxic to the brain, and this can result in a range of permanent neurological problems, including deafness, movement problems, and cognitive impairment. Fortunately, this outcome is extremely rare and is preventable.

When should we contact our doctor or local hospital?

If you think your baby appears yellow, you should have her assessed on an urgent basis.

▶▶ Jaundice Red Flags

Having one of these factors might indicate that your baby's jaundice is more than just a routine case, which means you should consult your child's doctor immediately:

- Jaundice that can be seen within the first 24 hours of life
- Not feeding well
- Not soiling diapers
- Not passing meconium (newborn baby stools)
- Fever
- Lethargy

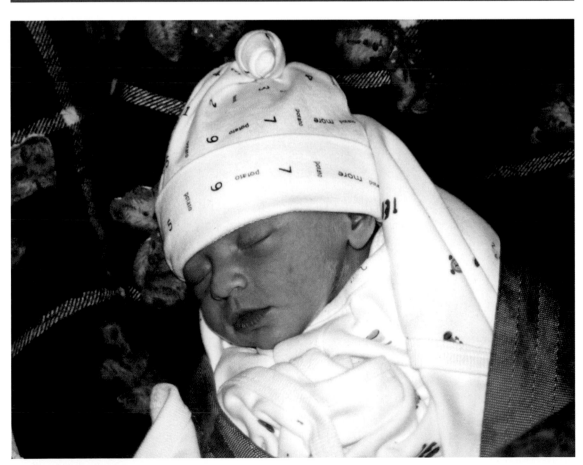

Jaundice (yellow skin) in a newborn

❷ What Causes Jaundice?

In some instances, jaundice in a newborn results from an underlying infection or disease. If the jaundice is severe or does not resolve quickly, further tests will be done to look for another cause.

Risk Factors

Babies with one or more of these factors are at an increased risk of developing severe jaundice:

- Prematurity (less than 38 weeks gestation)
- Having had a sibling with jaundice
- Mother with blood group O
- Bruising on the skin or under the scalp (cephalohematoma)
- Asian background

Babies who have a known risk factor for higher jaundice levels are more closely monitored and promptly treated in order to prevent any adverse consequences.

Newborn Testing

Although jaundice is often noted just by looking at the baby, diagnosing high bilirubin by this method alone is inadequate. The Canadian Paediatric Society and the American Academy of Pediatrics recommend that all babies be assessed by a health-care practitioner for high bilirubin during the first 72 hours of life. This can be done by taking a small blood sample (often along with other blood taken for the purposes of newborn screening) or by using a transcutaneous (through the skin) instrument that shines a light across the baby's skin to determine the bilirubin level. Depending on the level and your baby's individual risk factors, your doctor will determine if and when further testing is required.

❸ How Is Jaundice Treated?

Feeding and Hydration

Although most newborns do develop jaundice to some degree, the majority require no treatment. Since bilirubin is excreted in the stool, an important component of clearing jaundice is to ensure that babies are well hydrated and passing meconium stools, which is generally accomplished by establishing feeds.

Phototherapy

Some babies require special fluorescent lights, a treatment called phototherapy, to help bring the jaundice level down. If phototherapy is needed, your baby will be placed in an incubator with lights surrounding her, with her eyes covered for protection. Although this generally requires hospitalization, it is a safe and effective therapy that is commonly used. Given that dehydration can contribute to high bilirubin, and that hydration is an important part of clearing bilirubin from the body, it is important that your baby receive enough fluids. Breastfeeding should continue and — with appropriate support — is often enough in itself. If needed, additional fluids may be given either by mouth or sometimes with intravenous fluids.

FAQ

What is breast milk jaundice?

Toward the end of the first week of life, breastfed infants have higher levels of bilirubin compared with those who are formula-fed, a condition called breast milk jaundice. This type of jaundice begins slowly, peaks at approximately 2 to 3 weeks of age, and may persist up to 12 weeks. Though the reasons for this phenomenon are unclear, breast milk jaundice is not harmful. If the baby is being monitored by a doctor or midwife, is gaining weight, and is behaving normally, it is best to continue to breastfeed, allowing the jaundice to resolve on its own.

Doc Talk

Jaundice is not limited to babies! Jaundice can occur at any age due to infection, the breakdown (hemolysis) of red blood cells, or liver problems. You'll first notice jaundice affecting the whites of your child's eyes — this always warrants a trip to your doctor.

Knee Injuries

What Can I Do?

▶ Follow the R.I.C.E program for treating knee pain: Rest • Ice • Compression • Elevation

▶ Assess your child for any of the red flags which will require medical attention

▶ Work on strengthening and stretching the muscles supporting the knee after an injury to reduce the risk of recurrent injury.

❶ What Is Knee Pain?

RELATED CONDITIONS

• Osgood-Schlatter disease

The knee is the largest joint in the body. It is made up of three bones: the tibia (the shin bone), the femur (the thigh bone), and the patella (the kneecap). The knee is held together and stabilized by many ligaments and tendons. While providing stability, these supporting structures allow the knee to flex (bend) and extend (straighten). Ligaments are bands of tissue that connect bone to bone. Tendons connect muscles to bones. The inside of the knee joint is lined by cartilage (the meniscus), which acts as a cushion. See Limp (page 273) and Leg Aches (page 266).

When should we contact our doctor or local hospital?

Some knee injuries are more serious than others. Minor sprains and strains will heal quite readily and do not generally need a physician's asessment. More serious knee injuries with swelling, deformity, or severe pain require immediate medical attention.

⤞ Knee Injury Red Flags

Consult your child's doctor if your child has any of the following symptoms associated with a knee injury:

■ If the knee looks deformed or twisted

■ If the child cannot bear any weight on his leg

■ If the knee becomes extremely swollen or bruised immediately after the injury

■ If the leg or foot has any numbness or tingling

■ If the foot feels very cold or looks blue

Knee anatomy

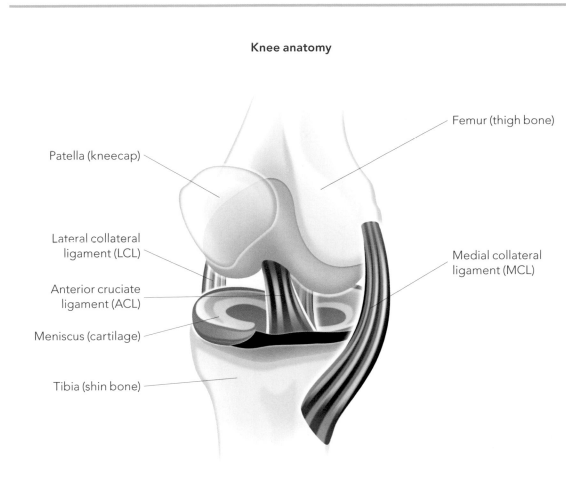

Patella (kneecap)

Femur (thigh bone)

Lateral collateral ligament (LCL)

Medial collateral ligament (MCL)

Anterior cruciate ligament (ACL)

Meniscus (cartilage)

Tibia (shin bone)

Common Knee Injuries

Because the knee is only designed to bend, straighten, and bear weight, it is susceptible to injury with any forceful twisting or turning motion. Acute injury or trauma and chronic injury from overuse can lead to pain, swelling, and warmth of the joint. Injuries to the ligaments, tendons, or cartilage of the knee are much more common than fractures (breaks/cracks) of the three bones making up the knee.

Sprains

A sprain occurs when a ligament is stretched or torn, often from twisting or stretching beyond a joint's normal range of motion. A sprain usually affects the anterior cruciate ligament (ACL) or the medial collateral ligament (MCL), though other ligaments can be affected too. A sprain can be mild, with a little bit of swelling and pain, or it can be severe, where the ligament is completely torn, resulting in significant pain and swelling.

Did You Know?

Flexion and Extension

The knee moves in two directions: flexion (bending) and extension. When the knee is twisted, compressed, or pushed sideways, knee injury can result.

A B C D E F G H I J **K** L M N O P Q R S T U V W X Y Z

Strains

This kind of injury occurs when a muscle or tendon is stretched or torn. A strain is usually due to a hyperflexion or hyperextension injury (stretching or bending beyond the normal range of the joint). A strain can range from mild to severe, with severe being a complete tear of the muscle or tendon. A strain may cause bruising around the knee.

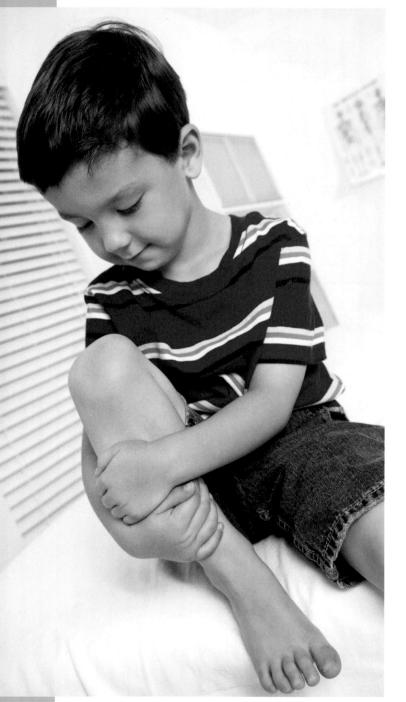

Cartilage (Meniscal) Tears

This kind of injury is common, and it usually happens during activities where sudden changes in speed or side-to-side movements occur (for example, soccer, football, and basketball). An injury to the meniscus often causes pain and swelling of the front part of the knee. Sometimes fluid collects around the knee joint.

Articular Cartilage Injuries

This kind of injury occurs when the cartilage in the knee joint gets soft because of injury or overuse. A small piece of cartilage or bone can break off, causing pain, swelling, joint stiffness, and sometimes locking of the joint. This is called osteochondritis dessicans.

If the cartilage on the patella softens, the bony surfaces of the patella and the femur may rub against each other, which causes pain, especially when walking up or down stairs or hills. This is called chondromalacia.

Fracture

This injury involves a cracked or broken bone. A fracture is usually caused by a direct blow to the knee. It is very painful, and it usually causes immediate swelling and bruising. Walking or moving the knee immediately after a fracture can be very difficult.

Patellar Dislocation

This happens when the kneecap (patella) is knocked sideways by a twisting injury or an impact. When this injury occurs, the patella usually moves toward the outside of the knee. It is a very painful injury, and it will be difficult to bend the knee or walk.

Bursitis

This injury involves inflammation of a bursa. Bursa are fluid-filled sacs lining the knee that help it to glide. Friction or overuse of the knee can cause swelling and inflammation of a bursa.

Testing for Knee Injury

No tests are required for most knee injuries. A good physical examination by your doctor is often all that is needed. Occasionally, however, your child's doctor may request one of the following tests to determine the diagnosis or severity of an injury:

- *X-rays:* are useful to look for fractures or dislocations. They do not show soft-tissue injuries (tendons, ligaments, or muscles), although some swelling can sometimes be seen on an X-ray.
- *Magnetic resonance imaging (MRI):* is a good test to look for tendon, ligament, or cartilage damage. It is not usually done urgently, but it may be necessary if a knee injury is not improving, especially if the child cannot resume his regular activities.
- *Arthroscopy:* is the most accurate test but is seldom necessary. An orthopedic surgeon inserts a scope (camera) into the knee joint to see which part of the knee is injured. The surgeon will usually repair any damage at the same time. Arthroscopy is usually done with a general anesthetic in children.

❷ How Is a Knee Injury Treated?

Most knee injuries get better with R.I.C.E.:

1. Rest
2. Ice
3. Compression (tensor bandage)
4. Elevation

How To: Apply a Compression Bandage to the Knee

- Begin wrapping the bandage around the leg in the middle of the calf.
- Circle the leg a few times to secure the bandage.

Did You Know?

Tendonitis
The term "tendonitis" means inflammation of the tendon. Most commonly, the patellar tendon (the tendon joining the kneecap to the femur) is affected. This is also known as patellar tendonitis, or jumper's knee. It can be caused by overuse of the knee or poor training, resulting in inflammation. Children with patellar tendonitis often complain of pain just below the kneecap while walking, bending, or jumping.

- It should be snug but not too tight; you should be able to slip a finger between the knee and the bandage
- Wrap the bandage up and diagonally behind the knee to above the knee joint.
- Continue wrapping diagonally (alternating above and below the knee) behind the knee joint in a figure eight.
- Repeat this several times.
- Secure with the clips provided or a safety pin. The final wrap should be above the knee joint.
- If more uncomfortable after application, or numbness/coolness or pain develops below the bandage, then release and reapply a little less snugly.
- Compression bandages are not required while in bed at night.

Note: Compression bandages do not generally affect the rate of healing but provide support for the knee and serve as a reminder to protect the injured area.

Pain management: Anti-inflammatory or pain medications, like acetaminophen or ibuprofen, are often helpful to reduce pain and swelling, and speed up the healing process.

Crutches: If the child is having difficulty walking, crutches can be useful to help rest the knee by reducing weight-bearing and stress on the joint.

Braces: Injuries to the ligaments or tendons may require a knee immobilizer or brace to keep the joint in place while it heals.

Surgery: Severe injuries to the ligaments (ACL or MCL) or cartilage (meniscus) sometimes require surgery. If surgery is required, it is usually performed weeks to months after the injury occurred.

Dislocation: A dislocated patella sometimes slips back into place on its own, but your doctor may need to put it back to its normal position.

Cast: Most fractures require a cast. Occasionally, surgery is needed.

Physiotherapy: Physiotherapy is often recommended after a knee injury that does not get better quickly. The goal of physiotherapy is to strengthen the muscles that support the knee.

❶ What Is Osgood-Schlatter Disease?

Osgood-Schlatter disease is a painful swelling of the tibial tubercle (the bump on the upper part of the front of the shinbone). This is where the tendon of the large upper leg muscles, the quadriceps, attaches to the lower leg. When the quadriceps muscles contract to straighten the leg, they pull on this tendon. In some children, especially if they are very active, repeated pulling on the tendon causes inflammation at the site of the tibial tubercle. Pain is most intense when putting large loads on the knee joint; for example, squatting or climbing stairs. Osgood-Schlatter disease is most common in active preteen and teenage boys.

Diagnosis of Osgood-Schlatter Disease

A good physical examination by your doctor is usually enough to make the diagnosis. X-rays can be normal or may show some swelling or inflammation of the tibial tubercle.

❷ How Is Osgood-Schlatter Disease Treated?

Osgood-Schlatter disease almost always disappears once the child stops growing. Until then, treatment consists of:

- Rest when the pain is severe
- Icing after activity
- Nonsteroidal anti-inflammatory medications, such as ibuprofen
- Knee pads to protect the area
- Low-impact strengthening and flexibility exercises

Ongoing athletic activity is generally not harmful to children with Osgood-Schlatter disease. You should encourage your child to continue to play sports as tolerated.

> **Doc Talk** After a knee injury, the knee is at a higher risk of re-injury, especially after a period of disuse. Strengthening and stretching the muscles supporting the knee after an injury are key factors in reducing the risk of recurrent injury. Take the time to do this to reduce recurrent knee injuries so that your child is able to play and eventually work without pain.

Knock-Knees and Bowlegs

What Can I Do?

▶ There is little you can do. Remember that very few children have perfectly straight legs. Some legs just curve more than others and few require medical treatment.

▶ See the list of red flags for knock-knees and bowlegs. If your child has any of these symptoms, then consult your doctor.

❶ What Are Knock-Knees and Bowlegs?

Most people's knees touch each other when they are standing. Usually, when a person stands with his knees together, his foot and ankle touch those of the opposite foot. In some people, when the knees are touching, the feet and ankles are wide apart. This is referred to as knock-knees (genu valgum). Bowlegs are when the legs are curved outward, and the knees are far apart (genu varum).

Children don't have perfectly straight legs. Some legs just curve more than others. Usually, children's legs get straighter with age and very few require medical treatment. In fact, doctors now believe that for the conditions described here, trying to straighten legs with

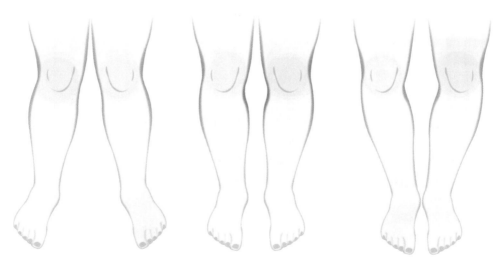

Knock-knees (genu valgum)   Normal   Bowlegs (genu varum)

braces, inserts, or orthopedic shoes may be unnecessary, ineffective, uncomfortable, expensive, and even harmful.

Bowing of the legs or knock-knees are often seen as a part of the normal stages of growth in children. Bowlegs are usually first noticed in infants and toddlers when they begin to walk. Bowlegs often overcorrect with time to become knock-knees. Knock-knees are usually seen in children between the ages of 2 and 5. The knock-knees then improve with further growth. They are usually not an issue by the time your child is 8 to 10.

When should we consult our doctor?

In most cases, knock-knees and bowlegs are part of normal development, but see your doctor if any red flags are present.

➤ Knock-Knees Red Flags

Consult your child's doctor if your infant or toddler has any of the following symptoms associated with knock-knees.

- Only knock-kneed on one side
- Pain
- Limping
- Leg swelling
- Delay in reaching developmental milestones, such as sitting, crawling, or walking

❷ What Causes Knock-Knees?

Most knock-knees are a normal part of the growth and development of a child's legs. Very rarely, knock-knees are caused by underlying nutritional problems (such as vitamin D deficiency/rickets) or inherited bone diseases.

❸ How Are Knock-Knees Treated?

Treatment is seldom needed because knock-knees usually get better on their own. If there is an underlying disease, medical or surgical treatment may be necessary.

➤➤ Bowlegs Red Flags

Consult your child's doctor if your infant or toddler has any of the following symptoms associated with bowlegs:

- One-sided bowing
- Pain
- Limping
- Leg swelling
- Delay in reaching developmental milestones, such as sitting, crawling, or walking
- Worsening of the bowing instead of the expected improvement that occurs between the ages of 1 and 2 years

❹ What Causes Bowlegs?

Did You Know?

Blount's Disease

Very rarely, bowlegs are due to a condition called Blount's disease. The bow tends to get worse with age, and surgery may be required.

Bowlegs are believed to be due to a baby's previous positioning in the womb, when the bones are still relatively soft. After children start to walk, the bowing straightens out. Some people will always have mild bowing of their legs. Sometimes bowing occurs after an infection or injury that damages the growth area of the bone. Bowlegs can also be caused by vitamin D deficiency and some rare bone diseases.

❺ How Are Bowlegs Treated?

Most bowlegs start to straighten out in the second year of life without any medical treatment. Time is often the number one cure. However, if there are any red flag symptoms, you should have your child assessed.

Doc Talk

In most cases, knock-knees and bowlegs will resolve themselves during normal growth and development. Children with "normal" knock-knees do not have difficulty walking or running, nor do they experience knee pain. Mild bowlegs do not interfere with walking or running, and they do not cause pain.

Learning Problems

What Can I Do?

▶ Review the 10 Ds of learning problems (below) and see if your child has any of them.

▶ If you suspect a serious learning problem, arrange with your doctor or your child's teachers to conduct psychoeducational testing.

▶ If your child shows red flag signs of a learning disability (LD), consult with your doctor for testing and treatment. Participate in your child's learning process regardless of whether he has a learning problem or not.

❶ What Is a Learning Disability (LD)?

A child is considered to have a learning disability if his ability to store, process, or produce information is impaired. If a child has great difficulty reading but excels in math (or vice versa), he probably has a learning disability. Sometimes the disability is less obvious (particularly when a child has more than one type of learning problem), and a special academic assessment, called psychoeducational testing, is required. Even when the disability is obvious, psychoeducational testing may best help teachers develop an individual education plan and also help your child get the resources he needs in the school setting (for example, a laptop and keyboarding training, an educational assistant, or an occupational therapist to help with writing). That said, children with normal intelligence (and even above-average intelligence) may have learning problems. See ADHD (page 58) and Autism (page 64).

When should we contact our doctor?

There are many reasons for learning problems. Most do not resolve on their own, so see your doctor if any of the signs and symptoms below seem to be present.

The 10 Ds of Learning Problems

Certain signs and symptoms may indicate a learning problem. Have your child tested if he is:

❶ **Distractible:** Children with attention deficit hyperactivity disorder (ADHD) are easily distracted, which causes learning problems. See ADHD (page 58).

Did You Know?

Dyslexia

A type of learning disability (LD) called developmental reading disability (or, using an older term, dyslexia) is an example of a learning disability that frequently runs in families with normal intelligence. Both Pablo Picasso and Leonardo da Vinci had dyslexia. If their learning disability had been assessed and treated earlier, they may not have spent so much time fooling around with all that painting!

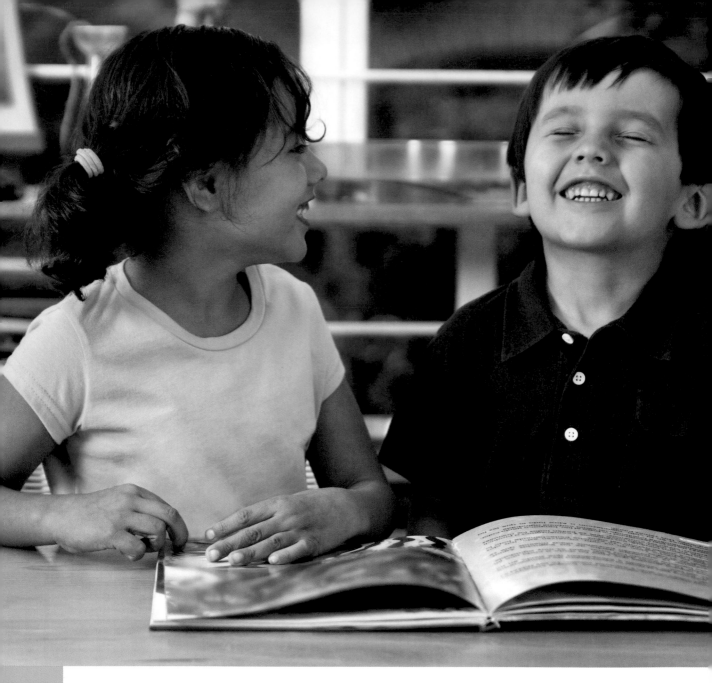

2 **Distracted:** Some children are distracted from their schoolwork by family problems (for example, the loss of a loved one).

3 **Depressed or anxious:** Children may be feeling depressed or anxious, focusing on their problems, not their schoolwork.

4 **Delayed:** Children may suffer from a delay in their growth and development that affects their ability to learn.

5 **Disconnected:** Some children may suffer from autism spectrum disorder, which teachers may not fully appreciate as a learning problem. See Autism (page 64).

6 **Dozy:** Children may find it hard to concentrate without a good night's sleep due to late night online gaming or sleep apnea, for example.

7 **Defiant:** Some children with oppositional defiant disorder (ODD) simply refuse to do the necessary schoolwork.

8 **Delinquent:** Some children are absent from, or late to, class so frequently that they fall behind and can't catch up.

9 **Drugged:** Many different drugs can cause drowsiness, not just illicit drugs. Prescribed and over-the-counter medications can also be sedating. Even so-called "nonsedating" antihistamines for allergies are a little sedating. Feeling sedated makes it hard to concentrate.

10 **Deaf or visually impaired:** Some children have moderate hearing or vision problems that can interfere with learning. However, subtle hearing problems caused by fluid in the ear are usually not the cause of school troubles.

2 How Are Learning Disabilities Treated?

Dietary therapy, special glasses, eye-training exercises, allergy treatment, biofeedback, and vitamin supplementation are examples of treatments that have not been found to be useful in properly conducted research. For children with learning disabilities, so far nothing has been found that can take the place of hard work, support, and individualized instruction.

FAQ

My child is smart but has a reading disability. How can I help at home?

Old-fashioned phonics helps the most (for example, "What is the name of this letter? What is its sound? Now let's blend them together"). Praise and rewards for extra time spent in tutoring may be helpful in getting your child through the hard work.

Doc Talk

Helping your child to learn more easily is one of the most challenging but most rewarding activities you will do as a parent — especially so if your child has a learning problem. However serious the problem may be, don't give up. In almost every case, children make great gains when parents participate in their learning process.

Leg Aches

What Can I Do?

▶ Start by comparing the symptoms for growing pains with your child's leg ache to determine if it is something more serious.

▶ Although 90% of cases resolve themselves, take leg aches seriously if you cannot easily manage your child's pain. See your physician if the pain persists or increases.

▶ Try muscle-stretching exercises, massage, and heating pads to relieve your child's pain. During more serious episodes, use over-the-counter pain medications (acetaminophen and ibuprofen).

❶ What Is a Leg Ache?

Discomfort in one or both legs that is unrelated to a known injury is a common occurrence in childhood and adolescence. In most children, these are temporary or mild discomforts due to muscle cramps or strains, viral illnesses, or a benign condition known as growing pains.

When should we contact our doctor or local hospital?

Leg aches typically resolve on their own, but occasionally there is a related problem that requires medical care. Persistent or recurrent leg pains should always prompt a visit to the doctor.

▶▶ Leg Ache Red Flags

Consult your child's doctor if your child has any of the following symptoms associated with leg ache:

- Inability to stand or walk
- Fever and pain in one leg only
- A swollen joint or an inability to move the leg at a joint
- Calf pain on one side that lasts several hours
- Red patch of skin over painful area
- Numbness (loss of sensation) that lasts longer than a few minutes
- Severe pain (or crying) when leg is touched or moved
- Appears ill

Growing Pains

Growing pains refers to a typical pattern of leg pains in childhood that have no known underlying abnormality of bone or muscle. The pain always goes away on its own without long-term consequences for the child's growth or development. Although the term is a misnomer because the pains are unrelated to periods of rapid growth, the term "growing pains" continues to be a useful way to refer to a very common and harmless type of leg pain (affecting about 1 in 10 children), and to distinguish it from serious illnesses that are much less common.

Comparing Growing Pains with Other Pains

Common Characteristics of Growing Pains	Characteristics That Are Not Typical of Growing Pains
• Onset from age 4 to 14 • Primarily located in the shins and thighs, and sometimes in the calves • Usually affects both legs (but sometimes affects only one side) • Often relieved by massaging the affected site • Typical onset of an episode is late in the day or at night, with complete resolution by morning • May awaken child from sleep and cause crying • Duration of each episode is minutes to hours • Episodes are separated by pain-free periods of days to months • Otherwise normal growth and development	• Onset at younger than 4 years or older than 14 years of age • Pain localized to any site other than the shins, thighs, calves • Pain episodes that continue beyond a few hours, or persist after the child wakes in the morning • Episodes that are worsening over time (getting longer, more intense, more frequent) • One-sided pain that persistently wakes the child from sleep • Pain in a joint • Swelling of joints or limbs, or changes in skin (for example, redness, warmth) • Reduction in the range of motion (arc) of the hips, knees, or ankles • Limp or another disturbance of walking or stance • Fever, general malaise, weight loss, or other unexplained symptoms • Slowed or stunted growth

❷ What Causes Growing Pains?

The reason why some children experience growing pains is unknown. Current theories include muscle overuse or fatigue (due to high levels of physical activity), joint hypermobility, a reduced pain threshold, lower bone strength, and emotional factors. However, it's likely that these factors have variable degrees of importance for each individual child. There are no specific tests that are routinely helpful for determining the cause of an individual child's growing pains.

❸ How Are Growing Pains Treated?

- Few medical or nutritional therapies for growing pains are supported by strong scientific evidence.
- Muscle-stretching routines, massage, and heating pads are the mainstays of therapy.
- Over-the-counter pain medications (acetaminophen and ibuprofen) may be used during more severe episodes.
- Occasionally shoe inserts (orthotics) may be useful. Ask your child's doctor about assessment.

Other Causes of Leg Aches

There are some serious conditions that can cause leg pain (for example, bone or joint infections, juvenile arthritis, deep vein clots, and tumors), but these are relatively rare and usually accompanied by other changes in the child's health or well-being. Here is a list of relatively more common causes of leg aches.

Apophysitis

This inflammation of the growth plates occurs when bone develops faster than muscle and tendon flexibility. It most commonly affects the knees and heels, and it can occur on and off during the two to three years of the growth spurt in puberty when growth is most rapid. Different names may be used to describe this condition, depending on its site; for example, Osgood-Schlatter disease for the knees, and Sever's disease for the heels. See Knee Injuries (page 254). These conditions, which truly are growing pains, generally go away without specific treatment.

Viral Infections

The influenza virus commonly causes leg aches in conjunction with other typical symptoms, including fever and general malaise. See Flu (page 207). Treatment for this is usually just comfort care, and it will be directed at the underlying infection, not just the leg pain.

Muscle Cramps and Strains

Pains that occur in the feet or calves and last only a few minutes are likely muscle cramps (spasms). In contrast, pain in an arm or leg that persists for hours to days following a strenuous activity on the preceding day is likely due to a muscle strain. Cramps and strains typically go away on their own, but if they persist beyond 1 week or recur frequently, they should be discussed with your child's physician.

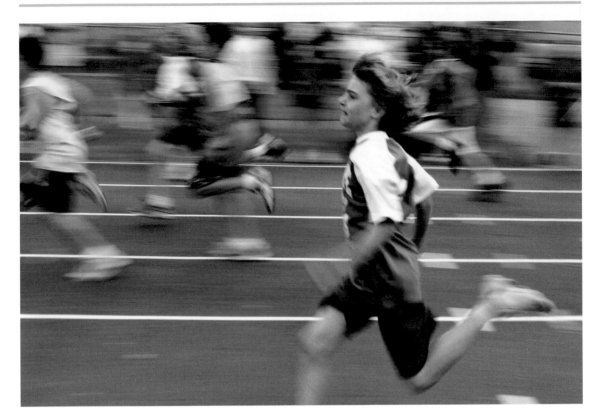

Treatment for Muscle Cramps and Strains

Simple comfort measures to address these bothersome but generally benign conditions are shown here.

Muscle Cramp	Muscle Strain
• During the attack, gently stretch the muscle in the opposite direction of the spasm (for example, for calf spasm, pull the foot and toes upward). • Apply a cold pack to the painful muscle. • For cramps during hot weather, provide adequate fluids to drink.	• Apply a cold pack to the sore muscle for about 20 minutes, several times daily, for the first 2 days. • If needed, administer acetaminophen or ibuprofen. • Try a hot bath to relieve muscle stiffness, and gently stretch the muscle under water.

Doc Talk Parents are often worried that leg pains signify a serious underlying disease. Discomfort that causes your child to stop or greatly reduce participation in regular activities is a signal that there may be a problem other than growing pains or muscle cramps and strains. In general, if you cannot easily explain and manage your child's pain, you should see a physician. It's important to talk to your child's physician about your concerns so that a proper assessment can be undertaken.

Lice

What Can I Do?

▶ Inspect your child's head for lice if your child has symptoms or has been in contact with other children who are infected. This takes time, patience, a knowledge of what to look for, and a good light!

▶ If your child is infected, wash toys, brushes, combs, bedding, hats, and clothes in hot soapy water. Store items that cannot be washed in a tight plastic bag for 10 to 14 days. Discourage sharing of hairbrushes, hats, towels, and pillows.

▶ Some strains of lice are resistant to standard treatment. If you suspect this might be the case with your child, see your child's doctor.

Case Study

Joseph's Lice

It is a new school year and all the students in Joseph's class have just been checked for lice by a nurse. Joseph's mother gets the dreaded phone call from the school office, asking her to please pick Joseph up at once because his hair is infested with lice. Joseph's mother is feeling guilty and ashamed and worries that no other mothers will allow their kids to play with Joseph. She rushes home and washes Joseph's hair with medicated lice shampoo.

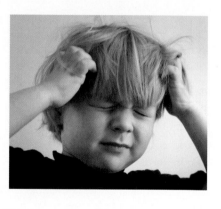

❶ What Are Lice?

Lice are tiny insects that live on the surface of the skin and feed by sucking blood. The infecting lice cause intense itching due to irritation from their saliva. Lice eggs are deposited on the hair shafts and are called nits.

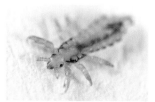

Adult lice (actual size 2–4 mm)

Adult Lice

Lice are $\frac{1}{16}$ to $\frac{1}{8}$ inch (2 to 4 mm) in length and dark grayish in color. In addition to intense itching, the presence of a louse is associated with small red bumps (papules) or scratch marks on the scalp. Lice are not easy to see at rest, but when they are moving, they may be a bit easier to spot.

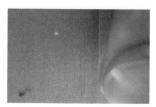

Nits

Nits

Nits are light gray and are firmly stuck to the hair shaft. This differentiates them from dandruff, which can be easily flicked off the hair shaft. They look like miniature cocoons firmly attached to a branch. They can be difficult to identify in many children. The persistence of lice is usually related to the inability to kill all the eggs. A good examination for lice and their nits requires very good light, lots of time, and persistence!

❷ What Causes Lice to Spread?

Lice infestation is spread by direct hair-to-hair contact. Sharing hairbrushes, hats, towels, and pillows contributes to their spread. Lice do not jump or fly but rather transfer from one head to another in close contact.

❸ How Are Lice Treated?

Check the hair of all members of the household and treat everyone who has lice or nits. Use lice shampoos and rinses. Often at least two applications 7 to 10 days apart are necessary. Treatment really has two components: environmental control and medicine to kill the lice and nits. Medicated treatments are highly effective in killing adult lice, but do a "lousy" job of killing nits.

Wash toys, brushes, combs, bedding, hats, and clothes in hot soapy water, and store items that cannot be washed in a tight plastic bag for 10 to 14 days.

Did You Know?

Social Stigma
A diagnosis of head lice can lead to embarrassment, frustration, and distress in many families because of the misconception that children with lice have poor hygiene. Lice, in fact, prefer clean hair and skin! In some warmer climates, lice infestation is very common and is associated with less social stigma.

Medical Treatment of Lice Infestation

Type of Treatment	Medicinal Ingredient	Some Examples	Comments
Pediculicide (insecticide)	Permethrin, pyrethrin, malathion	R&C shampoo and conditioner, Nix conditioner	• Treat at least twice, 7 to 10 days apart • May cause skin irritation • Consult your doctor for use in children younger than 2 years
Noninsecticide (dehydrates and asphyxiates lice)	Isopropyl myristate, cyclomethicone	Resultz	• Treat at least twice, 7 to 10 days apart • May cause skin irritation • Consult your doctor for use in children younger than 4 years

School Exclusion

Exclusion from school has not been demonstrated to reduce further lice infestation. The American Academy of Pediatrics and the Canadian Paediatric Society do not recommend school exclusion but rather avoidance of head-to-head contact until treatment for lice has been initiated. Families of infected children should be notified and counseled about treatment strategies and school "no-nit" policies should be discouraged.

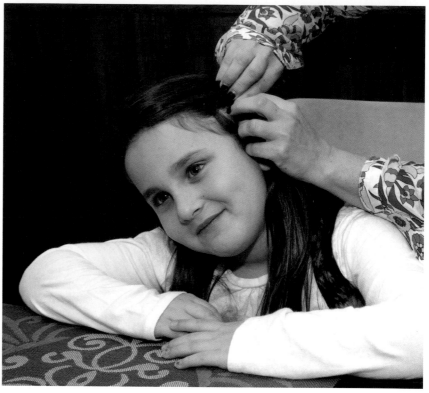
Checking for lice

FAQ

We followed the instructions given to us for handling a lice infestation in our family, but the lice are still alive. What do we do now?

Consider these common causes of treatment failure and start again:

- Insufficient application (too little, too short a time) of insecticide
- Failure to repeat treatment 7 to 10 days after the initial treatment
- Failure to remove all of the nits (this can be a painstaking job!)
- Lack of environmental eradication (pillows, sheets, combs)
- Reinfestation at school
- Resistance to treatment among some strains of lice

Doc Talk

Many home remedies exist for treating lice. Examples include applying mayonnaise, tea tree oil, coconut oil, or vinegar to the hair and scalp. Most of these are thought to act by clogging or occluding the respiratory spiracles (the "gills" or "lungs") of the louse, resulting in death. They have, unfortunately, not been proven to be effective.

Limp

What Can I Do?

▶ If there is no obvious cause for your child's limp, see your doctor to rule out causes one by one. See the list of possible causes by presence or absence of pain, and by age.

▶ Note that growing pains do not generally cause a limp.

▶ If your child is experiencing pain with his limping, try a simple analgesic or anti-inflammatory medication to ease his pain until the diagnosis is complete.

Case Study

Lyndsey's Limp

Lyndsey is a healthy 6-year-old girl. This morning, she woke up complaining of pain in her left hip and refused to walk. She doesn't remember falling or injuring her leg in any way. She is otherwise well but did have a cold and runny nose last week, from which she has now recovered. Her armpit temperature is 100.0°F (37.8°C). Her father notices that she only wants to keep her knee and hip bent and turned outward. Lyndsey's father takes her to the doctor to be assessed.

She was diagnosed with transient synovitis of the hip. Her doctor gave her ibuprofen to help relieve the inflammation and pain in her hip, and recommended that Lyndsey rest in a comfortable position and minimize weight-bearing on her affected leg until the pain improves. If Lyndsey develops a high-grade fever, she needs to be reassessed.

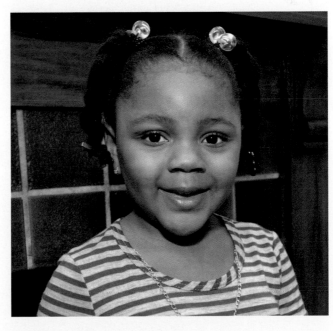

Transient synovitis is an inflammation of the membrane covering the hip joint. It is most often seen in children between 3 and 10 years of age and sometimes occurs 1 to 2 weeks after a cold. The hip joint is painful to move and the child may refuse to walk. Unlike an infection of the joint, the child generally feels well. Usually the child does not have a fever and, if present, it will be low-grade.

❶ What Is a Limp?

Limping refers to an abnormal walking pattern resulting from pain, weakness, injury, infection, and other abnormalities of the bones, muscles, or nerves involved in moving the leg. A limp in a child is never normal and should not be ignored. Possible causes of limp range from easily fixed nuisances, such as poorly fitting shoes or a splinter in the foot, to more serious problems, such as broken or infected bones.

When should we contact our doctor or local hospital?

Limping is not normal. Often there is a very straightforward reason for a child's limp, one that can be readily identified — for example, a cut on the foot or pebble in the shoe. In these cases, simple measures or first aid can be provided at home. However, a limp that cannot be immediately explained, lasts longer than a day, recurs, or is associated with severe pain or other concerns should prompt a visit to the doctor. A persistent limp in a young child who has just started to walk must be assessed by a physician.

▶▶ Limp Red Flags

- Sudden limp or refusal to walk with no obvious cause
- Fever with the limp
- Severe pain, especially if the child has pain at night or at rest
- Persistent pain or swelling of a bone or joint
- An infant who is not walking yet but refuses to use the leg to crawl or sit

❷ What Causes a Limp?

The list of possible causes of limp is quite long. Children tend to have high levels of activity yet relatively immature bones, which means there is a risk of several problems not seen in adults. Determining the cause of your child's limp involves some basic clinical reasoning:

- How old is the child? Causes of limp differ by age.
- What was the child doing before you noticed the limp? Injury to the muscles or bones is a common cause of acute limp in children.

However, sometimes an apparent injury is a "red herring," meaning that it coincidentally occurred at the same time as the emergence of another cause of limp.

- Has the limp or pain been worsening over the course of weeks or months? Worsening symptoms should always be a signal to seek medical attention.
- Does your child seem otherwise unwell to you? Symptoms other than limp, such as fever or general malaise, may point toward the likely cause. For example, children with bone or joint infections usually have a fever.
- Is there pain? Pain is a key sign used to determine the cause of the limp.
- Is the onset of the pain sudden (acute) or gradual (chronic)?

Painful (Acute)	Painful (Chronic)	Painless
• Broken bone • Ankle sprain • Infection of the bone or joint • Hip inflammation • Slipped capital femoral epiphysis	• Inflammation of growth plate (apophysitis) • Legg-Calve-Perthes disease • Slipped capital femoral epiphysis • Juvenile idiopathic arthritis • Cancer	• Developmental dysplasia of the hip • Leg length differences • Legg-Calve-Perthes disease • Rickets

It's useful to consider the more common causes of limp according to age. Note that many of the listed conditions happen in more than one age group.

Preschool-Age Children (Up to 5 Years)

Limp that is present when a young child is learning to walk can indicate a developmental abnormality of the hip or a disorder of the nerve supply to the leg muscles. Infections, inflammation, and injury are important considerations in this age group.

- *Developmental dysplasia of the hip* (formerly called congenital dislocation of the hip): This problem starts from birth. Doctors routinely look for it as part of their examination of newborn babies and at checkups throughout infancy. If you notice your baby has extra skin creases on one thigh or that one hip doesn't open as much as the other when you change the diaper, you should tell your child's physician. The limp, which is painless, may be noticed after the child starts to walk.

- *Toddler's fracture:* This injury can surprise parents because a fracture (broken bone) of the tibia (one of the two bones that goes from the knee to the ankle) in a young child can happen even after seemingly innocent jumping or twisting. The child might have only minimal swelling and a mild limp, and often she is too young to be able to recall exactly when she felt the initial pain.

- *Infections:* Infections of the joints (septic arthritis) or the bones (osteomyelitis) in the legs can result in a limp. More often than not, a child will completely refuse to walk or bear weight. The infection is usually caused by bacteria that spread through the bloodstream from elsewhere in the body. An affected child often has pain, fever, poor appetite, and may look unwell. The pain is usually quite severe. There may be swelling and redness over the sore area.

- *Juvenile idiopathic arthritis:* This disease of childhood involves chronic inflammation (swelling) of the joints. Symptoms will vary depending on the type of arthritis, but limp is a common characteristic. The inflammation can come and go, and it affects different joints throughout the body. The limp can be worse at the beginning of the day rather than at the end of the day. A joint, often the knee, can appear swollen or puffy. Young children may not complain of pain, but they may reduce their level of activity. In some types of arthritis, children can have a fever, swollen glands, and a rash.

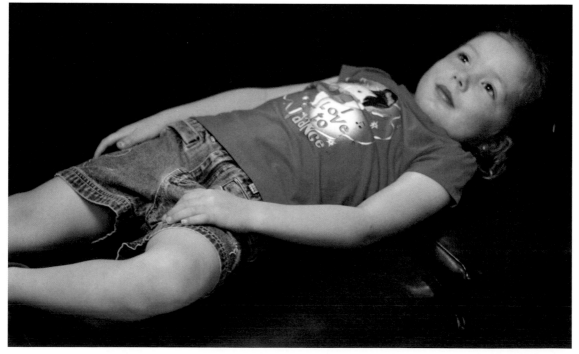

Painful left hip: frog-leg position

Young School-Age Children (5 to 10 Years)

Infections continue to occur in this age range, but this is the group in which sprains, strains, and fractures (bone breaks) become more predominant. Other less common conditions that are important in this age group are noninfectious diseases of the hips, particularly in boys.

- *Transient synovitis:* The cause of this inflammation of the membrane covering the hip joint is unknown, but it is not an infection. This condition is most often seen in children between 3 and 10 years of age and sometimes occurs 1 to 2 weeks after a cold. The hip joint is painful to move and the child may refuse to walk. Unlike an infection of the joint, the child generally feels well. Usually she does not have a fever and, if present, it will be low-grade (below 100.4°F/38°C).
- *Legg-Calve-Perthes disease:* The cause of this softening of the growing end of the femur (the bone between the pelvis and the knee) is also unknown. It tends to occur in children aged 4 to 8 years, and it is more common in boys. There may or may not be any hip or knee pain associated with the limp, which begins gradually and can involve both sides.

Older Children and Adolescents (10 Years and Older)

In this age group, overuse and athletic injuries predominate, particularly involving the hips and knees.

- *Ankle sprains:* These are common in older children and usually result from a fall when the foot is twisted onto its outside edge. This causes the ankle to swell up, and movement in any direction is painful. See Ankle Injuries (page 49).
- *Apophysitis:* This is one of the more common causes of limp and leg/foot discomfort during the adolescent growth spurt. The term literally refers to inflammation (swelling) of a bony outcropping, and it tends to occur at sites of active bone growth that are subjected to the substantial pulling forces of a large tendon (the fibrous connection of bone to muscle). When it affects the heel, it is called Sever's disease, and at the knee, it is called Osgood-Schlatter disease. A physician should make the diagnosis to ensure that other conditions are ruled out, a process that may involve taking some X rays. Treatment is usually focused on comfort measures (for example, stretching, resting, icing, and over-the-counter pain medication, such as ibuprofen or acetaminophen) and the reassurance that this problem will resolve with time.

Did You Know?

Growing Pains

Growing pains may explain a child's leg aches (see page 267), but they are not an adequate explanation for a limp.

Did You Know?

Cancer

There are several serious but rare causes of limp, such as cancers of the blood (leukemia) and of the bone (osteosarcoma). Children with these conditions tend to have changes in their energy level and behavior, pain at night, or other concerning symptoms over a prolonged period of time.

Nutritional Rickets

This bone disease is due to vitamin D deficiency. It is rare in the modern era, but it still occurs in young children who do not have vitamin D in their diet and lack adequate exposure to sunlight. This can also result in bowlegs, swelling of the wrists, and seizures.

- *Mechanical spine problems:* These problems (for example, spondylolysis, where a vertebra is defective, or spondylolisthesis, where a vertebra slips forward) may also develop during this period. These conditions usually also involve back pain. See Backache (page 67).
- *Slipped capital femoral epiphysis:* This is a rare condition of early adolescence in which the top part of the femur (thigh bone) "slips" into an abnormal position. The exact cause is unknown, but this usually affects overweight teenagers, boys more often than girls. The onset of the symptoms can be abrupt or gradual, but they typically involve complaints of a limp and pain in the hip.

❸ How Is a Limp Treated?

To treat children with a limp, the doctor will attempt to determine the specific cause and remove it or address it. Treatments vary depending on the specific cause. Remember, limping is a symptom, not a diagnosis.

Doc Talk Any child with a change in his ability to walk or bear weight requires a thorough medical assessment. Problems in the hip can cause pain in the knee due to the way that the nerves transmit messages from the leg to the brain. This may mislead parents and physicians about the true reason for a child's limp. You may also be surprised to know that abdominal problems can occasionally cause a limp.

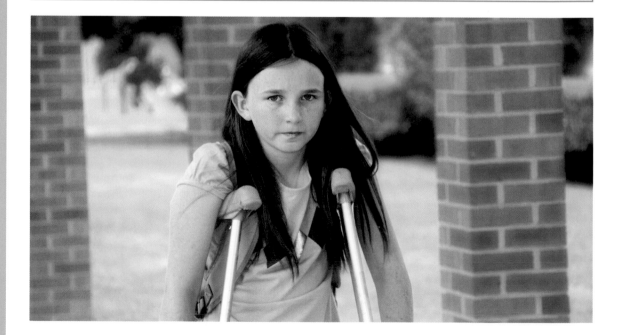

Mouth Sores

What Can I Do?

Soothe your child's mouth in the following ways:

▶ Minimize feeding your child acidic and spicy food and drinks.

▶ Apply a local anesthetic gel, generally available from pharmacies without a prescription.

▶ If your child refuses to drink or eat, seek medical advice because of the risk of dehydration, particularly in younger children.

❶ What Are Mouth Sores?

The term "mouth ulcers" refers to open sores affecting the mucus lining of the cheeks, gums, tongue, lips, roof and floor of the mouth, and upper throat. This is sometimes called stomatitis, which means inflammation of the mucus lining. The cause and type of mouth ulcer can often be diagnosed by determining the location and by examining the appearance of the ulcer.

RELATED CONDITIONS

- Canker sores
- Chapped lips
- Cold sores
- Hand, foot, and mouth disease (herpangina)

When should we contact our doctor or local hospital?

Mouth ulcers, in most cases, do not require emergency measures. Occasionally, the pain can cause the child to stop drinking, which can lead to dehydration (see page 150). If your child is not drinking despite the institution of home pain control measures, see her doctor.

⟩⟩ Mouth Sore Red Flags

Consult your child's doctor as soon as possible if your child is not able to drink fluids or eat due to mouth pain. Your child could be dehydrated.

Common Childhood Causes of Mouth Sores

Cause	Typical Age	Location	What They Look Like
Canker sores (aphthous ulcers)	Any age	Usually on the inside of the lips but can occur on gums or roof and floor of mouth	A $\frac{1}{16}$- to $\frac{1}{2}$-inch (2 to 12 mm) red base with a whitish-gray crater or ulcer
Cold sores (herpes simplex infection)	First presentation usually as a toddler; can experience symptoms throughout life	The first time, cold sores usually appear anywhere in the mouth or on the lips; in recurrences, on the lip or edge of the lip	The first time, symptoms include swollen gums and tongue, plus painful ulcers on gum, tongue, throat, and palate; in recurrences, cold sores appear as groups of blisters on a red base that burst and then crust on the lip edge
Hand, foot, and mouth disease (herpangina)	Toddler age	Back of the throat	Red sores are $\frac{1}{16}$ to $\frac{1}{8}$ inch (2 to 4 mm) in diameter, with a small fluid-filled blister that pops, leaving a tiny ulcer

❶ What Are Canker Sores?

Canker sores (aphthous ulcers) are sores affecting the lining of the mouth or the tongue. They are quite common in toddlers and children, but they are not serious, although they can be very painful. They are not contagious.

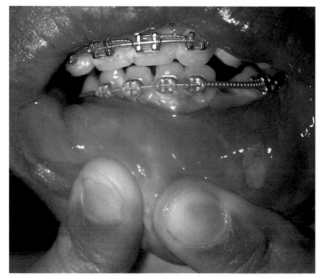

Canker sore (lower lip on right)

Signs and Symptoms of Canker Sores

- Canker sores usually start off as red bumps anywhere in the mouth.
- Red bumps progress to painful, whitish-gray ulcers with a raised, inflamed edge.
- Ulcers form, looking like small craters that vary in size from $\frac{1}{16}$ to $\frac{1}{2}$ inch (2 to 10 mm).
- Canker sores may appear alone or in small groups.
- Toddlers may drool or refuse to eat because of the pain.

❷ What Causes Canker Sores?

There is no known cause for this kind of mouth ulcer, but a long list of potential causes has been suggested:

- Trauma
- Diet
- Stress
- Nutritional deficiencies
- Infections
- Allergic or toxic drug reactions
- Immune system problems
- Genetics

❸ How Are Canker Sores Treated?

There is, unfortunately, no cure for canker sores. The goal of treatment is to minimize the pain until the canker sore resolves after a few days to a couple of weeks. In the meantime, you can soothe your child's mouth in the following ways:

- Minimize feeding your child acidic and spicy food and drinks.
- Apply a local anesthetic gel, generally available from pharmacies without a prescription.
- If child is cooperative and old enough, rinse and spit out with mouthwash or salt water.

See your child's doctor if the ulcers haven't settled after 10 days or recur frequently. Occasionally, your doctor may recommend an anti-inflammatory steroid cream to speed up healing. Your doctor may see if there is any identifiable contributing factor to recurrent canker sores, such as a vitamin or mineral deficiency.

❶ What Are Cold Sores?

Cold sores, sometimes called fever blisters, are little blisters that form on the lips. They are filled with fluid and are caused by a herpes simplex virus (HSV) infection. This is not usually the same herpes virus that causes genital infections. HSV infections are very common, with over 90% of adults showing evidence of a previous infection. The initial infection often begins in childhood through contact with oral secretions or an open lesion of an infected person.

A B C D E F G H I J K L **M** N O P Q R S T U V W X Y Z

Signs and Symptoms of Cold Sores

The first time a child is infected with HSV, the infection is usually the most severe. Your child may have:

- High fever
- Irritability
- Blisters that affect the gums and the tongue
- Swollen and very painful gums, palate, and tongue
- Difficulty eating and drinking due to pain

Following the initial infection, the virus lies inactive in the nerve cells around the lips. When reactivated (for whatever reason), a child might experience a variety of other symptoms:

- **Infection in the mouth:**
  - Shallow, white ulcers surrounded by a rim of redness
  - Gum swelling

- **Infection of the lips:**
  - Tingling at the site of where the blisters will form; this usually happens 4 to 12 hours prior to any lesion becoming visible.
  - Grouped blisters on a red background on the lip or edge of the lip; these can be itchy and painful.
  - The blisters burst in a couple of days, leading to crusting; this heals within about a week without any scarring.

FAQs

Are cold sores contagious?
Yes! Like most viruses, herpes simplex virus can be spread through saliva or contact with an open lesion. Children with active infections should avoid contact with newborns, people with immune system problems, and people with severe eczema because these populations are at particular risk of becoming very sick with infection.

Why do some people get frequent cold sores and others only get them once?
Recurrences of HSV infection are very common because the virus stays dormant in the nerve endings and tends to reactivate from time to time. Certain triggers can predispose individuals to frequent eruptions.

❷ What Causes Cold Sores?

Common Triggers

- Colds
- Fever
- Fatigue
- Sun exposure
- Wind exposure
- Stress
- Chapped lips
- Menstruation

Prevention

- Wear lip balm (minimum SPF 15).
- Avoid kissing or contact with blisters when present.
- Avoid sharing utensils and lip balm.
- Don't touch blisters and then other parts of the body — this can spread the virus.

❸ How Are Cold Sores Treated?

- Herpes lesions resolve in about a week, with crusting that tends to peel off with no long-term scarring. No treatment is usually required.
- Pain medication (acetaminophen or ibuprofen) can be offered.
- Prescription antiviral medication may be used at the onset of tingling or lip pain; this can sometimes reduce the severity of infection.

Did You Know?

Herpetic Whitlow

Herpes infections can affect almost all parts of the body. When affecting the fingers, this is termed herpetic whitlow. This particular location can lead to significant stretching of the tissues from swelling, leading to pain.

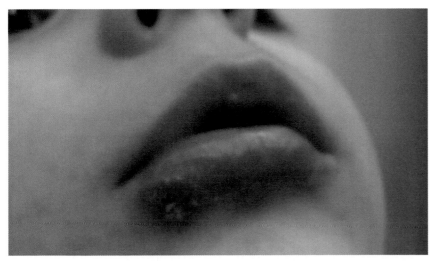

Cold sore

❶ What Is Hand, Foot, and Mouth Disease (Herpangina)?

This is a common viral infection that can occur at any age but most commonly affects young children during the summer and fall seasons. When it affects the mouth only, it is referred to as herpangina.

Signs and Symptoms of Hand, Foot, and Mouth Disease

- Small red dots at the back of the throat, with little fluid-filled blisters (vesicles)
- Vesicles quickly pop, leaving painful, red $1/16$- to $1/8$-inch (2 to 4 mm) ulcers in the mouth
- Skin rash of small blisters against a reddish base on the palms and soles
- Skin rash may also be seen in the diaper area or around the mouth
- Fever
- Decreased appetite
- Irritability and decreased energy

❷ What Causes Hand, Foot, and Mouth Disease?

Hand, foot, and mouth disease is an infection caused by a virus called coxsackievirus. Like most cold viruses, coxsackievirus is highly contagious and spreads from one child to another through coughing, saliva, and shared surfaces, such as toys.

❸ How Is Hand, Foot, and Mouth Disease Treated?

There is no specific treatment for hand, foot, and mouth disease. The illness subsides on its own within 7 to 10 days. Because it is caused by a virus, antibiotics don't work to treat it. You can provide supportive care at home by:

- Offering the child food and liquids, as tolerated (see your child's doctor if taking in only minimal amounts of fluid).
- Giving acetaminophen or ibuprofen for fever, as needed.

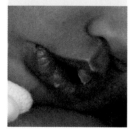

❶ What Are Chapped Lips?

Chapped lips result from excessive dryness of the lips. Lips can appear dry, swollen, or cracked, and they can peel and occasionally bleed. They may feel irritated or burn.

❷ What Causes Chapped Lips?

Chapped lips are caused by too much moisture evaporation from dry air or from decreased production or removal of the naturally occurring oils on the lips.

❸ How Are Chapped Lips Treated?

The goal is to increase and retain lip moisture:

- Apply lip balm regularly, especially in dry weather.
- Apply petroleum jelly (Vaseline), which helps hold moisture in.
- Keep a humidifier on in your child's room, especially in the winter months, when the air may be particularly dry.
- Discourage your child from licking her lips; licking removes the natural oils that are produced.

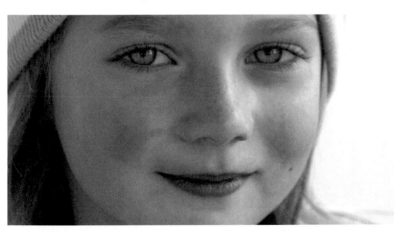

Doc Talk Hand, foot, and mouth disease is not to be confused with foot and mouth disease (also called hoof and mouth disease). This latter disease is caused by a similar virus but affects cattle, pigs, and sheep. Humans do not get infected with this virus — although we, as humans, are all guilty of putting our foot in our mouths from time to time!

Muscle Cramps

What Can I Do?

▶ If the cramp occurs during exercise or during sleep, try stretching and massaging the muscle to relieve pain.

▶ Provide your child with a sports drink when she is exercising strenuously.

▶ If the pain persists, try alternating cold and warm compresses on the affected area and give your child a nonsteroidal anti-inflammatory medication, like ibuprofen.

❶ What Is a Muscle Cramp?

A muscle cramp happens when a muscle tenses up (goes into spasm). Muscle cramps are often painful, and may last minutes or hours. They most commonly affect the calf and foot muscles, but any muscles, including those in the arms, neck, and abdomen (stomach), can be affected.

When should we contact our doctor or local hospital?

Muscle cramps caused by injury tend to resolve as the injury heals, but cramps caused by infection may need medical attention.

▶▶ Muscle Cramps Red Flags

Consult your child's doctor as soon as possible if your child has any of the following symptoms associated with a muscle cramp:

■ If your child looks very sick

■ If the muscle or joint looks swollen or very red

■ If your child cannot walk or seems very weak

■ If your child is limping

■ If the pain is not improving or there are other symptoms, like fever, a rash, or weakness

❷ What Causes a Muscle Cramp?

There are two common causes of muscle cramps — injury and infection — as well as some rare muscle diseases that cause muscle pain. These rare muscle diseases are almost always long-lasting and the child usually has other symptoms, such as fever, weakness, or rashes.

Injury or Overuse

Most muscle cramps are caused by injury or overuse (for example, excessive running, skipping, or jumping). They can occur during or immediately after exercise, or several hours later. Some children get leg or foot cramps at night, often after a very active day. Muscle cramps or pains that last a long time (hours or days) are usually due to overexertion or injuries.

Viral Infections

Viral infections, like influenza, can also cause muscle pains. This type of pain usually affects many muscles at the same time, and the child may have fever and appear unwell. See Flu (page 207).

❸ How Is a Muscle Cramp Treated?

Stretching and massaging the muscle usually provides relief to the child, especially if the pain occurs during or after exercise, or wakes him up at night. If the cramp occurs during strenuous exercise, especially if the weather is very hot, it may help to give your child extra water or a sports drink. If the pain persists, alternate holding cold and warm compresses on the affected area, and give your child a nonsteroidal anti-inflammatory medication, like ibuprofen.

Prevention

Encourage your child to drink lots of fluids, especially before and during exercising. Stretching before and after exercising and before going to bed may also be helpful.

> **Doc Talk** Muscle cramps at night are often mistakenly called growing pains, but they actually have nothing to do with growth. Strenuous exercise tends to be the culprit. See Leg Aches (page 266).

Nail-Biting

What Can I Do?

▶ Encourage your child to stop biting her nails by rewarding her, not criticizing her.

▶ Consider applying bitter solutions on her fingers, but not hot pepper products that use pain to deter nail-biting.

▶ If the nail-biting is serious, with damage to the surrounding skin, see your doctor for further assessment.

❶ What Is Nail-Biting?

Nail-biting is a very common habit that affects up to one-third of children 7 to 10 years old. Sometimes it is associated with stress or anxiety, but there is more commonly no obvious reason for nail-biting. The habit appears to run in families.

When should we contact our doctor?

Nail-biting is usually not harmful. Occasionally, however, the nail bed and cuticle can be damaged, or the skin surrounding the nail can become infected. Children whose fingers and nails are frequently in their mouths can spread germs to others, and they can pick up more germs from their surroundings.

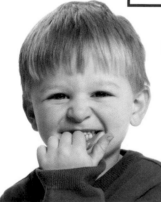

❷ How Is Nail-Biting Treated?

As with thumb-sucking, distraction and positive reinforcement are often helpful techniques. Punishing or criticizing will have the opposite effect. Applying bitter solutions to the fingernails may serve as a reminder and a deterrent to nail-biting. Ensure nails are kept trimmed and free from hangnails. See Thumb-Sucking (page 388).

Doc Talk

Many children will stop biting their nails of their own accord. However, it is estimated that the habit persists in up to 20% of adults. Help your child break this habit now before it becomes a lifelong behavior.

Nosebleeds

What Can I Do?

▶ Follow the guidelines on how to stop a nosebleed. You need to keep constant pressure on the nose for 10 minutes. No peeking!

▶ If this fails, or the nosebleed continues for more than 20 minutes (see red flag symptoms on page 290), contact your doctor or local hospital for further guidance.

▶ Help prevent nosebleeds by keeping the air in your home well humidified.

▶ Use a lubricant to keep the nasal septum moist, especially in cases of recurrent nosebleeds.

❶ What Is a Nosebleed?

The medical term for nosebleeds is "epistaxis." Nosebleeds are extremely common in children. They usually begin in the wall between the two nostrils, called the nasal septum, an area rich in blood vessels.

❷ What Causes a Nosebleed?

There are many causes for nosebleeds, the most common of which is digital trauma, a polite term for nose-picking.

Often colds and allergies lead to nosebleeds. When your child has a cold or is suffering from allergy symptoms, the veins in the congested nasal passages are dilated and thin-walled. Blowing the nose or sneezing raises the pressure inside the vein to the point that it pops, like a flat tire, causing bleeding.

It is much less likely, but possible, that a nosebleed is the result of a foreign body, injury, polyps, or a bleeding disorder, such as hemophilia.

When should we contact our doctor or local hospital?

Most nosebleeds will stop before 20 minutes and can be treated at home. However, if the bleeding continues, seek medical help. See the red flags on page 290 for further indications to seek medical attention.

➤➤ Nosebleed Red Flags

Seek immediate medical attention if your child has any of the following symptoms associated with a nosebleed:

- The bleeding hasn't stopped within 20 minutes.
- The nosebleed is part of a head injury.

Consult your child's doctor if your child has any of the following symptoms associated with a nosebleed:

- Your child has recurrent, severe nosebleeds.
- Your child has other sources of bleeding, such as from the gums during tooth brushing.
- Your child has more bruising anywhere on the body than you would normally expect.
- Your family has a history of bleeding tendencies.

❸ How Is a Nosebleed Treated?

Did You Know?

Swallowing Blood

Blood is sometimes swallowed with a nosebleed and may be vomited back up. This is usually not a cause for concern.

Simple nosebleeds can be treated at home.

How To: Stop a Nosebleed

- Tightly squeeze together the two sides of the soft part of the nose, just above the nostrils, below the hard, bony part.
- Apply firm pressure for at least 10 to 15 minutes.
- Because 10 to 15 minutes is a long time, you may want to provide some distraction for your child, such as reading a story or watching a TV program.
- Your child should be sitting with her head tilted forward to avoid blood trickling into the back of her throat.
- She should try not to sniff, pick, or blow her nose for the next few hours.

Prevention

You can often prevent recurrent nosebleeds by keeping the nasal septum moistened with lubricating creams or ointments. If the environment is very dry in your home, you might use a humidifier in your child's bedroom. In recurrent or severe cases, your child's doctor might treat the bleeding areas with cautery, a chemical burning of the bleeding site, to prevent further bleeding episodes.

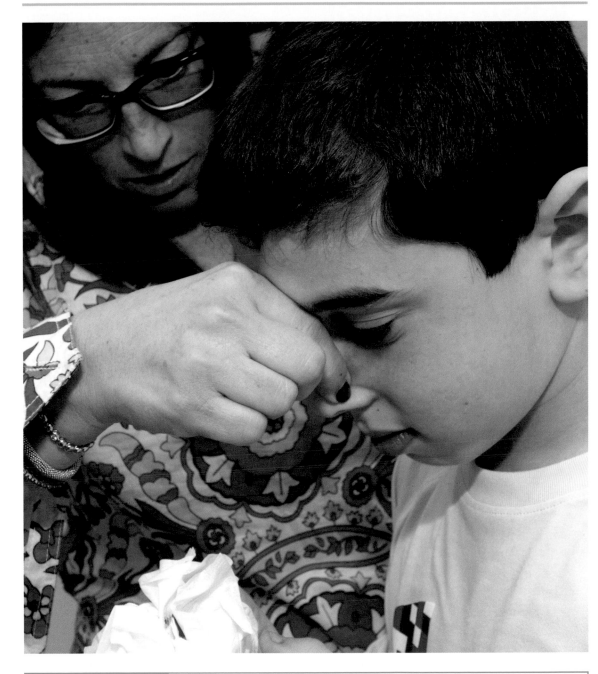

Doc Talk Although nosebleeds may feel frightening, remember that they are common and often completely harmless. The real amount of blood lost is usually much less than it appears. Nosebleeds tend to become less frequent as the child gets older.

Pallor (Anemia)

What Can I Do?

▶ Select iron-rich and enriched foods for your child's diet in consultation with your doctor.

▶ Limit your child's milk intake to 16–20 ounces (475–600 mL) daily, switching from a bottle to a cup.

▶ If your child has a vegan diet, ensure adequate intake of vitamin B_{12}; if you feed your child goat's milk, ensure that he has adequate sources of folic acid.

▶ Give your child an iron supplement if prescribed by your doctor. If your child is truly iron deficient, he will need to continue this for at least 6 months to replenish stores.

❶ What Is Pallor?

Every parent, at some point, thinks that their child appears pale. Sometimes this paleness is related to your child being acutely unwell, in which case his color returns as soon as he begins to feel better.

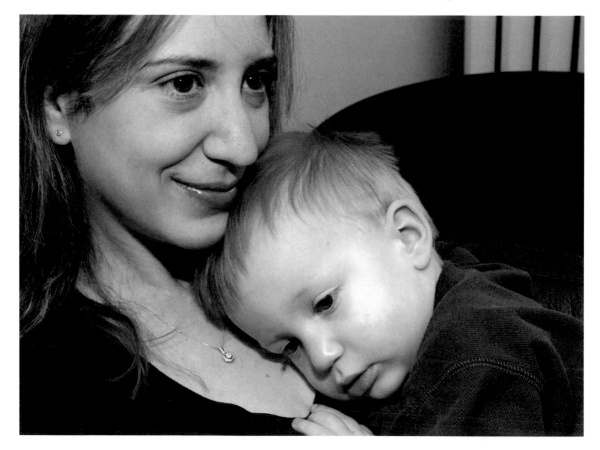

Other times it may just be your genetic makeup — were either you or your child's other parent considered to be pale kids when you were younger?

When should we contact our doctor?

Occasionally, pallor may be a sign of a medical problem called anemia. Anemia can result in many symptoms that will require medical attention. See the red flags below.

▶▶ Anemia Red Flags

Consult your child's doctor if your child has any of the following symptoms associated with pallor:

- Decreased pinkness of the lips, the inner lining of the eyelids, and the nail beds
- Persistent irritability
- Persistent sleepiness (more than usual)
- Dizziness
- Light-headedness
- Rapid heartbeat, especially when resting
- Trouble breathing
- Jaundice (yellow-tinged skin)
- Dark, tea-colored urine

If your child's color doesn't seem to be returning following a period of acute illness, it is important to have him checked by his doctor. If necessary, the doctor can order some blood tests to check for anemia and its different causes.

❷ What Causes Anemia?

Anemia occurs when the amount of hemoglobin in the blood is too low. Hemoglobin is the molecule in the red blood cells that helps deliver oxygen to the body. Anemia results when one of three situations occurs:

- Red blood cells aren't adequately produced.
- Red blood cells are destroyed to quickly (hemolysis).
- Blood is lost from the body.

A B C D E F G H I J K L M N O P Q R S T U V W X Y Z

Iron Deficiency Anemia

Iron, folic acid, and vitamin B_{12} are all essential for the production of hemoglobin in red blood cells. If your child is not getting enough of these in his diet, he could become anemic. Iron deficiency is by far the most common cause of anemia in children. It can affect children at any age, but it is most commonly seen in children younger than 2 years old and in adolescent girls who have started menstruating.

Adequate iron in the diet is crucial, especially for children who are still growing and developing. An anemic child may appear pale and fatigued, and may suffer from behavioral and developmental problems. There is evidence to suggest that iron deficiency during the important years of brain development can lead to permanent loss of points in the child's intelligence quotient (IQ) score.

❸ How Is Iron Deficiency Anemia Treated?

Although iron deficiency is best treated with the guidance of your health-care provider, you can help prevent this problem. Your child will feel better, have more energy, and be less likely to have related problems with his behavior, development, and cognitive function. Treatment often includes ensuring your child's diet has many iron-rich sources, as well as daily supplementation with iron to replenish depleted iron stores.

How To: Prevent Iron Deficiency Anemia

- Exclusively breastfeed your baby for the first 6 months of life. The iron in breast milk, combined with your baby's natural iron reserves, should provide sufficient iron until 6 months of age.
- If you choose to formula-feed, use an iron-fortified formula.
- Introduce iron-rich foods at 6 months of age. By this point, your baby has used up his natural reserves and requires iron from solid foods. As nature would have it, this is also the time when your baby is developmentally ready to start solids!
- Good iron-rich food choices include iron-fortified cereals, puréed meat, fish, tofu, legumes, and eggs.
- Introduce water in a sippy cup to quench your child's thirst with meals. Make the sippy cup available. At first, babies will play with it, but many will begin to drink from it between 6 and 9 months of age. This will prepare them well for the introduction of homogenized cow's milk.

- Introduce homogenized milk at 1 year of age, not earlier. Stick with breast milk or iron-fortified formula until that time.
- Offer milk in a cup, not in a bottle. Research shows that children who drink milk from a bottle are at higher risk for iron deficiency.
- Limit the intake of cow's milk to 16 to 20 ounces (475 to 600 mL) daily.

Iron Supplementation

Many children with iron deficiency will also need an oral iron supplement. If necessary, your doctor will prescribe this for your child and will monitor his progress. In general, your child's hemoglobin will return to normal after 2 months of iron therapy, but the supplements should be continued for at least another 6 months in order to replenish the body's iron stores. While taking iron supplements, your child's bowel movements will often look darker, or even black. This is expected and is harmless — don't be alarmed!

Did You Know?

Milk Interference

Milk can interfere with the absorption of iron; avoid taking iron supplements with a glass of milk!

FAQ

My child is 2 years old and loves her bottle. How can I possibly take it away?

As toddlers grow, they become increasingly stuck in their ways and resistant to change! There are a few different approaches to making the transition from bottle to cup. "Cold turkey" is one approach, which requires strength and determination on the part of the parent or caregiver! Be prepared for a few days of temper tantrums and a decreased intake of fluids (as your toddler refuses the cup). Both behaviors will resolve in time. The cold turkey option is a good one for younger toddlers, around 1 year of age, or for those not too attached. It will, however, prove challenging and may be increasingly difficult as your child gets older.

A gradual transition is more likely to be well accepted by both child and caregiver. Strategies include decreasing the amount of fluid in each bottle and decreasing the number of bottles offered each day; this is done while gradually increasing the presence of a cup. Substituting milk with water in the bottle — and offering milk in a cup — may work as well. Make one change at a time, and wait 3 or 4 days before trying something new. When you're making some progress, involve your child in a ceremony to say good-bye to her bottle, or help her give it to a younger baby, a rite of passage as she is growing up.

Did You Know?

Synergy

Vitamin C can increase the absorption of iron. Encourage your child to consume a citrus fruit or a small glass of 100% fruit juice when taking iron supplements.

FAQs

I'm worried that if I cut my toddler down to 2 cups (500 mL) of milk daily, she won't get enough calcium.

The recommended amount of calcium in the diet is 700 mg daily for children ages 1 to 3 years, 1000 mg daily for ages 4 to 8 years, and 1300 mg daily for ages 9 to 18 years. Given that one 8-ounce (250 mL) cup of milk contains 300 mg of calcium, you will need to pay attention to your child's calcium intake. Supplement milk with other dairy products, such as yogurt and cheese, and encourage the consumption of other calcium-rich foods, such as tofu, broccoli, almonds, and tinned salmon. Most children do not require a calcium supplement, but speak to your doctor if you are concerned.

My child refuses to eat meat. How can I get enough iron into his diet?

Children can be picky! Suggestions for getting a child to eat meat include:

- Serve small portions that are presented in an appealing manner.
- Introduce new foods at the beginning of the meal, when your child is hungry.
- Be a role model, ensuring that your child sees you and the rest of the family eating and enjoying the food.
- Avoid a pushy attitude, but don't give up. Making a fuss will almost certainly prompt your child to dig in his heels and be even more steadfast in his refusal. Be patient, wait a week, and try again.
- If this fails, talk to your doctor about your child's iron intake.

Doc Talk

Most of us were raised to believe that milk is a good thing — milk is chock-a-block full of calcium for strong bones, a good source of protein, and fortified with vitamin D. Indeed, it is important to include milk (or a calcium alternative) as part of a well-balanced diet. Like most good things, though, too much can cause problems. Milk contains minimal iron, so if toddlers fill up on too much milk, they lose their appetite for other iron-rich foods. On top of that, too much milk can actually cause microscopic blood loss from the gut, increasing further the child's risk for iron deficiency.

Penis Problems

What Can I Do?

▶ Don't try to retract a nonretractile foreskin. By the end of the first year of life, about half of all uncircumcised boys will have retractable foreskins, and most will by 4 to 7 years of age.

▶ If any of the red flags develop with the phimosis (nonretractile foreskin), then you will need to seek medical advice.

▶ Teach your child the basics of penis hygiene.

Case Study

Sanjeev's Phimosis

Sanjeev is 2 years old and his parents are concerned because they are unable to fully retract his foreskin to clean it while bathing. During the last couple of weeks, Sanjeev's parents have noticed the foreskin is a bit red, swollen, and irritated. When they took him to their family doctor, he diagnosed Sanjeev as having a normal physiologic phimosis with balanitis, which sounded serious. Their doctor assured them that these conditions were a normal part of growth and advised them not to try to retract Sanjeev's foreskin; the foreskin requires time to naturally separate from the head of the penis.

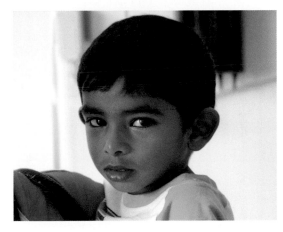

❶ What Is Phimosis (Nonretractile Foreskin)?

There are two types of phimosis: physiologic and pathologic.

Physiologic (Normal) Phimosis

As a fetus develops, the foreskin grows attached to the glans. At birth, many boys will have nonretractile foreskins. This is called physiologic (normal) phimosis because it occurs naturally and is not a medical problem.

RELATED CONDITIONS

- Balanitis
- Balanoposthitis
- Hypospadias
- Paraphimosis
- Phimosis

By the end of the first year of life, about half of all uncircumcised boys will have retractable foreskins, and most will by 4 to 7 years of age. A small percentage, roughly 1% to 2% of boys, will not be able to retract their foreskin until adolescence. This type of phimosis requires no treatment; it will resolve over time.

Phimosis can also occur when the foreskin is too tight and cannot be retracted, closing over the head of the penis. Some boys will have very mild phimosis, whereby the foreskin can be partially retracted; others will have more severe phimosis, where the foreskin is not able to be pulled back at all. Phimosis is most often painless and will usually improve with time.

Pathologic (Abnormal) Phimosis

Pathologic (abnormal) phimosis occurs when the foreskin becomes adherent to the glans from inflammation and scar tissue. This can be a result of poor hygiene, repeated infections, or forceful retraction of a foreskin that doesn't naturally retract.

When should we contact our doctor or local hospital?

Phimosis sounds serious, but in most cases this condition is physiologic and a normal part of growth. Look out for signs that the phimosis may be pathologic (see below).

➤➤ Pathologic Phimosis Red Flags

Consult your child's doctor if your child has any of the following symptoms associated with pathologic phimosis:

- Difficulty initiating the stream of urine
- Pain with peeing
- Ballooning of the foreskin while peeing
- Recurrent infections of the foreskin (see Balanitis, page 299)
- Pain, redness, swelling, or discharge from the penis
- Painful erections
- Bleeding from the tip of the penis
- Recurrent bladder or kidney infections (urinary tract infections)

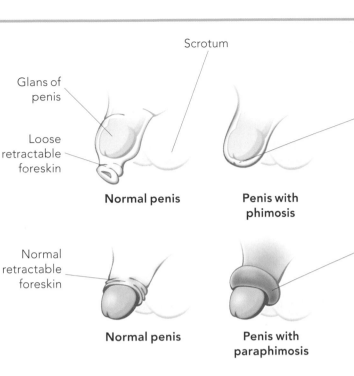

Scrotum

Glans of
penis

Loose
retractable
foreskin

Normal penis

Tight
unretractable
foreskin
adherent to
glans of penis

**Penis with
phimosis**

Normal
retractable
foreskin

Normal penis

Foreskin is
swollen and
cannot be
unretracted

**Penis with
paraphimosis**

❷ How Is Phimosis Treated?

A nonretractile foreskin is normal in young children and does not require medical treatment. Pathologic phimosis with symptoms will require some intervention.

How To: Treat Phimosis at Home

Gently wash the penis and scrotum with mild soap and water when bathing. With a nonretractile foreskin, trying to retract and clean under the foreskin is unnecessary and will only lead to inflammation and scarring.

If symptoms develop into pathological phimosis, your doctor might prescribe a topical steroid ointment to be applied to the tip of the penis twice daily for 4 to 6 weeks. If your child still has persistent or recurrent symptoms related to a phimosis, you might be advised to have him circumcised by a pediatric urologist or general surgeon.

❶ What Are Balanitis and Balanoposthitis?

Balanitis is an infection of the foreskin, and balanoposthitis is an infection of the foreskin and glans (head of the penis). These conditions can occur in children with phimosis and might be related to a difficulty cleaning under the foreskin. Balanitis can also occur as

Did You Know?

Paraphimosis
Paraphimosis occurs when the ring of phimosis tissue is pulled back behind the glans of the penis. This causes very painful swelling. Take your son to the nearest emergency room immediately! If the paraphimosis cannot be corrected, your child might need a surgical procedure to release the constriction.

a reaction to chemicals, for example in detergents or soaps, or due to contact with irritating materials.

FAQ

How should I care for my uncircumcised boy's penis?

Uncircumcised penises require no special care. To keep the area clean:

- Wash the penis and scrotum gently during your son's bath time.
- Avoid pulling back the foreskin; it is often not fully retractile.
- Once the foreskin is fully retractile, often by age 5, teach your son to retract the foreskin, gently wash the glans with mild soap and water, and then replace the foreskin each day while bathing.
- As the foreskin separates from the glans, dead skin cells collect and form white, cheesy lumps called smegma. If present, the smegma can be gently wiped away each day.
- Never forcefully retract an uncircumcised penis. This can lead to inflammation, infection, and scar tissue, turning what was once physiologic phimosis into pathologic phimosis.

Signs and Symptoms of Balanitis and Balanoposthitis

- Discomfort, especially around the tip of the penis
- Itchy penis
- Mild swelling of the tip of the penis
- Discharge from the tip of the penis
- Foreskin is nonretractile (phimosis — see above section)

❷ How Is Balanitis Treated?

If the balanitis is mild, you can try the following at home:

- Warm soaks in the bathtub
- Gentle cleaning of the penis with warm water
- Local antibiotic cream or ointment administered 2 to 3 times daily until symptoms resolve
- Regular, local hygiene with gentle retraction of the foreskin (only if easily retractile!)
- Application of lubricant, such as petroleum jelly, after cleaning — to prevent recurrences
- Avoid bubble baths and scented soaps, which can contribute to irritation
- Provide cotton underwear and ensure detergent has been rinsed out after washing clothes

If these measures fail or the symptoms do not improve within a couple of days, see your child's doctor. He may suggest oral antibiotics or a local steroid ointment. If a boy has recurrent, bothersome episodes, you might be advised to have him circumcised by a pediatric urologist or general surgeon.

❶ What Is Hypospadias?

Hypospadias is a common congenital (present from birth) malformation affecting almost 1% of boys. Rather than the opening of the urinary tract being located at the tip of the penis, it is on the underside.

Signs and Symptoms of Hypospadias

Hypospadias may be discovered as part of the examination of the newborn baby boy. This condition can be minor if the opening is located very close to the tip, or it can be severe if the opening is actually closest to the base of the penis. In hypospadias, part of the foreskin might be absent, forming a "hood" over the end of the penis.

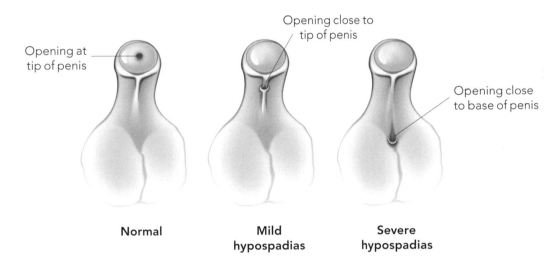

Opening at tip of penis

Opening close to tip of penis

Opening close to base of penis

Normal

Mild hypospadias

Severe hypospadias

Doc Talk The main concern with hypospadias is that it can make it challenging to pee with a direct stream while standing. As a boy gets older, this difference can be socially difficult. In addition, if he has significant chordee, this can have an impact on sexual function and satisfaction. For these reasons, severe hypospadias and chordee are generally repaired. Surgical correction might not be necessary for very minor degrees of hypospadias. Infants with hypospadias should not be circumcised prior to any other surgery because the foreskin is often required to be used as part of the hypospadias repair.

Poisonings and Ingestions

What Can I Do?

▶ Poison-proof your home. Lock poisonous substances in secure cabinets. Keep the phone number of your local poison information center handy.

▶ If you suspect that your child has ingested something toxic, do not hesitate to contact the local poison information center or seek immediate medical attention.

▶ Keep the following information ready for a 911 call: your child's estimated weight, the container or bottle of the product, the time that the child came in contact with the substance, and your name and telephone number.

❶ What Are Poisonings and Ingestions?

Young children and infants are curious little beings! When given the opportunity, they will mouth or eat objects; open containers and pour out, eat, or drink their contents; and get into boxes, drawers, and cupboards you didn't think they even knew about! This curiosity, although a natural and healthy part of a child's development, can be hazardous and even fatal for some children if proper precautions are not taken.

When should we contact our doctor or local hospital?

If you suspect that your child has ingested something toxic, then do not hesitate to contact the local poison information center or seek immediate medical attention. Keep the phone number of your local poison information center handy.

➤ Poisoning Red Flags

If your child is unconscious, having convulsions, or having difficulty swallowing or breathing, call 911.

Signs and Symptoms of Poisoning

- Clues or evidence of ingestion (for example, an open medicine container or household product) near the child

- A burn, stain, or discoloration around the mouth
- Sleepiness or unusual crankiness
- Vomiting or severe tummy pains
- Drooling or difficulty swallowing
- Unusual smell on breath
- Difficulty breathing
- Convulsions or loss of consciousness

Common Household Poisons

- Medicines (prescription and over-the-counter)
- Vitamins and herbal remedies (for example, iron and vitamin A)
- Household cleaners (for example, bleach, ammonia, and oven cleaner)
- Cosmetics (for example, nail polish, toothpaste, mouthwash, and perfume)
- Plants and garden products (for example, pesticides, berries, and houseplants)
- Alcohol
- Car products (for example, antifreeze and gasoline)

❷ How Is Poisoning Treated?

For All Suspected Poisonings

- Avoid exposing yourself to the poison — through touching, breathing, or ingesting.

For Suspected Swallowing of a Poisonous Substance

- Give small sips of water to the child.
- If there is still something in his mouth, then get him to spit it out or remove it yourself.
- Keep any material that is removed, spat out, or vomited. It may be of help later.
- Do not give him anything to make him vomit (for example, ipecac); caustic material can cause damage on the way back up.
- Call your local poison control center.

For Suspected Poison Exposure to the Eyes

- Pour lukewarm water over the eyes while trying to keep them open for at least 10 minutes.
- Call your local poison control center.

For Suspected Poison Exposure to the Skin

- Remove all clothing exposed to the poisonous substance.
- Rinse the area with lukewarm water for 10 to 15 minutes.
- Call your local poison control center.

Home Safety Do's and Don'ts

Do

- Keep medicines stored in bottles with child-resistant caps, but remember that some children can still open them.
- Store medicines in locked or inaccessible cabinets — including vitamins and herbal medicines that contain compounds like iron.
- Install safety latches on cupboards.
- Leave medicines and other products in their original containers — a child might think antifreeze stored in a pop bottle is pop!
- Teach children the meaning of warning labels (for example, poison, corrosive, explosive, and flammable).
- Learn the names of poisonous houseplants and what they look like. Do not keep them in your home.
- Read labels before using poisonous products (for example, oven cleaner and pesticide).
- Keep the number of your local poison information center handy.

Don't

- Call medicines "candy" or make a game out of taking medicine.
- Take your medicine in front of small children — they might imitate you!
- Give your child medicine that was prescribed for someone else.
- Leave any car, home, or garden products in containers that are unmarked or in unlocked areas of the garage, shed, or basement.

Key to warning labels

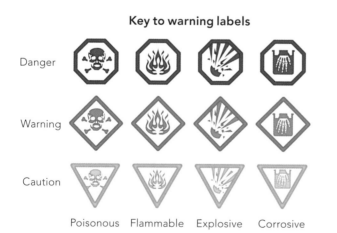

	Poisonous	Flammable	Explosive	Corrosive
Danger				
Warning				
Caution				

Doc Talk   Medicines, both prescription and over-the-counter, are the most common causes of poisoning in infants and young children. Some children can open child-resistant caps, so do not rely on this method of safety! Keep all medicines locked away.

Precocious Puberty

What Can I Do?

▶ Discuss with your doctor any signs of puberty before the age of 7 years in girls and 9 years in boys.

▶ If your child has signs of precocious puberty and develops significant headaches, vomiting or changes in vision, seek urgent medical attention.

▶ If no cause for the precocious puberty is found, weigh the risks and benefits of taking medications to stop the progression of puberty, in consultation with your doctor.

▶ Help your child to cope with any teasing or bullying she may receive as a result of precocious puberty.

Case Study

Janet's Precocious Puberty

Janet is 3 years old. Lately, her mother has noticed that her breasts are getting bigger. She has been very healthy and seems to be about the same height and weight as most of her friends at daycare. She has been doing well socially, and she is meeting all of her expected developmental milestones. Her mother asked their family doctor if this symptom was normal. The family doctor asked whether there were any other signs of early puberty, such as body odor or pubic or underarm hair. A careful look (and smell!) revealed that these were not present.

When Janet went to see her doctor, she was checked thoroughly for other signs of puberty and for the red flags that would point to a need for more extensive tests.

Thankfully, Janet's bone age was normal, based on an X-ray of her wrist compared to a normal wrist X-ray for a 3-year-old. She had no red flags or other signs of puberty. She was diagnosed with premature thelarche (breast development). Her doctor told Janet's mother that absolutely no treatment was needed at this time. However, Janet would need to return every 3 to 6 months to be reassessed for any signs that she may, in fact, be progressing into puberty and to confirm that her premature breast development was not a sign of another condition.

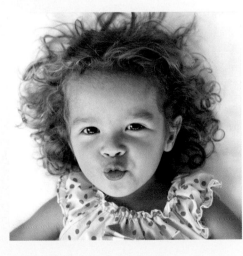

❶ What Is Precocious Puberty?

Although puberty begins at varying ages for both boys and girls, pubertal changes can begin before the typical age. Puberty that starts before 7 years of age in girls (or before 6 years of age in Black girls) and 9 years in boys is called precocious puberty. Early puberty is more commonly seen in girls.

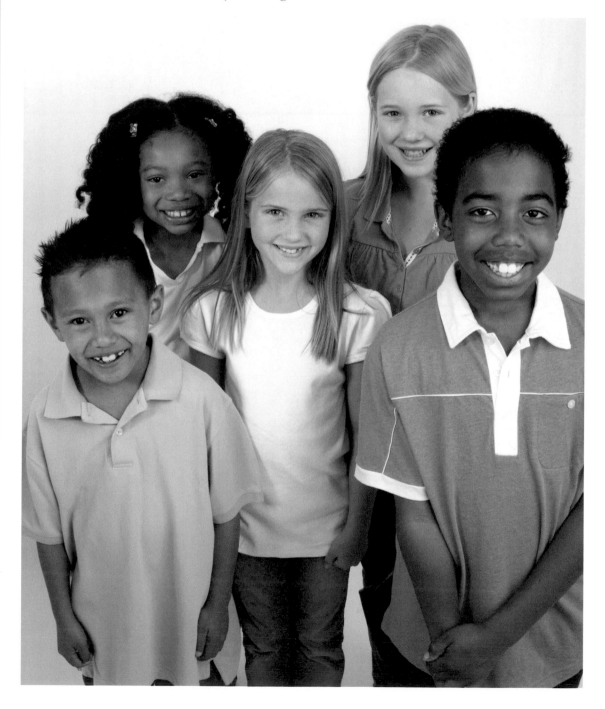

Demographics

Normal puberty is starting earlier than it did in prior generations. On average, it starts about 5 months earlier now than it did 30 or 40 years ago. Obesity and genetic factors are two of the causes of earlier puberty. Normal puberty begins earlier in some ethnic groups and in some families. Girls of Black and Hispanic descent, for instance, generally experience puberty earlier than girls of Caucasian or Asian descent.

Signs and Symptoms of Precocious Puberty

Girls (Prior to Age 7 Years)	Boys (Prior to Age 9 Years)
• Is there breast development? • Is there body odor? • Is there facial acne? • Is there pubic hair? • Is there underarm hair? • Has there been a growth spurt? • Is there discharge from the vagina?	• Is there enlargement of the testicles? • Is there body odor? • Is there enlargement of the penis? • Is there pubic hair? • Is there underarm hair? • Is there facial hair? • Is there facial acne? • Is there a deepening of the voice? • Has there been a growth spurt?

When should we contact our doctor?

Precocious puberty is not an emergency condition, but discuss any early changes you see with your doctor. Urgent attention is required for any of the red flags below in combination with early puberty.

▶▶ Precocious Puberty Red Flags

Consult your child's doctor if your child has any of the following symptoms accompanying the signs of precocious puberty:

- Severe headaches
- Vomiting
- Changes in vision
- Seizures
- Pubertal changes usually only seen in the opposite sex (for example, voice deepening in a girl)

❷ What Causes Precocious Puberty?

- In most cases of precocious puberty, the brain sets the normal process of puberty in motion earlier than usual for no known reason. This is by far the most common cause, especially in girls.
- An injury, infection, or tumor in the brain can jumpstart the process, causing early puberty.
- Increased levels of hormones that are being abnormally produced by the testicles, ovaries, or adrenal glands can set off precocious puberty.
- Brief increases in estrogen from the ovaries can cause breast development in toddlers or young girls without other signs of puberty. This resolves on its own and is not serious.
- The use of certain medications, creams, or supplements may cause precocious puberty.

❸ How Is Precocious Puberty Treated?

Often, isolated breast development with no other signs of puberty (as with Janet's case) will be monitored periodically by the doctor but will not need treatment.

Bone Development

Children who are showing signs of more pubertal changes should be treated to prevent their bones from finishing their growth too quickly due to premature closure of their growth plates. This is especially true if puberty starts very early.

Medications

These hormone-like drugs are given by injection. They prevent the release of the sex hormones in the body. Not all children require treatment — this is usually a decision made by the family and the doctor together. Your child will need to be closely monitored, with regular examinations, blood tests, and bone-age assessment.

Did You Know?

Tanner Staging
Physicians will evaluate the degree of puberty using a system called Tanner staging. This will make re-evaluating puberty easier at each visit. Previous height measurements are important to assess the pace of growth, which can increase with puberty. Children who have precocious puberty may grow quickly early on, but may stop growing because the bones mature too early.

Did You Know?

Social Stigma
There can be social consequences to early puberty. Children may get teased, or they may be treated as if they were older because of their advanced sexual maturity.

Doc Talk Children with precocious puberty who do not need treatment still need regular evaluation by a doctor. Treatment depends on the cause of the problem. If a cause for the precocious puberty is found, it needs to be treated accordingly. If no cause is found (idiopathic precocious puberty), your child can take medications to stop the progression of puberty, if appropriate.

Rashes in Newborns

What Can I Do?

▶ Be reassured that most infant rashes resolve on their own and don't need medical attention.

▶ If your baby has a fever, seems unwell, is hard to console, and/or is not feeding appropriately, then you should seek medical advice. These may be signs that you are not dealing with a simple newborn rash.

▶ As she grows older, your child will likely encounter more rashes. See Rashes in Children (page 312) for more information on these other rashes.

When should we contact our doctor?

Newborns can be affected by a number of different skin changes or rashes in the first month of life. Most are harmless and resolve on their own, but in some cases medical attention is needed. See the red flags below.

➤➤ Newborn Rash Red Flags

Consult your child's doctor if your child has any of the following symptoms accompanying the skin rash:

- ▪ Fever
- ▪ Looks unwell
- ▪ Inconsolable (cannot settle her down)
- ▪ Not feeding normally (too sleepy to feed or disinterested in feeding)

Baby Acne

Believe it or not, babies can get pimples too! These little red bumps with yellowish centers usually show up in the first weeks of life and disappear, without scarring, on their own within a few months. As with teenage acne, the cheeks, nose, and forehead are most commonly affected. No treatment is required.

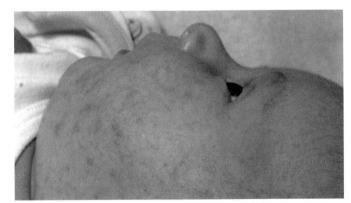
Baby acne

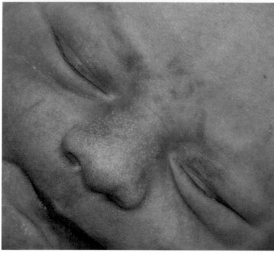

Milia

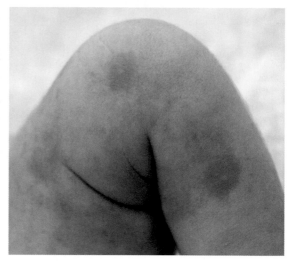

Erythema toxicum

Milia

Milia are tiny white bumps on the skin. They are most prominent over the bridge of the nose and on the cheeks. They are small cysts containing keratin (fibrous proteins from the outer skin layer). Milia appear on a newborn's face during the first few weeks of life. These are completely harmless and go away on their own within weeks to months.

Pearls

A baby can also have milia on the roof of her mouth. These are called Epstein's pearls when found in the mouth. In the same manner as milia in the skin, they are harmless and disappear on their own.

Miliaria

Also known as heat rash or prickly heat, these reddish bumps and blotches usually appear on areas that tend to be covered and therefore get sweaty, such as the upper back, chest, and neck. To prevent heat rash, avoid over-bundling your baby or exposing her to excessive heat and humidity. Cotton clothing allows heat and moisture to escape more easily.

Erythema Toxicum

Contrary to the name of this condition, this extremely common rash is by no means toxic! Often noted in the first few days of life, this rash presents as red, flat blotches with tiny white or yellow pustules (pus-filled bumps) in the center. You may see just a few spots or several over your baby's body. They come and go in different areas, almost before your eyes. No treatment is needed.

Cradle Cap

Cradle cap, also known as seborrheic dermatitis, is an oily, scaly, or crusting rash that affects the scalp in the first months of life. Occasionally it can extend to involve the forehead, eyebrows, neck, and around the ears. Cradle cap results from build-up of sebum (an oily substance produced by the body to lubricate the skin and hair); it is not caused by poor hygiene! Babies are typically not bothered by it, nor is it harmful.

The scales will often fall off on their own. If persistent, mineral or baby oil can be applied and left on 30 minutes before bath time, and this will soften the crust, allowing for easy removal during the bath. In very few cases, a medicated lotion, shampoo, or cream may be required.

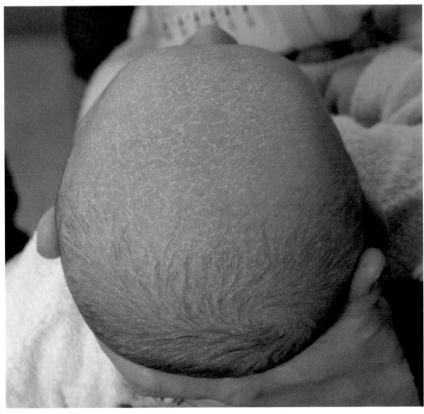

Cradle cap

> **Doc Talk** Rashes seem to be attracted to babies like magnets and cause no end of concern for parents. In most cases these skin conditions will resolve on their own. If you are concerned or your child has any red flag symptoms, then it is time to see your doctor.

Rashes in Children

What Can I Do?

▶ Recognize that many reddish, generalized nonspecific rashes are part of the common viral infections that children often pick up in their preschool years. Use acetaminophen or ibuprofen for high fevers or general discomfort that may accompany a viral infection.

▶ Moisturize the skin to manage eczema effectively.

▶ Keep your eyes open for the red flag symptoms accompanying eczema and hives that require urgent medical attention.

▶ If you want to avoid the chicken pox rash and its potential complications, get your child immunized.

RELATED CONDITIONS

- Chicken pox
- Eczema
- Hives
- Impetigo
- Molluscum contagiosum
- Ringworm

❶ What Is a Rash?

Rashes are one of the most common reasons for a child to be brought to the doctor. Often, a child will be suffering from a fever due to a viral infection and will develop a nonspecific reddish, generalized rash. These viral rashes do not require any treatment and usually go away along with the infection. But there are other kinds of rashes too.

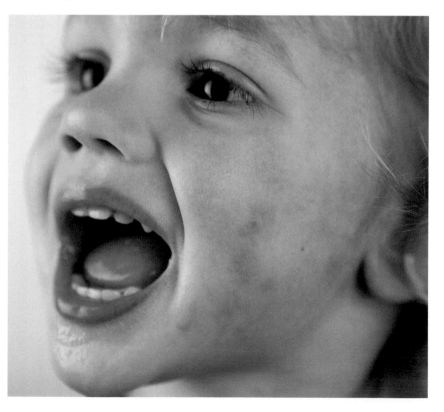

Common Childhood Rashes

Condition	Symptoms/Location	Appearance
Eczema	• Appears on cheeks in babies; appears inside of elbows and knees in older children • Itchy	• Scaly • Dry • Red
Hives (urticaria)	• Rash moves around • Usually itchy	• Pink, red, or white welts
Impetigo	• Appears around mouth and nose	• Honey-colored crusts
Molluscum contagiosum	• Appears on any part of the body	• Flesh-colored, dome-shaped bumps • Bumps have a central dimple
Chicken pox	• Very itchy • Fever • Headache • Aches and pains	• Small water blisters
Fungal infection (for example, ringworm, tinea)	• Usually itchy	• Ring-shaped • Pink, slightly raised border with pale center

❶ What Is Eczema (Atopic Dermatitis)?

Eczema, or atopic dermatitis, is a chronic, very common skin rash, affecting up to 20% of children. Children with eczema often have patches of dry, red, scaly, and very itchy skin. In babies, these patches are usually seen on the cheeks and the arms and legs, whereas in children, the rash is most common in the inner creases of the elbows and behind the knees. Children with more severe eczema might have more widespread areas of redness, crusting, and even bleeding due to scratching and skin breakdown. If your child has been scratching a particular area for a long time, the skin will become rough and thickened. Classically, the severity will fluctuate over time.

❷ What Causes Eczema?

We do not know exactly what causes eczema. Several factors, including genetics and the environment, play a role. Children with allergies (see Allergies and Food Intolerances, page 41 and Allergic Rhinitis, page 38), and asthma (see Wheezing, page 428) tend to be predisposed to eczema.

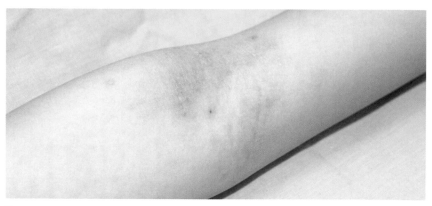

Eczema

Common Eczema Triggers

- Hot, humid weather
- Dry, cold temperatures
- Irritants on the skin (wool, excessive use of soap)
- Inhaled allergens (pollens in the spring, strong perfumes)

When should we contact our doctor or local hospital?

Eczema is a chronic problem that flares up from time to time. If your regular strategies are not working or if any of the red flag symptoms appear, see your doctor. Medicated ointment should get the flare-up under control fairly quickly.

⏵ Eczema Red Flags

Consult your child's doctor if your child has any of the following symptoms associated with her eczema:

- Extensive nighttime scratching that leads to poor sleep.
- Extensive crusting, blisters, weeping sores, or pus-like discharge from the skin. These are signs of infection and your child may need topical or oral antibiotics.
- Widespread redness and eczema over the whole body. This indicates poorly controlled eczema. If the redness is fairly sudden and/or your child has a fever, this might indicate a skin infection.

❸ How Is Eczema Treated?

Unfortunately, there is no cure for eczema. Current therapies are directed at controlling the disease to make it more manageable.

Approximately 60% of people who have eczema develop signs of this condition in the first year of life. Although eczema resolves by school age in about 50% of these cases, 25% of individuals continue to be affected into adulthood. Fortunately, the severity of disease often improves as a child ages.

There are a number of ways you can treat your child's eczema at home.

- *Avoid potential allergens and irritants:* Avoid harsh soaps, bleaches, fabric softener, bubble baths, and wool clothing.
- *Exercise environmental control:* Use a humidifier in dry environments, and keep your child's room temperature cool during both winter and summer months.
- *Bathe frequently:* Short (5 to 10 minutes) baths, once or twice daily, in lukewarm (not hot!) water improves the moisture of the skin.
- *Use oils in the bath:* Add a few drops of an emulsifying oil (for example, Aveeno, Alpha Keri oil, or Oilatum) to each bath to help hydrate the skin.
- *Moisturize, moisturize, moisturize!* Use a moisturizing ointment such as petroleum jelly (Vaseline) several times daily to help trap water into the skin. Ointments work better than creams, which work better than lotions, to retain moisture.
- *Limit scratching:* Skin breakdown from scratching leaves the skin even more irritated and itchy. It also promotes infection. An oral antihistamine, such as diphenhydramine (Benadryl) or hydroxyzine (Atarax), can reduce itchiness, especially at night. Keep fingernails trimmed to limit skin breakdown.
- *Treat skin inflammation:* Use topical steroid ointments on the inflamed and itchy areas. Application of medicated ointments 2 or 3 times daily is often necessary to get the inflammation under control.

❶ What Are Hives?

Hives, or urticaria, are raised welts on the skin. They appear pink, red, or white but blanch when you put pressure on them. Hives can range in size from $\frac{1}{2}$ inch (1 cm) to giant hives that can cover an entire extremity. They are often, though not always, itchy. Hives can be present on any part of the body, and they tend to move around. Each single lesion doesn't stay in the same place for more than 24 hours.

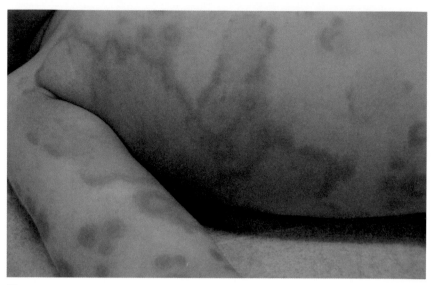

Hives

❷ What Causes Hives?

- Allergic reactions
- Viral infections
- Physical stimuli (cold, sunlight)
- Most causes are unknown

❸ How Are Hives Treated?

Most hives can be treated with an antihistamine, available without prescription — for example, diphenhydramine (Benadryl). If your child has a known cause for her hives, such as an allergy to a food, avoidance of the trigger is necessary. If you suspect an allergy, testing can be arranged through your health-care provider (see Allergies and Food Intolerances, page 41).

▶▶ Hives Red Flags

Consult your child's doctor if your child has any of the following symptoms associated with her hives:

- Hives that last for more than 6 weeks
- Hives in a newborn
- Hives that stay in one place for more than 24 to 48 hours, leaving a purplish color behind

❶ What Is Impetigo (Bacterial Skin Infection)?

Impetigo is a very common bacterial skin infection, most often affecting preschool and school-age children. It is a contagious condition and spreads easily.

❷ What Causes Impetigo?

Impetigo is caused by streptococcal bacteria. It typically occurs when the skin is broken down by insect bites or scrapes and the bacteria enter the body, but it can occur on normal skin as well. It is more common in the summertime.

Impetigo often starts out as a small bump around the mouth or nose. The bumps can be itchy and sore, leading to frequent picking and scratching. Impetigo is recognized by the location of the sores and by the pus and scabs that develop over the bumps. These reddish lesions can also ooze a honey-colored material that typically dries up and leaves a very characteristic crust behind.

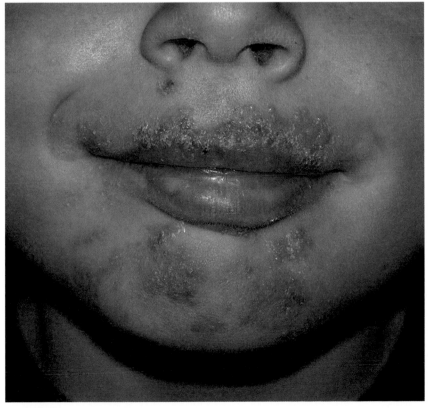

Impetigo

❸ How Is Impetigo Treated?

If the bacterial infection is mild (1 or 2 small bumps), an antibiotic ointment may be sufficient. With more extensive infections, an oral antibiotic, lasting 7 to 10 days, may be used.

How To: Treat Impetigo at Home

- Trim your child's nails to reduce irritation and local spreading.
- Impetigo is extremely contagious — avoid sharing washcloths or towels while infected.
- If the spots are extensive, children should not go to school or daycare for at least 24 hours after antibiotic treatment has been started.

❶ What Is Molluscum Contagiosum?

Molluscum contagiosum is a common contagious viral infection of the skin. It is most often seen in children between 2 and 5 years old. Molluscum contagiosum can present as a single bump or multiple shiny, flesh-colored, dome-shaped little bumps with a central dimple. These can be found on any part of the body.

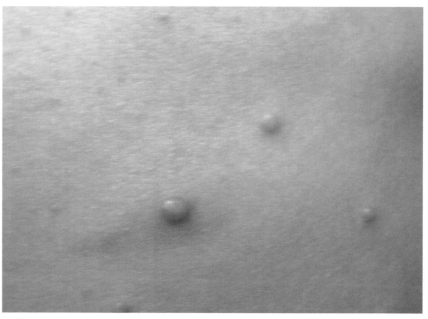

Molluscum contagiosum

❷ What Causes Molluscum Contagiosum?

Transmission occurs by contact with someone else who has the virus. Once a child has molluscum contagiosum, the infection spreads to other parts of the body by scratching existing lesions and then touching other parts of the skin. This is called auto-inoculation.

❸ How Is Molluscum Contagiosum Treated?

Molluscum contagiosum lesions often go away on their own, almost always without scarring. This can take several months. Other options for treatment involve a trip to the dermatologist (skin specialist) and can include curettage (scraping off the molluscum) or applying medicated irritants to the skin.

❶ What Is Chicken Pox (Varicella Virus)?

This infection, caused by the varicella virus, used to be contracted by almost all children until the chicken pox vaccine was developed. Ever since immunization programs have been in place, the numbers of cases have dropped dramatically.

Children with chicken pox often get a fever, headache, and muscle aches, followed by a very itchy rash. The red spots quickly become small water blisters that come out in crops over the course of a few days. They usually dry up to form scabs within 4 to 5 days.

❷ What Causes Chicken Pox?

Chicken pox is very contagious. If one child in the home gets the virus, it will usually spread to all the others who live there. Most daycare centers require children to stay at home until the last blisters have scabbed. Children are usually contagious from about 2 days before the rash appears until about 5 days after the rash has appeared.

Did You Know?

Chicken Pox Immunity

In most cases, people who have been immunized or people who have had chicken pox will not get chicken pox again. These individuals develop long-term immunity against the virus. In the rare case where a person develops the rash a second time or after immunizations, the illness is much less severe, with significantly less spots.

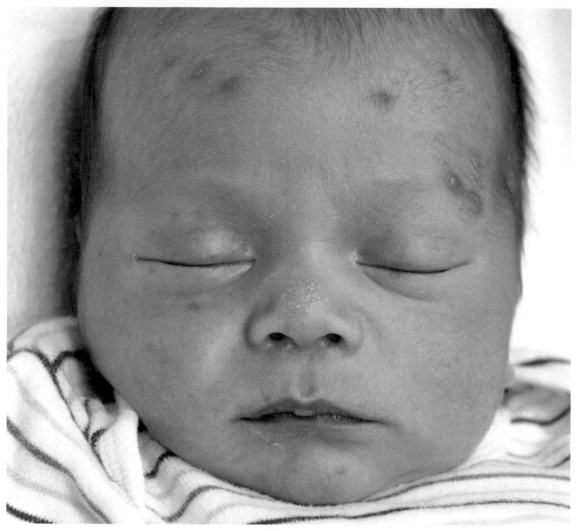

Chicken pox

❸ How Is Chicken Pox Treated?

The best treatment for chicken pox is prevention by immunizing against the virus. But if your child does develop symptoms, try the following:

- Administer acetaminophen or ibuprofen for aches and fever.
- Administer oral antihistamines and provide soothing oatmeal baths to relieve the itch.
- Keep nails short to minimize trauma from scratching.
- Keep an eye on the blisters to look for local skin infection. Redness, warmth, and swelling of a blister or a crop of lesions warrants assessment by a health-care provider.

❶ What Is Ringworm (Tinea)?

Ringworm is a fungal infection. On the body it is called tinea corporis; on the head it is called tinea capitis; and on the feet it is called tinea pedis (or athlete's foot). The infection appears as ring-shaped patches (hence the name of the condition) that are slightly raised and pink, with a clear center. The rash is usually itchy. On the scalp, hair tends to fall out, leaving little black dots of broken hairs.

❷ What Causes Ringworm?

Ringworm is caused by a fungus that is most commonly acquired from contact with a puppy or kitten, though human-to-human transmission is also common.

❸ How Is Ringworm Treated?

For the body and feet, topical antifungals, such as clotrimazole (Lotrimin) or tolnaftate (Tinactin), available without prescription, are effective. These creams should be used for 3 to 4 weeks and continued for a week beyond the disappearance of the rash. If the nails or scalp are infected, see your health-care provider for treatment with oral antifungals.

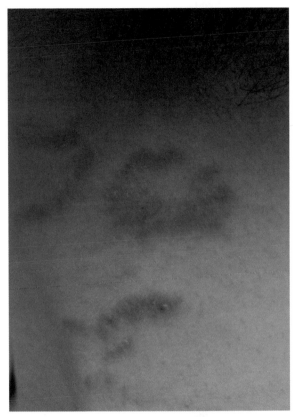

Ringworm

Doc Talk

A relatively common challenge for doctors is knowing how to manage the child with fever who has been started on an antibiotic and then develops a reddish nonspecific skin rash. Is the rash part of the natural course of the underlying viral infection that was causing the fever in the first place? Or is it an allergic reaction to the antibiotic prescribed? Sometimes it is impossible to distinguish. One of the solutions is to try not to prescribe antibiotic therapy for viral sore throats or other fevers unless there is a clear bacterial cause, for example a positive throat swab for strep.

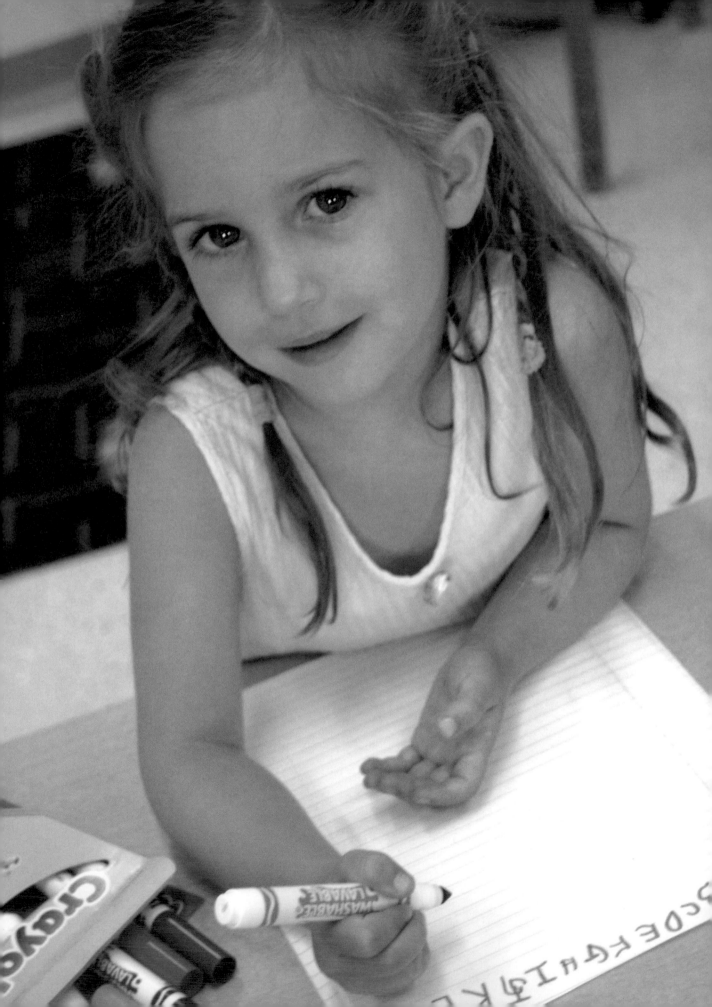

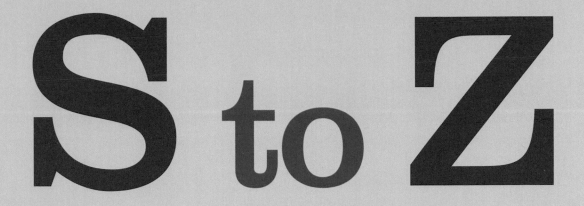

S to Z

School Phobia and School Avoidance

What Can I Do?

▶ If your child refuses to go to school because of frequent vague physical symptoms, consider a school phobia. You may notice these complaints occur only on school days.

▶ Support and believe your child. The underlying stressors causing the symptoms need to be addressed.

▶ Transition your child back to school as soon as possible. The longer the absence, the harder it will be for him to return.

❶ What Is a School Phobia or School Avoidance?

Children often complain about having to go to school, at least some of the time. Parents expect those comments and should view them as normal. Sometimes, instead of the occasional complaint about attending class, a child will either refuse to attend school or create reasons not to go. This is called school avoidance. It's a common problem, occurring in approximately 5% of school-age children. The term "school phobia" refers to a real anxiety about attending school and falls in the spectrum of school avoidance.

Signs and Symptoms of School Phobia

- Frequent school absences for extensive periods of time.
- Complaints of various, vague physical symptoms (such as abdominal pain, nausea, or headaches) that are actually related to stress or anxiety. The child is usually unaware of what is truly making him feel unwell, and he may be unable to label his feelings or understand and articulate the cause.
- Symptoms occur on school days and improve on weekends.
- Symptoms that would accompany significant medical illnesses — such as weight loss, fever, and vomiting — are absent.
- When you seek medical attention for your child, it becomes evident that the pattern of symptoms and the physical examination findings do not fit with the severity of symptoms described.

❷ What Causes School Phobia or School Avoidance?

School phobia or avoidance results from anxiety or stress related to attending school. Young children might not find the class environment is as secure and loving as at home. In some situations, it is related to a recent loss of a family member, or there is conflict between family members in the home. Your child's reluctance to attend school might be due to difficulty with schoolwork. Teasing or bullying sometimes leads to school phobia or avoidance, and sometimes no clear explanation for the child's anxiety can be found.

❸ How Are School Phobia and School Avoidance Treated?

School phobia and avoidance can be difficult problems to solve and require patience and perseverance.

Steps for Managing School Avoidance

❶ Obtain a medical assessment to ensure there is no underlying physical illness.

❷ Once physical illness has been ruled out, explore with your doctor the underlying reasons for the school avoidance.

❸ Engage the whole family, school personnel, and health-care professionals to develop a transition-to-school plan that makes sense for your individual child. In many cases, an immediate return to full-time school attendance can be accomplished; in other situations, a more graduated return is required.

❹ Remain firm in helping your child, who will likely continue to complain about symptoms upon his return to school.

| Doc Talk | Just like adults who feel true pain with their stress headaches, children with these symptoms are not "faking" their pain; rather, they generally truly feel unwell. In some cases, the symptoms can be quite severe and cause you, and even your doctor, concern that a medical diagnosis is being missed. Eventually, with appropriate exploration of psychosocial stressors, the underlying issues causing the symptoms may be found. |

Scrotum Pain and Swelling

What Can I Do?

▶ Minor trauma to the scrotum is not uncommon, especially in sports, and can be very painful. The discomfort should settle fairly quickly within minutes. If it doesn't or the scrotum swells up, then seek medical attention.

▶ Most painless swellings are not urgent, but sudden or severe pain is a medical emergency. See your doctor to rule out a testicular torsion or incarcerated hernia.

Case Study

Samuel's Scrotal Mass

Samuel was seen by his family doctor at 2 months of age for a checkup. His parents reported he has been growing and developing well but that they have noticed a persistent bulge in his left scrotum. They report the bulge is relatively unchanged since birth and it doesn't seem to bother Sam. Their doctor reviewed her notes from previous visits and confirmed that this bulge has been present since birth. When she examines Sam, he has a moderate-sized left scrotal mass. It is relatively smooth, non-tender, and soft. She shines a light through it and it lights up. When she gently compresses it, she can feel both testicles.

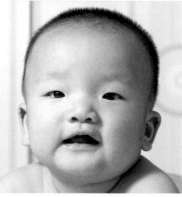

At his 6-month checkup, his doctor notes again that the scrotal mass is unchanged or perhaps even slightly smaller than in previous examinations. Sam's parents report it does not seem to change in size with coughing or crying, or when Sam is having a bowel movement. It continues to be painless. Their doctor explains that this is a noncommunicating hydrocele that Sam was born with. It will likely disappear on its own by 12 months of age as the fluid naturally reabsorbs. This condition needs no treatment.

❶ What Is the Scrotum?

The scrotum is a skin sac beneath the penis that contains the most important structures involved in puberty and, eventually, sexual function. It contains two testicles, a system of related ducts called the epididymis, the tube that carries the sperm to the penis (the vas deferens), and the blood supply (arteries and veins).

➤➤ Scrotum Red Flags

Seek immediate medical attention if your child has any of the following symptoms associated with a swollen scrotum:

- Sudden onset scrotal pain on one side of the scrotum can indicate a serious problem.
- A suddenly swollen or tender scrotum may indicate that there is torsion of the testicle.
- A painful swelling in the groin that extends toward the scrotum may be an incarcerated hernia in which the bowel has become trapped.

❷ What Causes Scrotal Pain and Swelling?

A variety of conditions can cause a boy's scrotum to enlarge or be painful. To determine the cause of the problem, it is important to distinguish between situations in which there is pain (with or without swelling) versus those in which there is painless swelling.

The major causes of scrotal pain are: the mechanical twisting of the testicle (testicular torsion) or infections of the structures inside the scrotum (orchitis and epididymitis). These conditions require medical attention.

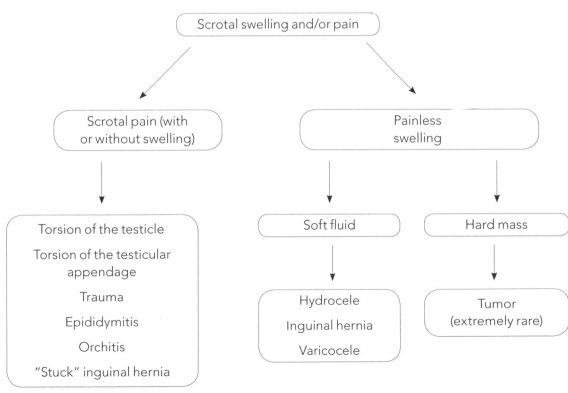

Scrotal swelling and/or pain

Scrotal pain (with or without swelling)
- Torsion of the testicle
- Torsion of the testicular appendage
- Trauma
- Epididymitis
- Orchitis
- "Stuck" inguinal hernia

Painless swelling

Soft fluid
- Hydrocele
- Inguinal hernia
- Varicocele

Hard mass
- Tumor (extremely rare)

A B C D E F G H I J K L M N O P Q R S T U V W X Y Z

Testicular Torsion

This occurs when the spermatic cord twists tightly, interfering with the blood supply to the testicle. This twisting can most commonly occur in newborns (in the first month of life) or in early puberty. In the older age group, sudden severe testicular pain is present, often with nausea or vomiting. Initially, there is swelling and, later, redness of the scrotum.

▶▶ Testicular Torsion Red Flags

- Torsion of the testicle is a medical emergency.
- A child with suspected testicular torsion should be taken immediately to an emergency department, where the diagnosis can be confirmed by physical examination and a specialized ultrasound test. In order to save the testicle, surgery is required as soon as possible, ideally within 6 hours.

Trauma

As most boys eventually find out at one time or another, a hit to the scrotum can produce pain, even when the force of impact is relatively low. Pain resulting from trauma is usually transient and subsides in a few minutes. However, if the discomfort persists or significant swelling occurs, a medical evaluation is indicated.

Epididymitis

This is the name for inflammation of the epididymis, a tubular structure attached to the testicle. Epididymitis can be associated with a bladder infection or due to a viral illness. In teenagers, epididymitis may be the result of sexually transmitted infections. The symptoms of epididymitis may include painful or frequent urination, followed by increasing scrotal discomfort. The scrotum may appear swollen or red. Because epididymitis can look like testicular torsion, these symptoms should prompt medical evaluation. However, unlike testicular torsion, epididymitis does not require surgery and is treated with pain relievers and antibiotics.

Inguinal Hernias

Occasionally these hernias can become "stuck" and lead to a painful swelling in the groin and scrotum. However, inguinal hernias usually cause painless swelling. See Inguinal Hernia (page 330).

Did You Know?

Testicular Torsion Surgery

A surgeon performs a special procedure to fix the testicle to the inside of the scrotum in the proper position. Having the surgery performed within 6 hours of the onset of symptoms gives the highest chance that the testicle will retain its sperm-producing function.

Torsion of the Testicular Appendage

A small structure related to the testicle, called the testicular appendix, can also twist on its stalk. When this happens, the situation is called torsion of the testicular appendage. Boys aged 7 to 11 years (prepubertal) are most likely to be affected. They will have pain, but it is not as severe or rapid in onset as the pain of testicular torsion. Although swelling and redness of the scrotum eventually may appear, initially there may only be a blue dot of discoloration apparent beneath the scrotal skin. The symptoms settle down after about a week, during which time rest and pain relievers will help. It may take a little longer for the swelling to completely subside.

❶ What Is Painless Scrotal Swelling?

To understand the cause of a boy's painless scrotal swelling, it is useful to separate soft fluid swellings (typically a hydrocele, varicocele, or hernia) from firm, solid masses.

❷ What Causes Swollen Painless Scrotum?

Hydrocele

A hydrocele is a collection of fluid surrounding the testicle. Hydroceles are quite common in early infancy. Usually, these swellings disappear spontaneously in the first year of life. However, if they persist beyond about 2 years of age, they may be treated by a simple surgical procedure.

Did You Know?

Orchitis
This is an infection or inflammation of the testicle itself. It often happens in conjunction with — and for the same reasons as — epididymitis, but can sometimes occur on its own, often involving both testicles at the same time. The treatment of orchitis is similar to that for epididymitis.

Did You Know?

Most Common Cause
Hydrocele is the most common cause of scrotal swelling in little boys in the first year of life.

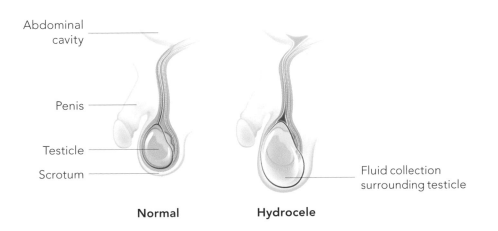

Abdominal cavity

Penis

Testicle

Scrotum

Fluid collection surrounding testicle

Normal   **Hydrocele**

Inguinal Hernia

In an infant, this involves the appearance of a soft bulge in the groin or a scrotal swelling. This is created when a loop of bowel enters the groin or scrotum through an opening that did not fully close during the baby's development in the womb. A physician's examination is required to distinguish an inguinal hernia from a hydrocele or undescended testicle in an infant. An inguinal hernia is usually a painless swelling, but if the bowel gets stuck ("incarcerated"), it can make the scrotum feel hard, tender, and painful. All hernias in

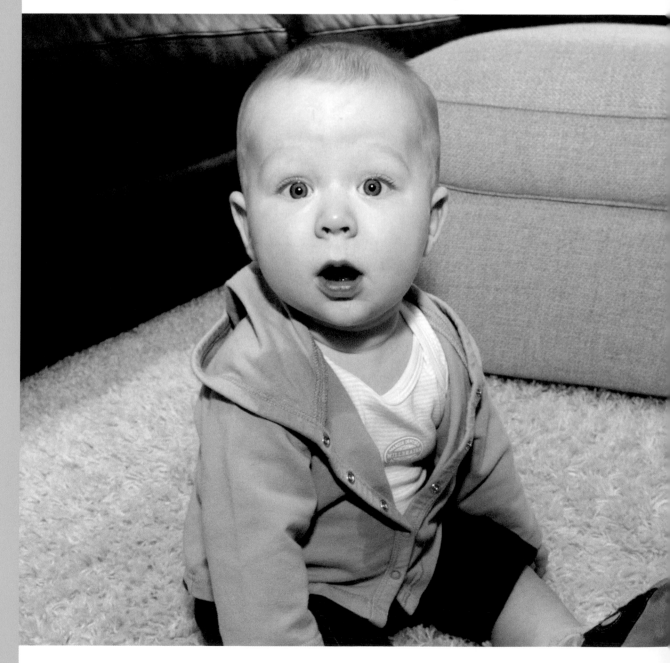

infants require surgical correction, but this is not usually performed urgently. However, incarcerated hernias require immediate assessment by a surgeon.

Varicocele

This collection of varicose, or dilated, veins in the scrotum is somewhat unpleasantly described as feeling like a "bag of worms." These are rare before puberty but quite common in adolescence; in fact, about 15% of teenage boys will have one, almost always on their left side. Although many adolescents are understandably uncomfortable with a genital examination, it is partly for this reason that they should consent to being thoroughly checked at their annual checkup.

Tumor

Hard, painless scrotal masses might be the result of a tumor in the testicle. Both benign (innocent) and malignant (cancerous) scrotal tumors occur, although rarely. While worrisome to parents, it is important to remember that these tumors can often be very successfully treated.

Did You Know?

Enlarging
Both hernias and hydroceles can appear to be getting larger (although still painless) when a baby is crying, coughing, or straining to pass stool.

❸ How Is Swelling of the Scrotum Treated?

Understandably, discovering that your child has a scrotal mass or swelling can be alarming. Any new painful or tender swelling requires urgent medical evaluation at a hospital emergency department because of the possibility of testicular torsion. However, most of the conditions causing painless swellings are not urgent. Still, all scrotal concerns need to be reported to your child's physician.

Doc Talk Health authorities do not currently recommend that healthy teenage boys or young men be counseled to perform testicular self-examination for cancer detection because of the lack of scientific evidence that doing so improves health. However, adolescents with an undescended testicle, previous testicular cancer, or a family member who has had testicular cancer should discuss the potential role of self-examination with their physician. Also, all young men should be counseled to see a physician immediately if they find a lump in their scrotum.

Seizures (Convulsions)

What Can I Do?

▶ If your child has abnormal movements or behaviors, try to videotape them to show to your health-care provider.

▶ In the event of a seizure, place your child on her side out of harm's way. Do not restrain or place anything in her mouth. Call emergency services (911).

Case Study

Ella's Seizures

It seemed like just another night in the McKenzie home. Ella, a very active 1-year-old, had seemed a bit cranky that evening before going to bed, and she had had a cold over the last few days. In the early hours of the evening, Ella's mom was alerted by a strange noise coming from Ella's bedroom. When she popped in to check on her, Ella's whole body was jerking, causing the crib to bang against the wooden floor. It was terrifying. The rhythmic jerking continued for about a minute before stopping on its own. When she lifted Ella up, it felt like Ella was burning up with a fever and she seemed to flop limply, like a rag doll, in her arms. The McKenzies rushed her to their neighborhood hospital. By the time they arrived, Ella appeared to be waking up. Although still very warm and sleepy, Ella was looking like her normal self again.

The emergency room doctor took a detailed history about her developmental milestones, as well as information about the events of the previous 24 hours, especially about the "spell." He thoroughly examined Ella from head to toe, by which time she was starting to play with his stethoscope and charming him with her sparkly, albeit somewhat subdued, personality. He checked her carefully for any specific signs of serious infection and any signs of an underlying brain problem. He concluded that the event was due to a febrile convulsion, likely secondary to a viral illness. He advised the McKenzies to treat her fever with acetaminophen or ibuprofen if it appeared to be bothering her. He gave them an information sheet explaining all the facts about febrile convulsions.

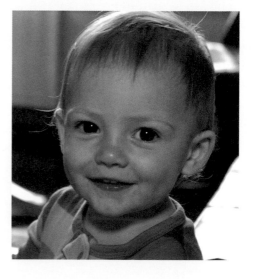

❶ What Are Seizures (Convulsions)?

Young children often have some very strange (but normal) movements or body behaviors, especially while falling asleep or in the process of waking up. Sometimes, these movements indicate a seizure. There are not many things scarier than seeing your child have a seizure. Although it is frightening to see, in many cases it is actually quite harmless. Seizures are caused by abnormal electrical activity in the brain. The effects of these abnormal electrical discharges vary depending upon which part of the brain is involved. Seizures can involve a decreased level of consciousness, abnormal or uncontrollable movements, behavioral or emotional abnormalities, or changes in sensation. Seizure disorders occur in 4 to 6 children in 1,000 (febrile convulsions are much more common, usually about 4 children in 100).

Kinds of Seizures

There are a number of different types of seizures. These can involve the whole body, a single limb, or even simple staring spells. Seizures can be rhythmic or include only stiffening. In many cases, the cause of the seizure is unknown.

Seizure Type	Typical Features
Generalized tonic-clonic seizure (grand mal seizure)	• Sudden loss of consciousness • Stiffening of the arms and legs followed by rhythmic jerking that generally involves the whole body • Might urinate or defecate • Often quite sleepy following the seizure
Tonic or clonic seizure	• Stiffening (tonic) • Rhythmic, jerking (clonic) movements
Absence seizure (previously called petit mal)	• Brief staring spell during which the child is unresponsive, with no speech or movement • May have flickering of the eyes • Episodes usually last 5 to 20 seconds
Myoclonic seizure	• Brief, symmetric jerking movements of the muscles
Partial seizure (involves only one part or side of the body)	• Can include abnormal limb movements • Is usually conscious and somewhat aware • May include automatisms, which are semi-purposeful actions, such as lip-smacking, chewing movements of the mouth, or picking or pulling at clothing • Might move head or eyes to one side or have shaking movements on only one side of the body

❷ What Causes a Seizure?

- Febrile convulsions
- Infection (for example, meningitis)
- Poisoning or drug overdose
- Head trauma
- Brain tumor
- Low blood sugar
- Abnormalities in the brain's structure

Febrile Convulsions

Febrile convulsions are by far the most common form of seizures in young children. They affect approximately 4% of North American children and typically occur between the age of 6 months and 6 years. A febrile convulsion is a seizure that occurs only in the presence of fever. It is commonly believed that the convulsion occurs as part of a young brain's response to a rising temperature.

Typical Features of a Febrile Convulsion

- Family history of someone having febrile convulsions
- Usually only one seizure within the first 24 hours of the febrile illness
- Brief duration (less than 15 minutes)
- Whole body shaking (versus only one body part or half the body shaking)
- Child may temporarily lose control of bowel or bladder
- Age 6 months to 6 years
- Developmentally normal child
- Child will be very sleepy for several hours after the seizure but will eventually return to normal

Risk of Epilepsy

The terms "epilepsy" and "seizure disorder" are sometimes used to describe those seizures that recur in the absence of fever. Fortunately, most children with febrile seizures (more than 95%) will never develop epilepsy, nor do they seem at greater risk for neurological problems. Children with febrile seizures generally develop normally, meaning they will reach their developmental milestones as projected. Although these seizures are extremely frightening to witness, they are generally not dangerous to the child and, unless the seizure is extremely long, there is no risk of brain damage.

Did You Know?

A Picture Is Worth a Thousand Words

Not all abnormal-looking movements are seizures. In fact, young children often have some very strange (but normal) movements or body behaviors, especially while falling asleep or in the process of waking up. Fainting, night terrors, breath-holding spells, and tics can sometimes look like seizures. If you are not sure, try to catch the activity on video to show to your health-care provider. A picture is usually worth a thousand words!

Did You Know?

Supervision

Don't ever leave a child with a known seizure disorder unsupervised in a bathtub or swimming pool! If they have a seizure, they may drown.

> ### When should we contact our doctor or local hospital?
>
> Seizures are very frightening for anyone to see. If this is the first episode, you should call 911 immediately. If your child is having a seizure, try to remain calm in spite of the sense of alarm and helplessness.

❸ How Are Seizures Treated?

Immediate Care

Here are a few tips on immediate care:

- Do not attempt to restrain her movements.
- If possible, place your child on her side.
- Do not put anything in her mouth.
- Ensure that she cannot be injured by the convulsions; for example, do not put her on a bed where she could fall off.
- Loosen any clothing around her head or neck.
- Unless you are very familiar with your child's seizures and are comfortable with their management, call an ambulance immediately.
- Even if you are familiar with her seizures, if the seizure continues for more than 1 to 2 minutes, your child has difficulty breathing, or is turning blue, call for emergency help right away.

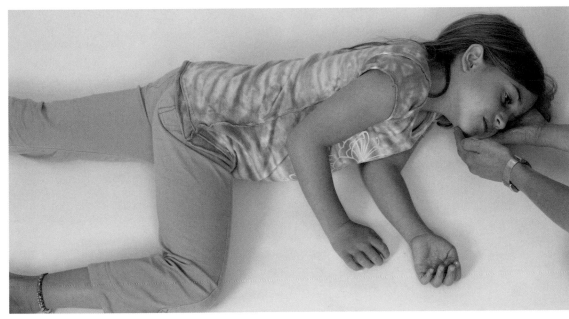

Place your child on her side during a seizure

Hospital Care

If the seizure is prolonged, doctors or paramedics might need to administer medication to stop the seizure. These medicines can be given by mouth or nose, syringed into the rectum, or injected. Once the seizure is over, the doctor treating your child will order a number of tests to determine the cause of the seizure.

Infection

If your child has a fever, the doctor might suggest tests to determine if an infection caused the seizure.

Lumbar Puncture

One of these tests is a lumbar puncture, which tests for meningitis. If meningitis is suspected, your child will be started on antibiotics.

Blood Tests

Blood tests might be ordered to check for low blood sugar or other problems with the body's electrolytes. If you suspect your child might have ingested a poison or medication, blood or urine tests can be done to look for this.

Imaging

A computed tomography (CT) scan or magnetic resonance imaging (MRI) of the brain would look for a brain tumor, a bleed inside the head, or anything else that may be putting pressure on the brain.

EEG

A special test called an electroencephalogram (EEG) records brain wave activity and can detect seizure activity in the brain. This test is done by placing sticky electrodes on your child's head, which collect and analyze electrical data. It can be useful for trying to detect which part of the brain is causing the seizure or to detect underlying abnormal brain waves.

Did You Know?

Recurrence

Approximately one-third of children who experience one febrile convulsion will have a recurrence with subsequent febrile illnesses. This is more likely if the initial convulsion was prolonged (longer than 10 to 15 minutes), occurred in a younger infant (younger than 1 year), or involved only one side of the body.

Doc Talk Unfortunately, there is no evidence to suggest that lowering the temperature during a fever will prevent a febrile seizure. However, most physicians still recommend treating fever with anti-fever medications (antipyretics), such as acetaminophen or ibuprofen. This will help lower the fever and, more importantly, make your child more comfortable. In most cases, doctors do not recommend administering anti-seizure medications to prevent recurrence of typical febrile convulsions.

Short Stature

What Can I Do?

▶ If you are concerned about your child's height, make sure that your health-care provider measures him accurately and plots his height on the appropriate growth chart on a regular basis.

▶ In the case of the two most common causes of short stature (familial short stature and constitutional delay), no particular action is required.

▶ If the rate of growth is very slow, especially if there is a drop-off in appetite, weight gain, and/or energy, then discuss this with your regular health-care provider.

Case Study

Simon's Stature

Simon is a 2-year-old boy who is an active and rather rambunctious toddler. He has always been shorter than his brother at the same age, and his mom noticed that he was the shortest of the boys his age in his daycare. She is worried that he isn't growing well and takes him to the doctor to be assessed. Simon was born about average size, and although he fell to the bottom percentile on the growth chart within a few months, he has been gaining weight and growing along that line steadily since then. He eats a healthy, varied diet, easily keeps up with his bigger friends, and his daycare has no concerns about him. Notably, his parents are relatively short — his mother is 5 feet 2 inches (1.55 m), his father 5 feet 9 inches (1.75 m).

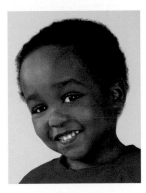

The doctor diagnosed Simon with having familial short stature. Simon is perfectly healthy, and he is small because his mom is small. His parents don't need to worry; he is growing steadily along his genetically predetermined growth curve and he is developing normally — even though he is smaller than his peers. He will likely grow to a height in between that of his mom and dad.

❶ What Is Short Stature?

There is a wide range of "normal" in childhood height. A child's height will depend mainly on how tall his parents are, as well as his nutritional and general health status. Your child's doctor will accurately measure your child and plot him on an appropriate graph, called a growth chart. There are separate graphs for boys and girls of different ages. (You can find growth charts on pages 339–344.) There is a slight difference in the growth charts recommended in different countries. For example, in Canada the World Health Organization (WHO) charts are now used, whereas in the United States the Centers for Disease Control (CDC) have slightly different growth charts. All children should have their growth and development monitored on a regular basis.

How To: Read a Growth Chart

The growth chart displays a pattern of growth over time. The growth velocity is an important clue as to whether there is a growth problem or not. There are normal values for the tempo of growth. We grow at different rates at different times in our life, with big spurts in the first year of life and during the teenage years.

Normal Growth Patterns

Age	Expected Growth (Per Year)
0 to 12 months	10 inches (25 cm)
1 to 2 years	5 inches (12.5 cm)
2 to 3 years	3½ inches (8.5 cm)
3 years to puberty	2 to 3 inches (5 to 7.5 cm)
Puberty	4 to 5 inches (10 to 12.5 cm)

Estimating Your Child's Final Height

A child's final height is often a reflection of his parents' heights. To estimate your child's final height, use the following calculation:

Girls

1 Add mother's height (inches) plus father's height (inches).
2 Subtract 5 inches.
3 Divide the total by 2.
4 This represents the average estimated final height (in inches) for your daughter. Your child should grow to within 2.5 inches (6 cm) above or below this height.

Boys

1 Add mother's height (inches) plus father's height (inches).
2 Add 5 inches.
3 Divide the above total by 2.
4 This represents the average estimated final height (in inches) for your son. Your child should grow to within 2.5 inches (6 cm) above or below this height.

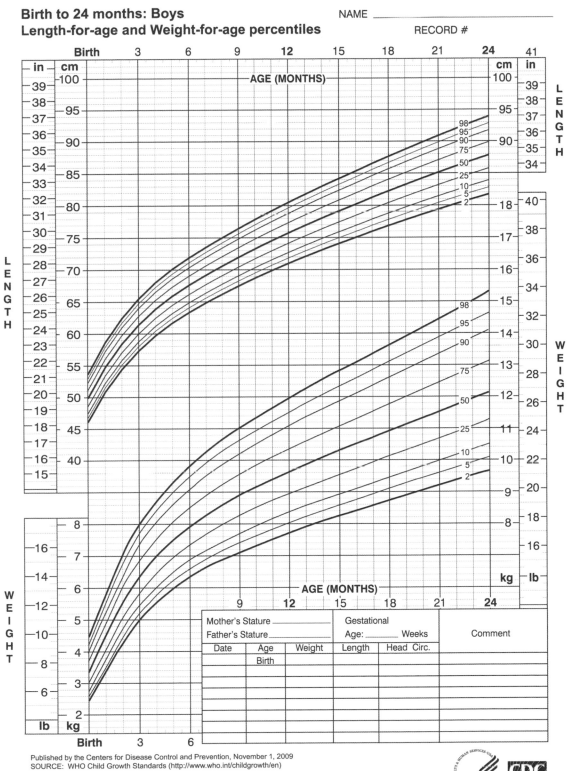

Birth to 24 months: Boys
Length-for-age and Weight-for-age percentiles

NAME _____

RECORD # _____

Published by the Centers for Disease Control and Prevention, November 1, 2009
SOURCE: WHO Child Growth Standards (http://www.who.int/childgrowth/en)

SAFER · HEALTHIER · PEOPLE™

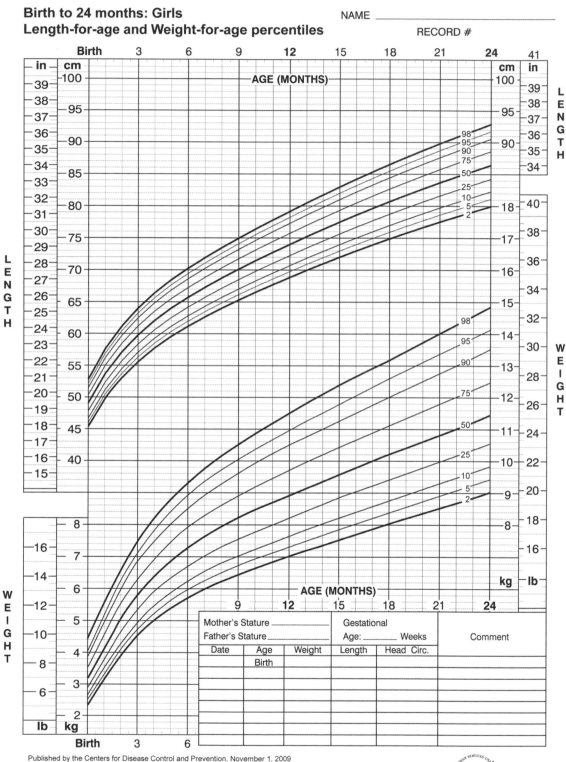

Birth to 24 months: Girls
Length-for-age and Weight-for-age percentiles

NAME _____

RECORD # _____

Published by the Centers for Disease Control and Prevention, November 1, 2009
SOURCE: WHO Child Growth Standards (http://www.who.int/childgrowth/en)

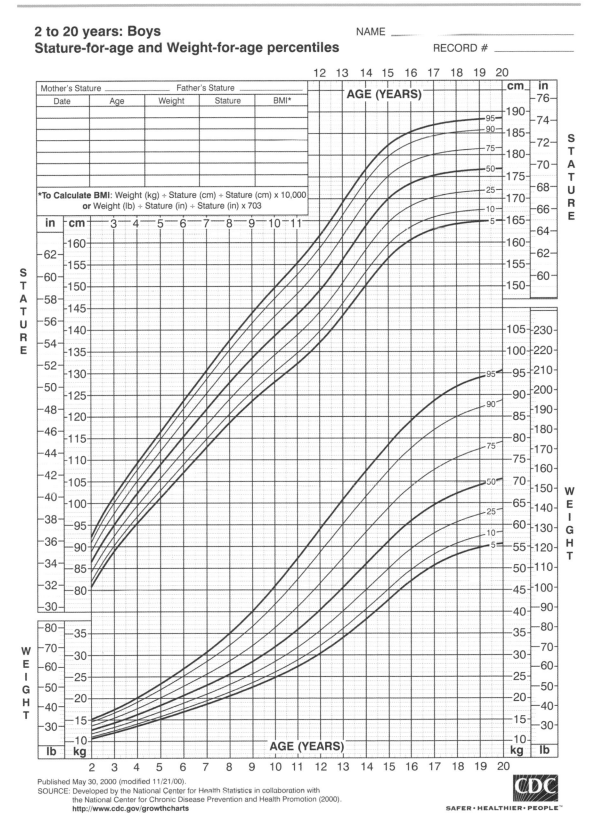

2 to 20 years: Boys
Stature-for-age and Weight-for-age percentiles

NAME _____

RECORD # _____

Published May 30, 2000 (modified 11/21/00).

SOURCE: Developed by the National Center for Health Statistics in collaboration with
the National Center for Chronic Disease Prevention and Health Promotion (2000).
http://www.cdc.gov/growthcharts

CDC
SAFER · HEALTHIER · PEOPLE™

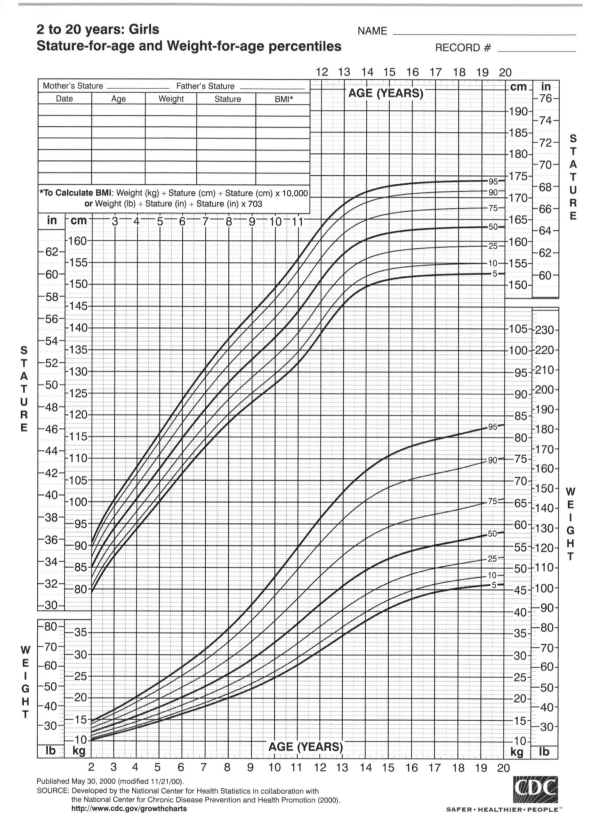

2 to 20 years: Girls
Stature-for-age and Weight-for-age percentiles

NAME _____

RECORD # _____

WHO GROWTH CHARTS FOR CANADA

BOYS

2 TO 19 YEARS: BOYS
Height-for-age and Weight-for-age percentiles

NAME: _____

DOB: _____   RECORD # _____

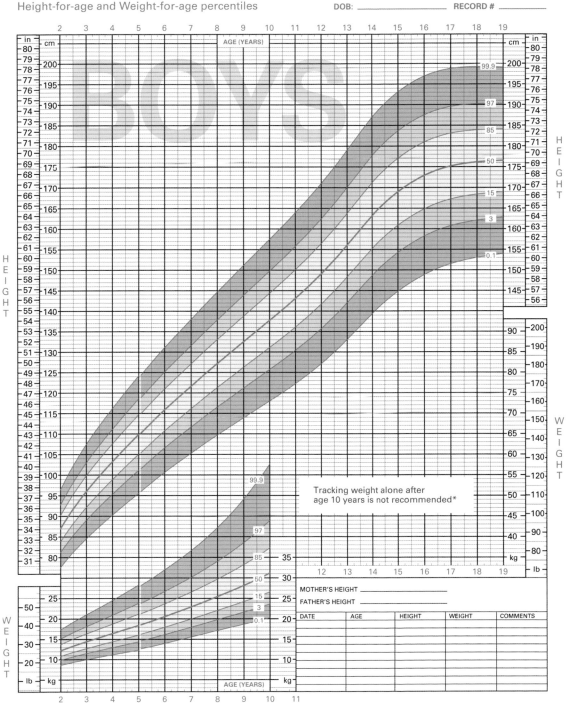

Tracking weight alone after
age 10 years is not recommended*

MOTHER'S HEIGHT _____
FATHER'S HEIGHT _____

DATE	AGE	HEIGHT	WEIGHT	COMMENTS

SOURCE: Based on the World Health Organization (WHO) Child Growth Standards (2006) and WHO Reference (2007) adapted for Canada by Dietitians of Canada, Canadian Paediatric Society, the College of Family Physicians of Canada and Community Health Nurses of Canada.

© Dietitians of Canada. 2010. May be reproduced in its entirety (i.e. no changes) for educational purposes only. www.dietitians.ca/growthcharts
*BMI is a better measure due to variable age of puberty.

WHO GROWTH CHARTS FOR CANADA

GIRLS

2 TO 19 YEARS: GIRLS
Height-for-age and Weight-for-age percentiles

NAME: _____

DOB: _____ RECORD # _____

Tracking weight alone after age 10 years is not recommended*

MOTHER'S HEIGHT _____
FATHER'S HEIGHT _____

DATE	AGE	HEIGHT	WEIGHT	COMMENTS

SOURCE: Based on the World Health Organization (WHO) Child Growth Standards (2006) and WHO Reference (2007) adapted for Canada by Dietitians of Canada, Canadian Paediatric Society, the College of Family Physicians of Canada and Community Health Nurses of Canada.

© Dietitians of Canada. 2010. May be reproduced in its entirety (i.e. no changes) for educational purposes only. **www.dietitians.ca/growthcharts**
*BMI is a better measure due to variable age of puberty.

When should we contact our doctor or local hospital?

There are no growth "emergencies," but if your child has any of the red flags below, then discuss with your doctor.

⏩ Short Stature Red Flags

If your child appears to be much shorter than most children his age, or if the growth rate has decreased or stopped, discuss with your health-care provider. Consult your child's doctor if your child has any of the following symptoms associated with short stature:

- Plots below the bottom curve on the growth chart
- Is inappropriately short when compared to the parents' heights
- Used to plot on a much higher percentile curve but has dropped down (except if your child is younger than 2 years; this can be normal)

- Has a consistently slow growth velocity for age (generally, less than 2 inches/5 cm yearly)
- Has weight loss or unusual weight gain
- Has very poor nutrition or loss of appetite
- Has poor energy and is not able to keep up with his peers

❷ What Causes Short Stature?

The term "short stature" describes height that is significantly below the average height for a person's age, sex, or family. Short stature is a variant of normal. The two most common reasons for short stature are familial short stature and constitutional delay of growth.

Familial Short Stature

In this case (as with Simon above), one or both parents are also short. These children are short compared to the general public, but not compared to their parents and family. They have normal growth spurts and enter puberty at a normal age. They will reach an adult height similar to one or both parents. Children with familial short stature do not have any symptoms related to diseases that affect growth.

Constitutional Growth Delay

In this case, children are small for their age but are growing at a normal rate. They may be short compared to both the general public and their family. These children enter puberty later than their peers. However, because they continue to grow for a longer period of time, they catch up to their peers as they reach their adult height, which is normal and comparable to their parents.

Doc Talk

In both familial short stature and constitutional growth delay, children are otherwise healthy, well nourished, and have no symptoms or signs of illness. Growth failure, on the other hand, is due to an underlying medical condition, and it may be caused by many chronic diseases.

There is not much you can do to help a healthy, well-nourished child grow taller more quickly. Growth hormone, a medication sometimes used in children with growth failure due to an underlying medical condition, does not help children with familial short stature or constitutional growth delay. Children may be self-conscious about their height, and short children are often teased. These children may benefit from the support of a health-care professional.

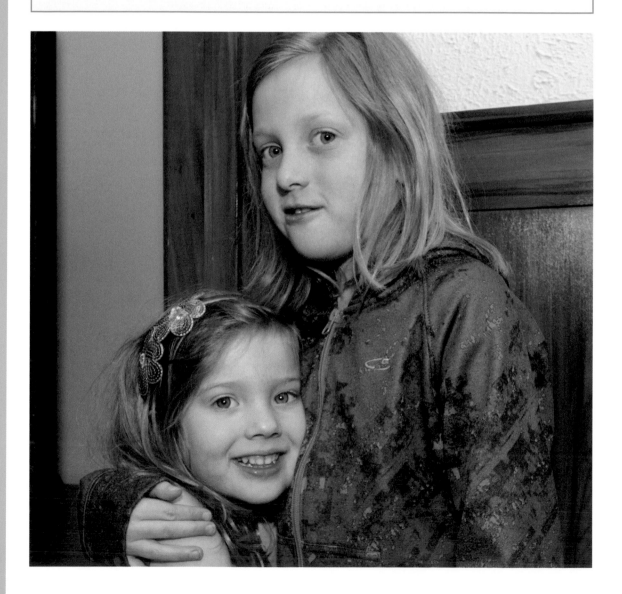

Sibling Rivalry

What Can I Do?

► Accept the fact that there will be rivalry between your children. When reasonable, let your children solve their own problems.

► Model your behavior. Show your children how you treat others with respect.

► Help your children understand what you expect from them. It is their character you love, not their accomplishments.

❶ What Is Sibling Rivalry?

Siblings may be jealous and competitive with each other. A little of this behavior is normal; a lot can be a problem. Good "chemistry" between siblings requires a little luck and is probably influenced by temperament, birth order, age, and gender.

How To: Manage Sibling Rivalry

❶ Teach your kids that being fair is not the same as being equal. It's okay to set different expectations based on each child's age (different bedtimes, for example), their unique personality traits, and abilities. Avoid comparing your kids, and if sibling rivalry is a problem, avoid competitive activities between them.

❷ When reasonable, let your children solve their own problems. There may be times when you'll need to intervene, especially if they become violent or cruel. It is often difficult for a parent to determine who "started it," and many children accuse a parent of taking sides. You might try removing the source of conflict, such as a particular toy, if they refuse to share or take turns.

❸ Praise your children when they interact well and support each other. Try to find time to spend alone with each of your children, on a regular basis, even if it is only for a few minutes a day.

❹ Remember to role model. Treat your partner and your kids in the way you would like them to treat each other. If they hear a lot of yelling, you can't expect them to behave differently!

Some circumstances are more challenging; for example, if one child is disabled and requires a lot of extra time and attention, the other child might feel resentful and ignored. It might be helpful to develop pride in the healthier sibling by encouraging him to assist in the care of the unwell sibling (but not if the care is so difficult to provide that he feels resentful for this too).

Did You Know?

Ongoing Rivalry

Approximately one-third of adults report having ongoing rivalry with their siblings. However, this does improve over time. At least 80% of siblings over the age of 60 report a close relationship with their siblings. So if you wait long enough, you may become friends!

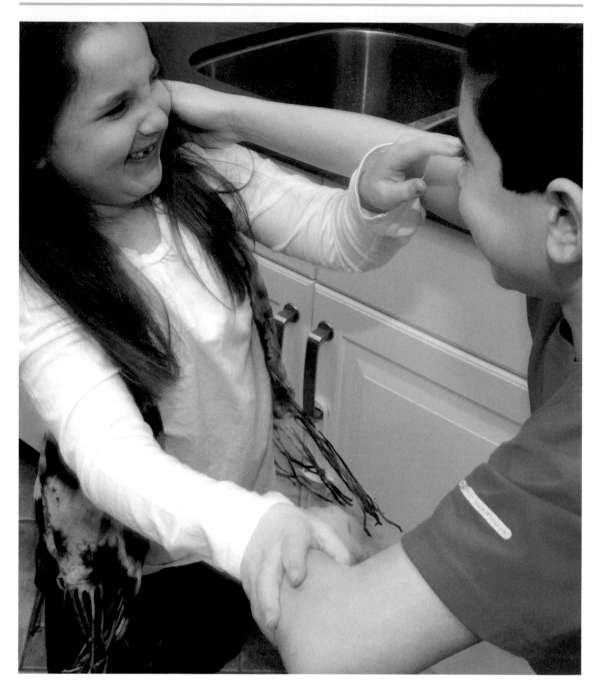

Doc Talk If one child is more capable and more successful than the other, jealousy is understandable. Your children should understand that you expect effort from each but it is their character you love, not their accomplishments.

Sinusitis

What Can I Do?

▶ Suspect sinusitis if cough and nasal congestion last longer than a week, especially if associated with thick green nasal discharge, headache, facial pain, and bad breath.

▶ If you suspect sinusitis, take your child to be assessed by his health-care provider.

▶ In addition to prescribed antibiotics, give your child some medication for pain relief, such as acetaminophen or ibuprofen.

Case Study

Oliver's Sinusitis

Oliver is a 12-year-old boy who had a cold 3 weeks ago. During the last 10 days, he has had foul-smelling breath and green discharge from his nose. He is coughing and complaining of a headache on the left side of his forehead. He tells his mother that his "eyes hurt." She is wondering what might be going on and takes him to the doctor for assessment. Their doctor explains that Oliver has sinusitis. Sinusitis is more common in a child over 10 years old because the sinuses become more developed as children grow, but sinusitis can occur in younger children as well.

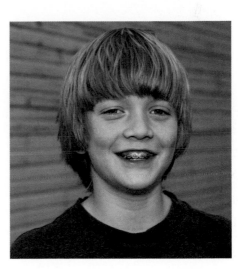

❶ What Is Sinusitis?

The sinuses are the air-filled cavities on both sides of the face — beside the nose and around the eye. These facial sinuses are connected with the nasal passages. Sinusitis occurs when the lining of these cavities becomes inflamed or swollen because of a bacterial infection.

Signs and Symptoms of Sinusitis
- Cough
- Nasal congestion with little improvement, lasting longer than 10 days

- Fever
- Thick, greenish-yellow mucus coming out of the nose for at least 3 days
- Headache
- Facial pain and/or swelling, especially around the eyes
- Sore throat
- Bad breath (halitosis)

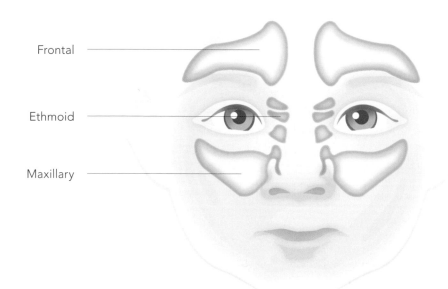

Frontal

Ethmoid

Maxillary

Location of the facial sinuses

When should we contact our doctor or local hospital?

If you suspect sinusitis based on the symptoms listed above, then you will need to seek medical advice. Rarely, bacteria causing sinusitis will spread beyond the sinuses, causing more serious complications, such as periorbital or orbital cellulitis (infection around or behind the eye; see page 183) or a blood clot in the veins or an infection around the brain. These complications, as suggested by the red flags opposite, require immediate assessment and treatment.

⇒ Sinusitis Red Flags

Consult your child's doctor or local hospital immediately if your child has any of the following symptoms associated with sinusitis:

- Swelling and redness around the eye
- Headache with vomiting
- Change in level of consciousness
- Stiff neck
- One-sided facial weakness
- Bulging of one or both eyes

❷ What Causes Sinusitis?

Sinusitis can happen whenever the drainage of secretions from the sinuses into the nasal passage is impaired, usually as a result of nasal congestion due to viral infections or allergies. When the secretions remain trapped in the sinuses, bacteria can then multiply, causing an infection.

❸ How Is Sinusitis Treated?

- *Antibiotics:* Sinusitis usually responds best to a course of antibiotics. With antibiotics, symptoms should improve within 48 to 72 hours.
- *Pain relief:* Initially, medication for pain relief, such as acetaminophen or ibuprofen, may be required as well.
- *Decongestants:* Although some doctors may recommend decongestants that are sprayed into the nose, their use in children is controversial and they are not routinely used.

Doc Talk Your doctor can usually diagnose sinusitis from symptoms and signs without any tests. CT (computed tomography) scans may occasionally be useful for children with suspected severe complications of sinusitis (such as an infection that has spread to around the eyeball or brain), but they are not considered routine for the diagnosis of sinusitis. Sinus X-rays are not helpful in diagnosing childhood sinusitis.

Sleep Problems

Case Study

Chloe's Sleep Problems

Chloe is a 4-year-old girl who has been sleeping in her parent's bed every night since she was born. Her mother is pregnant and would like to transition Chloe to her own room so that there is room for the new baby in her parents' room. Chloe's mom has tried asking Chloe to sleep in her own bed and has even slept with Chloe in her room to get her to do so. The problem is that Chloe usually wakes up a couple of hours later, crying for her mom.

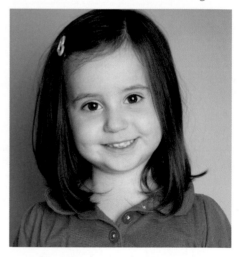

When they next visited their doctor, she listened to Chloe's mother's description of her predicament and diagnosed Chloe with sleep onset association disorder and night awakening, two very common sleep disorders. Chloe has never learned to fall asleep alone without her mother being present and cannot put herself back to sleep. Their doctor recommended the "chair-sitting" method to solve this problem.

❶ What Are Sleep Problems?

Most often, the sleep problems that infants and toddlers — and their families — experience revolve around difficulty settling down to sleep or waking up throughout the night. Sleep problems are extremely common in children and can lead to parental exhaustion and family disruption.

When should we contact our doctor?

Generally speaking, sleep problems are not emergencies, although parents may feel desperate when sleep-deprived! Your health-care provider will likely discuss your child's regular sleep patterns at most routine checkups. Different families will have different levels of tolerance for their children's sleep issues; when you have decided that your child and/or you and your partner are being sufficiently impacted by sleep problems, then the time is right to ask for some helpful strategies to deal with them. While there are reasonable solutions to many of these problems, they all require some effort, motivation, and consistency from all caregivers, so are unlikely to work until you feel like you really need to deal with them.

Common Childhood Sleep Problems

Symptoms	Problem	Treatment
• Child wakes up several times during the night • Child requires rocking or holding to fall asleep initially and during the night • Child requires parental presence or the presence of an object (for example, the TV) to fall asleep	**Sleep onset association disorder**	• Teach your child appropriate sleep association and to fall asleep alone (see page 357)
• Child uses various tactics to avoid going to bed at night (for example, wants a glass of water, wants another story)	**Limit-setting disorder**	• Set consistent limits and follow through with consequences
• Child wakes up screaming or confused in the first third of the night or in the early morning • It is difficult to comfort child • May be talking to you, but it feels as if she doesn't appreciate your presence • Has no recollection of this event the following morning	**Night terrors**	• Do not disturb the child or try to wake her up • Make sure she can't hurt herself
• Child wakes up scared in the middle of the night • Can recount to you a scary dream she just had • May feel that this dream was real	**Nightmares**	• Reassure your child that she is safe • Discuss the event during daylight hours • Avoid scary images (for example, stories about monsters)
• Child rocks herself to sleep • Bangs her head on the wall, crib, or headboard to fall asleep	**Rhythmic movements**	• Most of these movements tend to be normal and will disappear on their own
• Snoring, with periods of no breathing between snores • Can be either tired or restless or hyperactive during the day	**Sleep apnea** (see page 364)	• See your health-care provider for further evaluation

> ## FAQ
>
> ***How many hours should my child sleep in a night?***
> Depending on a child's age and developmental stage, there is considerable variation in the amount of sleep needed, as well as in the pattern and cycles of sleep. At each age, there is a range of normal; some children seem to require more sleep and others less.

Average Sleep Needs

Bear in mind that these are just averages and certainly may not apply to every child. Nevertheless, you may want to record your child's sleep duration and compare it with the average amount of time other children of a similar age spend sleeping.

Age	Average Hours of Sleep
0 to 2 months	16 to 18
2 to 6 months	14 to 16
6 to 12 months	13 to 15
1 to 3 years	12 to 14
3 to 5 years	11 to 13
5 to 12 years	10 to 11
12 to 18 years	8.5 to 9.5

Did You Know?

Normal Fussiness

Most infants have a normal period of fussiness while they make the transition from wakefulness to sleeping. In fact, it is normal for them to cry for 10 to 20 minutes as they fall asleep.

Sleep Cycles

Sleep consists of cycles that include periods of light sleep leading to deeper sleep, then to dreaming, and, finally, waking. These cycles repeat themselves regularly throughout the night. Dreams occur during a stage of sleep called rapid eye movement, or REM sleep. Rest, the restorative phase of sleeping, occurs during non-REM sleep. Non-REM sleep tends to happen earlier in the night and REM sleep occurs later. Most of us awaken during very light stages of sleep. In adults, these awakenings are usually brief: we usually turn over and go back to sleep without really being aware of waking up. However, many children have some difficulty settling back down to sleep and may need to be taught how to do so.

❶ What Are Sleep Onset Problems?

A sleep onset problem (also called sleep onset association disorder) is a fancy term for a child who has trouble falling asleep alone at night without being held or rocked. This is an extremely common problem. Up to one-third of children have some difficulty getting to sleep.

❷ What Causes Sleep Onset Problems?

It seems easiest for most young infants to fall asleep when they are held, rocked, or stroked, particularly when sucking on the breast or a pacifier. Toddlers and older children seem to fall asleep more easily when a parent lies beside them, singing or talking to them. Children easily become accustomed to these "sleep associations" and develop a dependency. They fail to learn to fall asleep without these associations.

❶ What Is Night Awakening?

Night awakenings are also extremely common in children. As children cycle through periods of lighter sleep, they often wake up. Children who have not learned to fall asleep by themselves might fully awaken and cry, call out for parents, or get out of bed and request that the parent rock or sing them back to sleep. Whether or not night waking is viewed as a problem is really a matter of personal perspective. Nevertheless, fragmented sleep is generally not beneficial for parents or children, especially in the long term.

❷ What Causes Night Awakening?

All children and adults have periods of deep and light sleep. When in a period of light sleep, there is a greater probability of awakening, especially if something in the immediate environment has changed — for example, if your daughter fell asleep with you lying beside her, but now, 1 hour later, she realizes you are gone. The more consistent the environment you fall asleep in is, the less likely you will be to reawaken.

❸ How Are Sleep Onset Problems and Night Awakening Treated?

Tips for Treating Inappropriate Sleep Associations

- Start with creating a regular sleep routine (consistent nap and bedtime).
- Stick to the times you have proposed — don't let a child who has stayed awake all night nap all day.
- Once you have consistent sleep times, wean your child off any nighttime feeds.
- Assess your child's sleep onset associations — where/how does she fall asleep, and with whom?
- Write out a list of the sleep onset associations.
- Choose a time to start eliminating inappropriate sleep associations (may start during a daytime nap, when you may have more energy).
- Eliminate associations one at a time.
- Be consistent. All caregivers must have the same approach.
- Don't implement something you cannot follow through on; this will only confuse your child and worsen her already challenging sleep habits.

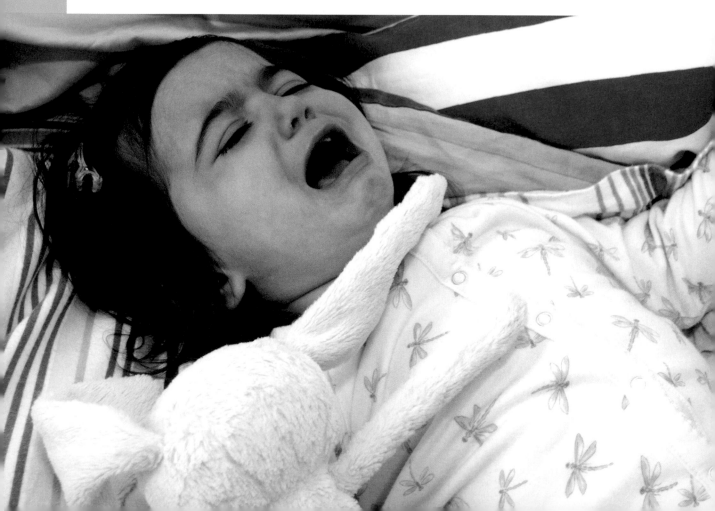

How To: Teach Your Child to Fall Asleep By Herself

Do

- Establish a predictable bedtime routine.
- Maintain a consistent bedtime.
- Encourage your child to fall asleep in her own bedroom every night.
- Create a dark and quiet environment.
- Leave the room while child is still awake.

Don't

- Neglect the importance of a bedtime routine.
- Allow a variable bedtime.
- Allow her to fall asleep in another room.
- Allow bright light, loud TV, or music that might disturb her sleep.
- Stay in the room until she is sound asleep.
- Breastfeed or bottle-feed to help her fall asleep.
- Provide drinks through the night.
- Hold your child until she falls asleep.

Timed Absence Technique

Some parents have real difficulty ignoring their child's cries at night. If your child has become conditioned to needing a parent's presence to settle down, you can reduce the acquired parental dependency. You might try responding to the night crying by gradually decreasing contact. One way to do this uses timed absences from the room while your child is crying and resisting separation. Another option is using the chair-sitting method.

How To: Use the Timed Absence Technique

This process may last from a few minutes to a few hours, and it may take several days before your child is able to go to bed without a fuss.

- Ensure that your child's bedroom is safe. Because she may get out of her bed when you're not in the room, there shouldn't be anything that she can pull down or climb onto that could injure her.
- Put your child down in her crib or bed following your normal bedtime routine (bath, brush teeth, read a book, give her a hug and kiss, etc.). Explain to her that you will leave her door open and will be outside her room. Explain that if she tries to leave her bed or her room, you will close her door.
- Leave the room. This may evoke many responses from your child, including protests and crying.

- Leave the door open, if this is your normal routine, as long as your child doesn't leave her room. If she tries to get out of bed and leave her room, you will need to use the door-closing technique (see below).

- If your child is in bed and keeps getting up and trying to leave her room, implement the following door-closing technique: First, escort her back to her bed and remind her that if she tries to leave her room, you will have to close her door. Tell her that if she returns to her bed, you will open it. If she leaves her bed, close her door. You may open it once she returns to her bed. If your toddler tries to open the door, you may even need to hold it shut. This may upset your toddler, who does not want to sleep alone in her room. Remind her that you will open her door if she returns to her bed. In the beginning, she may actually fall asleep on her floor rather than in her bed. This is okay. It may continue for a few nights until she learns to fall asleep alone.

- Continue to return to your child's room at timed intervals (gradually increasing the interval by 2 minutes per night) until she is calm or asleep. When you return to her room, if she's still awake, remind her that you are still there, that it is her bedtime, that she should be sleeping, and that you love her. You can escort her back to bed if she'll go, but this isn't essential. Then leave the room.

- Do not pick her up or cuddle her, because this will serve as positive reinforcement of inappropriate behavior. This should be a businesslike interaction, reassuring but not particularly desirable. When you check in on your child, do not introduce any new sleep associations.

How To: Use the Chair-Sitting Method

This method works well for parents who do not feel comfortable with the timed absence technique and usually takes about 3 weeks to implement.

- Ensure that your child's bedroom is safe. Because she may get out of her bed when you're not in the room, there shouldn't be anything that she can pull down or climb onto that could injure her.

- Sit on a chair that can be easily moved, such as a dining-room chair, while she falls asleep and then leave when she is asleep.

- During the first week of the process, place the chair beside the bed, and, if you usually touch your child when she's falling asleep, you can do this initially, but don't lie on the bed with her. Discourage talking and eye contact — it is now time for sleep.

- Let her know that you will always be around and that if she wakes up, she can call you and you will return to the chair and sit there until she falls asleep. (If this is the middle of the night, chances are that you will fall asleep before she does!)
- Every couple of nights, move the chair gradually closer to the bedroom door. Once you start to do this, you should discontinue physical contact with your child while she's falling asleep. You should also stop having conversations. You can turn the chair so that you're not looking directly at your child but she can still see you and know that you're there. By the end of the first week, your chair should be at your child's door.
- At the start of the second week, position the chair outside your child's door so that she can see you (but not necessarily your face). For the next week, sit in the chair while your child falls asleep, day or night.
- At the start of the third week, inform her that you will no longer be sitting in the chair while she falls asleep but that you will be close by, and if she calls out to you, you will come to her doorway. Find a quiet activity (e.g., reading a book) that you can do near her room so that she knows you're close by. By the end of the three weeks, your child should be able to fall asleep without you. She will have progressed from falling asleep with you to doing it all by herself.

> **Did You Know?**
>
> **Stimulation**
> TV and stimulating video games just before bed may hinder your child's ability to fall asleep. Try to stick to quiet activities (for example, reading books) before bed, and don't allow your child to have a TV (or computer) in her bedroom. Caffeine, a stimulant, is found in many foods, including chocolate. Avoid caffeine-containing products in the afternoon and evening.

FAQ

What medication can I use to keep my child asleep?
Medications, such as sleeping pills, are almost never required to treat sleep problems in children. Behavioral approaches are almost always successful when implemented consistently.

❶ What Is a Nightmare?

Nightmares are frightening dreams. They are very common and typically happen in the second half of the night in children aged three to six years. Children are often very scared and may feel that their dream was "real." When children are sufficiently frightened, they will have difficulty falling back to sleep after a nightmare. They can usually be reassured by your presence and a brief period of comforting.

❷ What Causes a Nightmare?

Daily Life

Children's nightmares can be related to things happening in their daily life, to TV shows they watch, or to books they read. Evaluating what your child's daytime stresses are, as well as what they are reading and watching, is essential.

No one knows exactly what causes nightmares. But they seem to start as the stage of development coincides with a normal but very active imagination. They may get worse if your child isn't getting enough sleep and may be related to images that your child is exposed to before bed, for example scary monsters in a book or TV show.

How To: Manage Nightmares

- Go to your child and reassure her as quickly as possible.
- Try to find ways your child can feel safe and comfortable in her own bed at night. Ask her what would make her feel safe; for example, leaving the bedroom light on for a short period or leaving the bedroom door open.
- The next day, evaluate the situation and see if you can identify a cause. Has your child suffered a traumatic event? Does your child watch scary TV shows or programs that are not age-appropriate? Does she look at books with scary pictures?
- The next day, discuss your child's dream with her. Don't do this at the time of the nightmare or it may only increase her anxiety.

When should we contact our doctor?

If nightmares are persistent or very frequent, you should consult your health-care provider.

❶ What Is a Night Terror?

Night terrors are a phenomenon that occurs when your child partially wakes up during the transition from deeper sleep to lighter sleep. They happen most commonly in children aged 2 to 4 years, usually 1 to 2 hours after falling sleep or in the early-morning hours.

During a night terror, your child might appear frightened, pale, and sweaty. Although her eyes may be wide open, she is not responsive to others in the room and might speak incoherently or scream. She might push a parent away, walk around, or appear to see something that is not there. The episode can last as long as 20 to 30 minutes. Parents tend to find this to be a very frightening experience. However, your child is not really awake and will typically fall asleep quickly afterward. She will not remember the event in the morning.

❷ What Causes a Night Terror?

Night terrors occur in normal children and do not indicate an underlying problem. Stress, fatigue, a full bladder, or loud noises can trigger a night terror in children who have them. Often, there is a family history of night terrors, sleepwalking, or sleep talking.

❸ How Is a Night Terror Managed?

- Ensure the environment is safe, particularly for children who walk around during the night terror.
- Don't try to wake your child up, talk to her, or pick her up. This will not stop or shorten the episode and may actually lengthen it. Furthermore, if your child does wake up while you hold her, she may be scared because she might not understand why you have your arms around her.
- Don't remind your child about this event the next day. Because children do not usually remember night terrors, talking to them about it or asking what happened is unlikely to be beneficial and may provoke anxiety.
- If the night terrors continue to be a problem, you can try to alter the child's sleep cycle. Arousing the youngster about 30 minutes before the night terror typically occurs (usually around 1 hour after falling asleep) for 1 week might correct things. A 30- to 60-minute afternoon nap might also decrease the frequency of night terrors. Only very rarely are sleep-altering medications needed.
- If night terrors persist in children older than 8 years old, you should have the problem assessed by her doctor.
- Rhythmic movements, such as jerking of the arms or legs, could rarely be a sign of seizures. If these movements occur during the episodes, this is a sign that your child needs further assessment. Video recording these episodes to show your health-care provider will be helpful. See Seizures (page 332).

> **Doc Talk** If you find yourself becoming angry with your child when she will not fall asleep, put her in her crib or bed, close the door, and take a break. Having someone available to help, if possible, may make things more manageable, particularly if you have more than one child.

Slivers

What Can I Do?

▶ In most cases, remove the sliver. A common exception is tiny fragments of wood superficially, and painlessly, embedded in the skin. They can be left alone.

▶ Watch out for any signs of infection — increasing redness, swelling, pain, or pussy discharge.

❶ What Is a Sliver?

It is one of life's annoying realities that kids get slivers. For that matter, so do their parents. Slivers can be large or small, superficial or deep, or lie horizontally or vertically, and they can be easy to remove or clearly difficult to do so. Most slivers are visible and can be adequately assessed just by looking at them. Some embedded objects, like a thorn in the foot, may only be noticed because a toddler starts limping.

When should we contact our doctor or local hospital?

Most slivers can be removed at home. Seek medical assistance if the splinter is deep or looks infected, or if you aren't sure that your child has had a tetanus shot in the preceding 5 years. Also, it is a good idea to get help if you don't think you'll be able to remove the splinter easily, or if you try but find removal more difficult than anticipated.

❷ How Is a Sliver Treated?

Generally, slivers should be removed. A common exception is the situation in which numerous tiny fragments of wood are superficially, and painlessly, embedded in the skin: removal would cause more trouble than the splinters. Clean the area involved with antiseptic, and the tiny fragments will eventually come out with the normal shedding of the skin.

How To: Remove a Sliver

1 Assemble the right equipment: tweezers, needle, antiseptic, a good source of light.

2 Sterilize the tweezers and needle by dipping them in rubbing alcohol or antiseptic solution. Let them dry.

3 Wash the area thoroughly and apply some antiseptic solution.

4 Firmly grasp the exposed end of the sliver with the tweezers and pull it out along the angle of entry.

5 If the splinter is just below the skin, a light feathering stroke with the needle will often expose the sliver so that it can then be removed with tweezers.

6 Horizontal, shallow splinters can be removed by using a needle or sharply pointed blade to stroke the overlying skin along the long axis of the sliver, exposing the fragment and then flicking it out.

7 Fiberglass pieces or plant spines that might be crushed by tweezers can often be removed by applying duct tape or even some wax hair remover, if available, and then peeling off the fragments.

8 Once the splinter has been removed, wash the area again and apply an antiseptic or antibiotic ointment.

9 It's also wise to periodically check the wound for a few days to make sure an infection hasn't developed.

FAQ

How do I know if the sliver has become infected?

These symptoms indicate infection:

- Increasing redness
- Increasing swelling
- Increasing pain
- Creamy discharge (pus)

Doc Talk

In the emergency department, certain foreign bodies (for example, metal and glass) are usually visible on simple X-rays, but other foreign bodies (for example, a piece of wood deep in a wound) may not be detected except by an ultrasound examination.

Snoring and Obstructive Sleep Apnea

What Can I Do?

▶ Videotape your child sleeping and snoring to show your doctor what he looks and sounds like.

▶ If your child has pauses in his breathing while sleeping, often followed by a gasp, he may have obstructive sleep apnea (OSA). See your doctor for this.

▶ Remember that snoring is common, tends to get worse with colds and allergies, and usually settles on its own.

Case Study

Joey's Snoring

Joey is a happy 6-year-old boy. His parents always joke that they can hear him snoring from the basement of their house. He enjoys school and is always glad to go. At a recent parent-teacher interview, his teacher reported concerns about his ability to learn. She felt that he has trouble concentrating, and his reading level is below his peers.

On a trip to the doctor, Joey's mother explains that he is an active kid who sleeps from 8 p.m. to 6 a.m. She has noticed that he is quite restless when he sleeps, a bit sweaty, and bends his neck backward in what looks like an uncomfortable posture while sleeping.

He snores loudly at night, with occasional pauses. This tends to be worse during allergy season and when he has a cold. His father is also a big snorer. Despite being very active, whenever he is in the car, he falls asleep almost immediately. Their family doctor thought this might be a case of sleep apnea and referred Joey to a sleep specialist for a possible overnight sleep study.

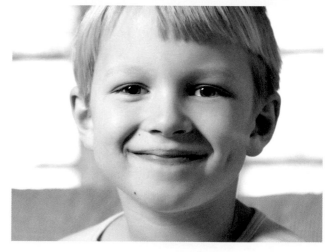

❶ What Is Snoring and Obstructive Sleep Apnea?

Snoring is a sound we all hope we don't make when we go to sleep! It is created by the vibration of the soft palate as you breathe in and out when you sleep. Anything that causes blockage of airflow through the nose — seasonal allergies, common colds, obesity, and enlarged adenoids — can contribute to snoring. Snoring is common. By some estimates, it affects 10% of children at some stage.

When should we contact our doctor?

Most instances of snoring are not worrisome and get better on their own. Often, when children are suffering from seasonal allergies or a common cold, they may start to snore when they have not done this before. This usually resolves on its own without any tests or treatments.

However, snoring can be associated with a condition called obstructive sleep apnea (OSA). This refers to episodes of a partial or complete blockage of the upper air passages during sleep, which leads to abnormal breathing and sleep patterns. Snoring related to OSA is concerning and warrants further evaluation. See your doctor if any red flag symptoms appear.

▶▶ Obstructive Sleep Apnea Red Flags

Consult your child's doctor as soon as possible if your child has any of the following symptoms associated with obstructive sleep apnea:

- Daytime sleepiness
- Behavioral and attention problems
- Growth problems
- High blood pressure
- Sleeping in an unusual position; for example, sitting up or with his neck bent backward
- New onset bedwetting (where previously the child was dry throughout the night)
- Morning headaches

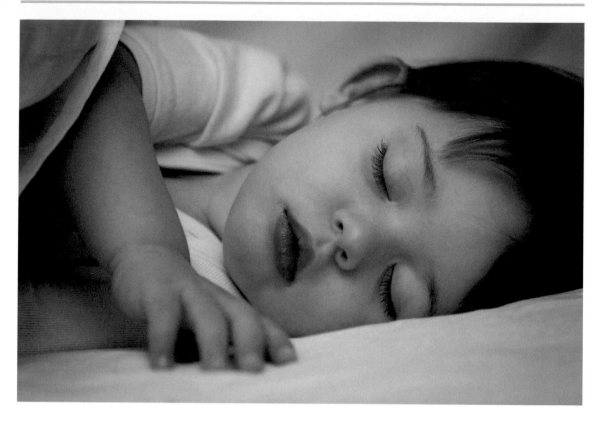

Adenoids

Adenoids (similar to tonsils) are part of the body's immune system, for filtering and fighting off infections. Adenoids are found at the back of the nasal cavity, so you cannot see them (unlike tonsils, which can be seen at the back of the throat). After the first year of life, they tend to grow, especially in response to infections and allergens. Normally they shrink in late childhood and adolescence. Enlarged adenoids can contribute to snoring.

Signs and Symptoms of Obstructive Sleep Apnea

If your child has OSA, he might have pauses in his breathing, where you cannot hear any noise due to a complete blockage of airflow, and then he may have a big gasp for air. In addition, your child may also be restless and sweat excessively during sleep. Sometimes children with OSA sleep in unusual positions — for example, sitting up or with their neck bent back — in order to open their airways when they are asleep.

Testing for Obstructive Sleep Apnea

The best tool for assessing sleep apnea is a sleep study (also called a polysomnogram, or PSG). This test is done in a special sleep lab while your child sleeps. Unfortunately, sleep studies are difficult to perform and interpret, and they are expensive. If you are concerned, you can start by video-recording your child during sleep so that your health-care provider can watch and decide whether any further testing is required.

❷ How Is Obstructive Sleep Apnea Treated?

Snoring itself requires no treatment and usually settles or improves on its own. It may require earplugs for other family members in the interim! True OSA will require intervention. The treatment for OSA caused by enlarged tonsils and adenoids is usually the surgical removal of the tonsils and adenoids in an operation called a tonsillectomy and adenoidectomy. If the OSA is related to a child's weight, a weight-loss strategy may be implemented, with or without a tonsillectomy and adenoidectomy. Very rarely, a CPAP (continuous positive airway pressure) machine may be required. This is a mask that blows air into the child's nose and mouth and helps to keep the airway open.

FAQ

My child snores. Does he need his tonsils and adenoids out?
Young children have relatively large tonsils and adenoids compared with adults. The adenoids usually grow in the first few years of life and begin to shrink by the time a child is 5 years old. This poses two major problems. First, enlarged adenoids can block the ventilating tubes to the middle ears and lead to recurrent ear infections. Second, enlarged adenoids can cause nasal obstruction leading to mouth breathing, snoring, and OSA. In a child with OSA without an obvious cause (non-obese, absence of allergies), he should be evaluated by an ear, nose, and throat specialist for possible removal of his tonsils and adenoids.

Doc Talk

Young children with obstructive sleep apnea do not always appear to be tired during the day; instead, they may be active or overactive. It is not until they become older that the effects of obstructive sleep apnea syndrome present as tiredness.

Soiling (Encopresis)

What Can I Do?

▶ Do not punish your child's behavior. It is not his fault. Consider setting up a reward system that encourages your child not to soil himself.

▶ Be patient. It will take some time for the rectum to return to normal.

▶ Encourage regular toilet sitting first thing in the morning and for at least a few minutes after meals.

❶ What Is Encopresis?

Encopresis is a condition defined by a toilet-trained child's inability to control bowel movements. He may be able to control going to pee but often doesn't make it to the toilet on time to pass stool. Most young children will have an accident or two at some point. This is perfectly normal. Soiling becomes a problem when it happens regularly after a child has been toilet trained and hasn't had accidents for a while.

When should we contact our doctor?

The occasional episode of soiling is not a problem and does not need any special attention. Most recurrent soiling, however, should be managed with the guidance and support of your doctor.

➤➤ Encopresis Red Flags

Consult your child's doctor if your child has any of the following symptoms associated with encopresis:

- Produces small, formed stools and has leakage of stool day or night
- Has a history of infrequent, hard stools
- Is having difficulty walking or balancing or has leg weakness
- Has urinary incontinence
- Is passing stool deliberately in places other than the toilet
- Is hiding soiled underwear or clothing
- Is soiling frequently after toilet training

❷ What Causes Encopresis?

There are two patterns of encopresis. The most common soiling is associated with constipation and fecal retention. See Constipation (page 124). In this situation, the rectum is so stretched that your child has difficulty sensing the need to defecate. Overflow leakage also tends to occur. The second pattern of encopresis occurs without constipation. Typically, a battle of wills has developed between the parents, who want their child to be bowel trained, and the child, who, for whatever reason, defiantly resists being told what to do. It can sometimes be from problems related to attention and impulsivity. Occasionally, soiling occurs with diarrhea due to the stomach flu and resolves on its own. See Diarrhea (page 164). Very rarely, it occurs because of a neurological problem.

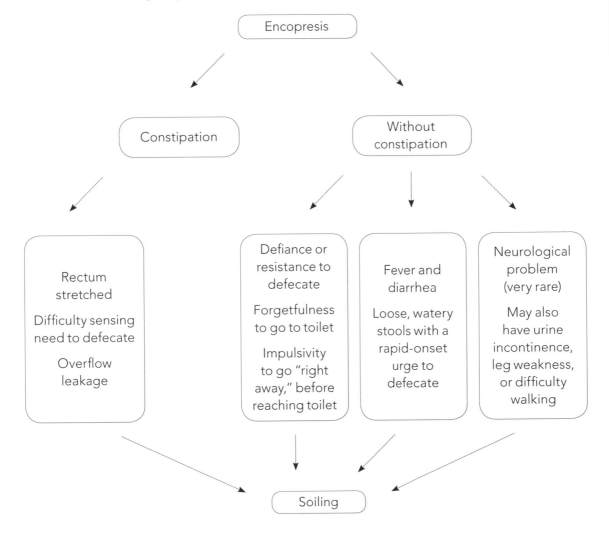

❸ How Is Encopresis Treated?

❶ Treat and prevent constipation. Soiling will end only when the rectum is no longer stretched with excess stool and normal bowel sensation is restored. See Constipation (page 124).

❷ Establish a routine. Encourage regular toilet sitting for at least a few minutes. The most "productive" times to sit are after meals or first thing in the morning.

❸ Manage behavior. The emphasis should be positive, not punitive. Encourage family members to be supportive.

Doc Talk There is a subtle psychological factor involved in the development of encopresis. Use a similar factor to break this cycle. Reward achievement. Once the constipation improves, begin a star chart or a calendar that records successful days with a star or sticker. When a particular target has been reached, a suitable reward can follow.

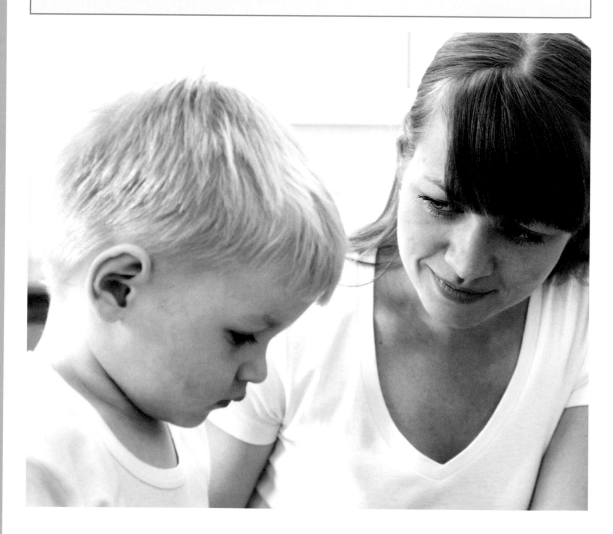

Sore Throat
(Pharyngitis and Tonsillitis)

What Can I Do?

▶ If your child has a high fever with white patches on the tonsils, especially if she doesn't have a lot of cold symptoms (runny nose, congestion), she will require a throat swab to test for strep throat. If positive, antibiotics are required.

▶ For sore throats with cold-like symptoms and associated with a virus, encourage lots of rest and fluids. Use pain relievers, if necessary.

Case Study

Mary's Sore Throat

Mary is 3 years old. Yesterday, she began complaining that her throat was sore. Today, she refused to eat anything, saying it hurt to swallow. When her doctor examined Mary, she found a low-grade fever, a red throat, a runny nose, reddened eyes, and a mild cough. Mary's mom wonders if she has tonsillitis or strep throat.

The doctor told Mary's mother that it was likely just a sore throat, which he called a viral pharyngitis. He suggested to give her plenty of fluids to drink, and not to worry if Mary didn't want to eat much for a few days. She could use acetaminophen or ibuprofen for the pain, but antibiotics were not necessary. Mary's sore throat was likely caused by a virus and would go away on its own.

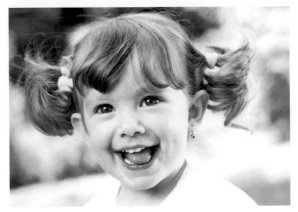

❶ What Is a Sore Throat?

Sore throat is a common condition among children. Symptoms of a sore throat usually indicate a viral pharyngitis or tonsillitis. Several clues can help distinguish between the most common viral pharyngitis/tonsillitis and a bacterial type (for example, strep throat).

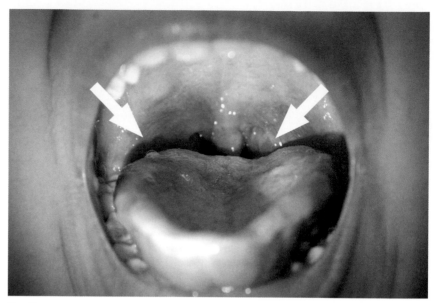

Tonsils

Viral Pharyngitis and Tonsillitis

The tonsils are the two fleshy lymph tissues at the sides of the throat that help fight off infections as part of the immune system. Tonsillitis is an infection of the tonsils at the back of the throat that results in pain and inflammation. Bacteria and viruses can cause tonsillitis, although viral causes are much more common in children. In tonsillitis, the rest of the back of the throat, called the pharynx, is frequently also infected. This is known as pharyngitis. Often, the words "tonsillitis" and "pharyngitis" are used interchangeably.

Sign, Symptom, or Clue	Bacterial Tonsillitis/ Pharyngitis	Viral Tonsillitis/ Pharyngitis
Age of child	Usually older than 3 years	Any age
Cough	Not usually	Common
Runny nose	Not usually	Very common
Sneezing	Not usually	Very common
Pain with swallowing	Common	Common
Fever	Common (may be high)	Common (may be low-grade)
Diarrhea	Not usually	Sometimes
Headache	Sometimes	Often
White patches/pus on back of throat	Common	Rare (except with infectious mononucleosis)

Sign, Symptom, or Clue	Bacterial Tonsillitis/ Pharyngitis	Viral Tonsillitis/ Pharyngitis
Mouth sores or ulcers	Rare	Very common
Pink eye (conjunctivitis)	Rare	Common
Hoarseness	Rare	Common
Enlarged lymph glands in neck	Common	Common

When should we contact our doctor or local hospital?

Most viral sore throats tend to resolve as the associated condition, such as a common cold (page 120), resolves. Occasionally, a sore throat can indicate a more serious condition, such as strep throat, requiring antibiotic treatment. See your doctor if your child shows signs of bacterial tonsillitis or pharyngitis.

▶▶ Sore Throat Red Flags

Consult your child's doctor if your child has any of the following symptoms associated with a sore throat:

- Has a sore throat that lasts more than 24 hours, especially with fever
- Has difficulty swallowing or breathing
- Has difficulty opening his mouth
- Has excessive drooling (young children)
- Has pus or white spots on the back of the throat
- Has a rash
- Has blood in her saliva or phlegm
- Has neck stiffness
- Is not drinking enough liquids and looks "dry"
- Has recurrent sore throats

❷ What Causes a Sore Throat?

Sore throat is usually caused by a virus or bacterium. The most definitive way to determine the cause of a sore throat is with a throat swab or a rapid strep swab done by your doctor.

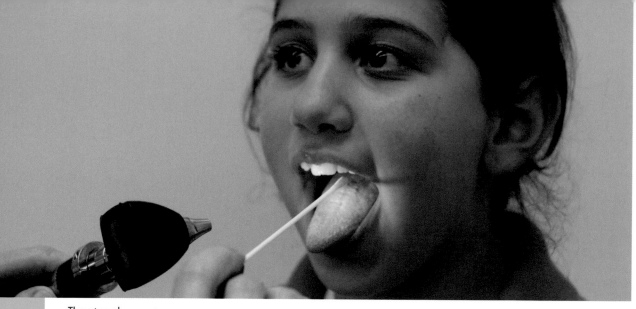

Throat swab

❸ How Is a Sore Throat Treated?

In most cases, a sore throat can be treated at home. Make sure your child gets some rest and drinks plenty of fluids. It is okay if she doesn't want to eat much. Acetaminophen or ibuprofen may help with the pain. Some people find a humidifier helpful as well.

- Because most sore throats are due to viruses, the majority do not need to be treated with antibiotics.
- However, if your child has symptoms of bacterial tonsillitis/pharyngitis, a throat swab should be performed. Only if the swab tests positive should antibiotics be used for treatment.
- If the throat swab is positive, your child should stay away from other children until she has been taking antibiotics for at least 24 hours.

How To: Prevent a Sore Throat
- Wash your child's hands often.
- Avoid close contact with people who have colds and sore throats.
- Avoid secondhand smoke.

Doc Talk

Some children seem prone to recurrent episodes of tonsillitis with sore throat. In the previous generation, many children had their tonsils removed to decrease the frequency of tonsillitis. These days, doctors are much more reluctant to remove a child's tonsils on the basis of frequent sore throats alone. As you get older, your tonsils tend to shrink in size by themselves. Nevertheless, if your child has extreme problems with tonsillitis or they are so big as to cause a blockage (for example, sleep apnea), then you may be referred to an otolaryngologist for an opinion regarding tonsillectomy.

Speech and Language Problems

What Can I Do?

▶ If your child doesn't seem to understand or has poor non-verbal communication (for example, eye contact, gestures, or pointing), discuss this promptly with your health-care provider.

▶ If you are concerned about stuttering or unclear speech, consider getting an opinion from a speech and language therapist. See below for some tips on how to help develop your child's speech.

❶ What Are Speech and Language Development Problems?

Speech and language development is complex and wonderful to behold in your child. If difficulties arise, it is important to distinguish which aspect of speech or language is affected and to be precise when seeking help,

Types of Speech and Language Disorders

There are several types of speech disorders with their own characteristics.

- **Receptive language (what the child understands):** A delay in receptive language development is the most concerning type of speech problem and often suggests a true developmental delay or even autism. (See pages 155 and 64.) However, it might be something else. If you are not sure that your child's hearing is normal, hurry and get it tested!
- **Expressive language (what the child says, or "speech"):** An isolated delay in expressive language development with normal receptive language (normal understanding of speech) is the least concerning type of speech problem — these kids tend to do really well.
- **Articulation (how the child pronounces words):** If your child is difficult to understand because his speech is unclear, but he understands your speech, he will usually do just fine with speech therapy and time.
- **Fluency ("smoothness" of speech):** Stuttering is a kind of "dysfluency." (See page 377.)
- **Non-verbal communication:** We also communicate in ways that do not include words. Examples of this would be the use of eye

contact, gestures such as nodding, shaking the head, shrugging shoulders, pointing, and facial expressions. Infants should look at an adult's face and be able to follow it with their eyes by 1 month. Eye contact should be well developed in infancy. Diminished eye contact and avoiding eye contact are two different things (the former indicating disinterest and the latter, normal shyness). Pointing typically begins around 1 year of age and is used both to make requests and to share interest.

- **Dysarticulation (trouble pronouncing) and dysfluency (stuttering):** Both of these conditions are usually temporary. Working with a speech therapist will be helpful. You will learn specific strategies that you and your child will work on together.

When should we contact our doctor?

If you are worried about a true language delay (a delay in receptive language) or worried about a delay in non-verbal communication development, then you should seek an assessment by your physician and by a speech therapist. You should request a hearing test. Your physician may also suggest an assessment by a developmental pediatrician or a psychologist. See Developmental Delay (page 155) and Autism (page 64).

How To: Treat an Expressive Speech Delay

- When talking to your child, use simplified language that is at, or just above, your child's own language level. If your 2-year-old is using only a few single words, lengthy explanations won't help as much.
- Simplify stories and prompt labeling of common pictures in a book ("Look at the dog!" "What's that?"). This may stimulate more talking.
- Sing songs with your child, with pauses to see if he asks for more or fills in the gap. This will be fun for you and your child and can help with language development.
- Name body parts or clothing as you dress, undress, or bathe your child to introduce language into everyday activities.
- Repeat back what you hear your child say. This helps reinforce your child's language development.

Doc Talk

Children's speech production typically ramps up when they are around other kids their own age. Consider increasing the time they spend in drop-in or daycare centers.

Stuttering

❶ What Is Stuttering?

Stuttering refers to a disruption in the flow of speech due to involuntary pauses, extra syllables, or repetition of all or part of a word. It is common and quite normal for children between 2 and 5 years of age to stutter. Up to 5% of children are affected by stuttering for a while, but it persists in less than 1% of children. Stuttering is three times more common in boys than in girls, and it sometimes runs in families.

Stuttering after 4 years old, if it upsets your child, or if it really interferes with his ability to communicate, is considered to be a dysfluency. This is a type of communication disorder in which the rate, rhythm, and flow of speech is interrupted.

Types of Stuttering

- Your child might repeat frequent sounds or syllables (for example, "L-l-l-l-l-like").
- Your child might substitute a weak vowel (for example, "Luh-luh-luh-like").
- Your child might prolong a sound (for example, "Sssssssssssnake").
- Sometimes, the stuttering child just appears to get "stuck" on a word.

When should we contact our doctor?

Stuttering is not an emergency situation. Most children who stutter are healthy and developing at an appropriate rate for their age. Seek medical attention if any of the red flags on page 378 are present.

➤➤ Stuttering Red Flags

Consult a speech and language pathologist if your child is older than 5 years old and has any of the following symptoms associated with stuttering:

- Your child's stuttering persists or worsens over a period of several months.
- Your child demonstrates anxiety or frustration about his speech.
- Your child starts to avoid situations where he is required to speak.

---

❷ What Causes Stuttering?

The actual cause and mechanism of stuttering is not well understood. It is believed that genetics and neurophysiology both play a role. Stress and anxiety are not felt to cause stuttering, but they can certainly make it much worse in those prone to the problem.

❸ How Is Stuttering Treated?

There are several simple ways in which you can help:

- Always allow your child to complete her thoughts or sentences — without interruption, prompting, or correction.
- Model slow and clear speech patterns.
- Encourage non-verbal activities if your child has more severe difficulties.
- Ask your family doctor for a referral to a speech pathologist if you feel your child's stuttering is not improving or is becoming worse.

Doc Talk   Some stuttering around the time of rapid increases in your child's vocabulary before age 5 is common. As long as your child is not upset by it, this is considered to be normal.

The good news is that stuttering gets better in the majority of children!

Teething

What Can I Do?

▶ Try massaging the swollen gum with a clean finger for a few minutes.

▶ Let your baby bite on a cold, wet facecloth.

▶ Don't use homeopathic teething remedies (potential toxicity).

▶ Don't automatically blame fevers or irritability on teething — think of other potential reasons for these symptoms.

❶ What Is Teething?

Teething refers to the normal appearance of new teeth erupting through the gums. This developmental process is highly variable, but most children will start to acquire their first tooth between a few months of age and 1 year. Most commonly, teething starts at 6 or 7 months, when the lower incisors appear. Thereafter, more baby teeth erupt every month or two, starting with the incisors, then the first molars, followed by the canines, and, finally, the second molars.

Sign and Symptoms of Teething

- Increased drooling
- Desire to gum objects
- Swollen gum where tooth will soon break through
- Reddish/blue discoloration over the molars

When should we contact our doctor?

In most cases, teething does not require medical attention. Many parents tend to blame a child's fever on teething, but it is doubtful that teething produces a fever. Rather, the age of teething coincides with a child's susceptibility to common childhood viruses. Many parents also believe that teething can be associated with diarrhea and diaper rashes, but these are actually myths too. If your child looks or seems unwell, do not blame it on teething; seek medical attention.

▶▶ Teething Red Flags

Fever or significant irritability in an infant should not be attributed to a tooth erupting but rather should be evaluated for other causes.

Normal Eruption Pattern

	Tooth	Eruption	Falls Out
Upper jaw	central incisor	7 to 12 months	6 to 8 years
	lateral incisor	9 to 13 months	7 to 8 years
	canine	16 to 22 months	10 to 12 years
	first molar	13 to 19 months	9 to 11 years
	second molar	25 to 33 months	10 to 12 years
Lower jaw	central incisor	6 to 10 months	6 to 8 years
	lateral incisor	7 to 16 months	7 to 8 years
	canine	16 to 23 months	9 to 12 years
	first molar	12 to 18 months	9 to 11 years
	second molar	20 to 31 months	10 to 12 years

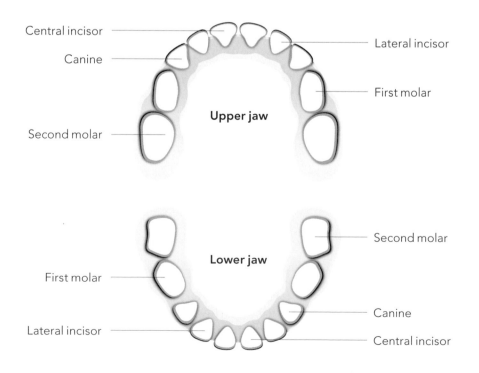

Central incisor — Lateral incisor
Canine — First molar

Upper jaw

Second molar

Second molar
Lower jaw
First molar
Canine
Lateral incisor — Central incisor

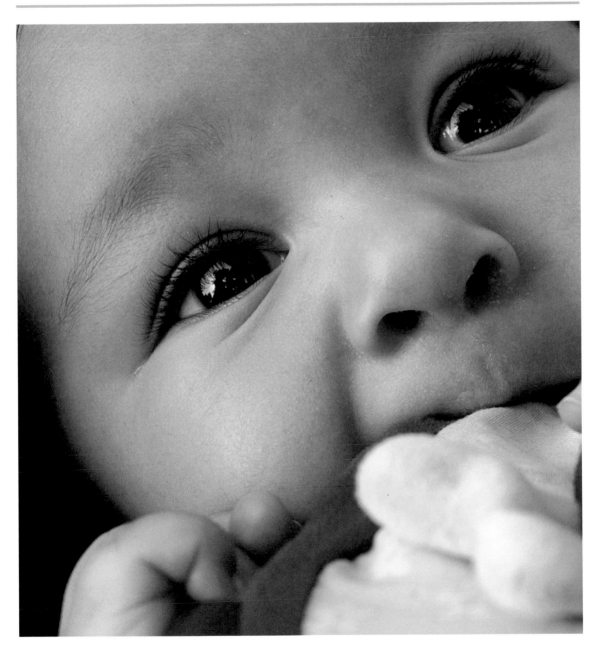

❷ How Is Teething Treated?

Most of the time, no treatment is needed. However, you can help soothe your child.

- If the gums are swollen and the baby seems fussy, try massaging the gum with a clean finger for a minute or two. If this brings relief, you can repeat the massage as needed.

- Babies can massage their own gums when they are provided with a teething ring or some safe object to gum. A cold wet washcloth or teething biscuit will do, but foods that may cause choking, such as a carrot stick, should be avoided.
- If your child seems unsettled because of teething, try some oral pain medication. You can give your baby a dose or two of acetaminophen or ibuprofen, but persistent irritability is probably caused by something else. You may need to seek help to investigate this further..

FAQ

My 11-month-old doesn't have any teeth yet. When should I worry that his first tooth eruption is late?

Late tooth eruption refers to the emergence of a tooth at a time significantly later than the expected time. The precise timing of when a tooth is "late" is based roughly on the chart at the beginning of this chapter. Most children who have delayed tooth eruption are perfectly normal, healthy kids, with normal dentition. Generally, if your infant has no teeth by 12 months, he should be assessed.

Doc Talk

Unexplained fever in a young child should be assessed by a health-care provider; don't simply attribute this to teething. Irritability and fever are not commonly seen with teething. If present and persistent, have your child assessed to look for other causes. For more information on children's teeth, see the chapter on Toothache (page 393).

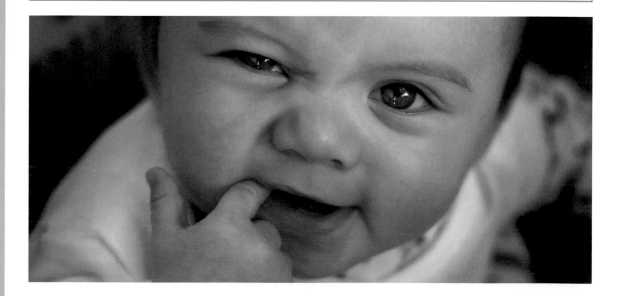

Temper Tantrums

Case Study

Taylor's Tantrums

Taylor is 3 years old and is terrorizing her mother with temper tantrums at the grocery store. Before going shopping, her mother makes it clear that Taylor cannot have all the treats she wants. She praises her for good behavior as they enter the store, but soon after, Taylor demands a treat (and doesn't get it). Taylor has a temper tantrum, and everybody watches her pound her fists on the aisle floor and scream. Her mother is embarrassed about the scene Taylor has caused, and she wishes to herself that Taylor would just stop all the fuss.

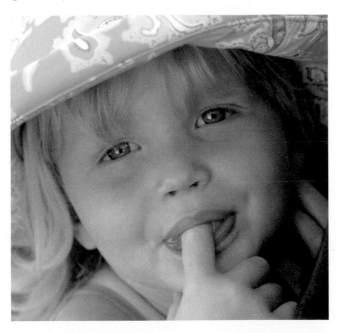

At her wit's end, Taylor's mother consults with their family doctor, who encourages her not to give in and explains that sensible onlookers will be more impressed if she doesn't. Eventually, Taylor will learn that temper tantrums don't get her what she wants and the tantrums will stop.

❶ What Is a Temper Tantrum?

Most toddlers have tantrums at some point, but some kids are more "strong-willed" than others and may be more likely to scream and throw themselves on the floor to try to get their way. Temper tantrums among children in their "terrible twos" are common and predictable. They usually begin after the age of 12 months, peak between 2 and 3 years of age, and settle down after the age of 4.

When should we contact our doctor?

Most temper tantrums will end when your child discovers they are not effective, and should be viewed as a normal developmental phase. Seek medical attention if any red flags are present.

❱❱ Temper Tantrum Red Flags

Consult your child's doctor if:

- Your child's temper tantrums continue to get worse after the age of 4.
- Your child injures herself, or others, during tantrums, or destroys property.
- Your child holds her breath or faints during tantrums (if these are deemed simple "breath-holding spells" by your doctor, still don't give in to the tantrums!).
- You are concerned about other issues, such as a delay or regression in development, headaches, abdominal pain, anxiety, or excessive clinginess.

❷ What Causes a Temper Tantrum?

Tantrums are often set off by frustration when your child does not get what she wants. They tend to be more likely to occur when she is anxious, tired, or hungry. Temper tantrums can also occur simply because a child is seeking attention or testing the rules.

❸ How Are Temper Tantrums Managed?

There is a great deal you can do to manage and even prevent temper tantrums at home.

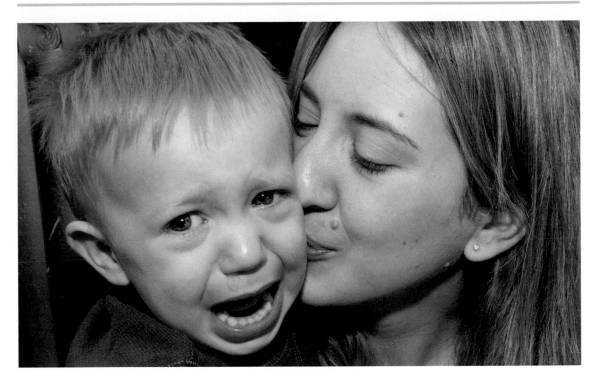

How To: Manage a Temper Tantrum

- Try to stay calm.
- Make sure that your child does not hurt herself, or anybody else.
- Appear to ignore the tantrum until she calms down. A short period of "time out" can help her regain control. Some children need to be held, gently but firmly, until they settle down.
- Do not try to reason with your child during the outburst. Later, when she has calmed down, it may be constructive to discuss her behavior and the consequences.
- Do not reward or punish your child. Neither rewards nor spankings stop temper tantrums! Do not reward the behavior by giving in to the tantrums. Rewarding a tantrum teaches her that it works and she'll do it again. Hitting or spanking teaches her that violence is a good way to deal with anger, and she may start to hit during a tantrum.
- Ignore the behavior and don't give in. She'll learn that this behavior doesn't work and will stop doing it (eventually).

Doc Talk You can help prevent temper tantrums by making sure your child gets enough sleep and eats as soon as she starts to feel hungry (overtired children and hungry children are more likely to have a tantrum). Stick to routines as much as possible, and have realistic expectations. Prepare your child for change or new situations. Establish the rules and enforce them consistently.

Thrush

What Can I Do?

▶ Look for white patches on the gums, cheeks, tongue, or roof of your baby's mouth that cannot be wiped away. This indicates that your child likely has thrush.

▶ Treat thrush by cleaning all pacifiers, bottles, and nipples that enter an infant's mouth. Failure to do so can lead to recurrent thrush.

❶ What Is Thrush?

Thrush is a common infection in a baby's mouth caused by a yeast called *Candida albicans*. It can appear as early as the first week of life and is common in the first months of life.

Signs and Symptoms of Thrush
- White patches on the gums, inner cheeks, tongue, and roof of the mouth
- Unlike milk curds, these patches are difficult to wipe off
- Fussiness (but may have absolutely no symptoms at all)
- Feeding difficulties (this symptom is not always present)

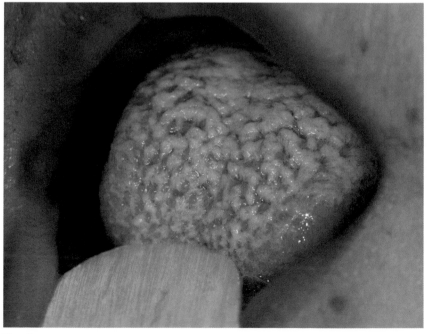

Thrush

- If infection spreads to the diaper area, the diaper rash looks red and irritated and doesn't seem to go away on its own. See Diaper Rash (page 160).
- If infection spreads to the mother's nipples, she may feel nipple pain, increased sensitivity, itching, irritation, and stabbing pain deep within the breast

When should we contact our doctor?

Thrush is not an emergency. If you notice whitish spots on your child's tongue or in her mouth that don't wipe away easily and if your baby is feeding poorly or is fussy, see your doctor.

❷ What Causes Thrush?

Thrush is caused by an overgrowth of naturally occurring *Candida albicans* (a type of yeast). It very commonly occurs for no apparent reason in young infants. In some children, the yeast overgrowth can occur after taking antibiotics or steroid medications, which disrupt the natural balance of bacteria and yeast in the mouth.

❸ How Is Thrush Treated?

If your doctor suspects thrush, he will prescribe an antifungal medication (for example, nystatin drops or fluconazole) for about a week. The medication will help restore the normal levels of *Candida* in her mouth. If her mother is breastfeeding, the doctor may suggest applying an antifungal cream to the nipple area.

Doc Talk

In babies with recurrent thrush, reinfection commonly occurs when the infection is passed back and forth from a baby to a mother's nipples or an infected pacifier that has not been properly cleaned. If your baby develops thrush, all pacifiers and bottles should be thoroughly sterilized and breastfeeding mothers should also be treated with a topical antifungal medication used on the nipples.

Thumb-Sucking

What Can I Do?

▶ If you try to stop your child's thumb-sucking by using a pacifier instead, do not put anything sweet (sugar, honey, corn syrup) on the soother as a way to entice your child to use the soother. This will cause significant tooth decay.

▶ After 2 to 3 years, children do not feel the need to suck as much. If your child is still sucking her thumb, work on eliminating the habit before her permanent teeth emerge at 5 years.

▶ See the tips below for some strategies to stop thumb-sucking.

❶ What Is Thumb-Sucking?

Did you know that many infants suck their thumbs even before they are born? Sucking provides comfort for infants, but thumb-sucking can become a prolonged habit as your child gets older. If thumb-sucking persists, pressure on the emerging permanent upper front teeth may cause the teeth to protrude, resulting in problems with your child's bite as he gets older.

When should we contact our doctor?

The American Academy of Pediatric Dentistry and the Canadian Dental Association state that thumb-sucking is not a concern until the permanent front teeth begin to emerge (usually after 5 years of age). Sometimes, children who suck their thumbs develop calluses, lacerations (cuts), or infections where their teeth contact the skin of the thumb.

❷ How Is Thumb-Sucking Treated?

Most thumb-sucking children actually stop on their own. Behavioral techniques, such as distraction and encouragement, may be helpful. Some parents apply bad-tasting (nontoxic) solutions to the thumb or thumbnail as a deterrent. Very rarely, the dentist can insert an oral device, which interferes with sucking, into the child's mouth. For similar treatments, see Nail-Biting (page 288).

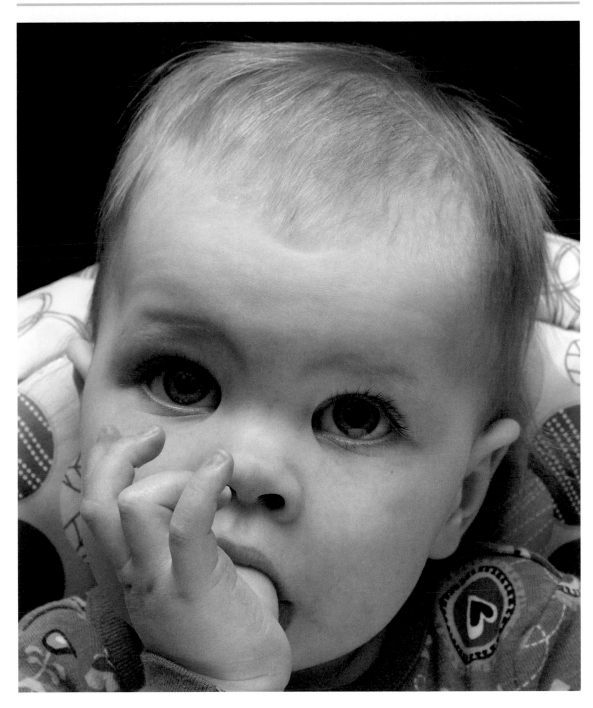

Doc Talk Is sucking a pacifier preferable to sucking a thumb? Thumb-, finger-, and pacifier-sucking all have similar effects on dentition. The only advantage of sucking a pacifier is that it is an easier habit to break because it can be physically removed from the child — it's not very practical to remove the thumb!

Tics and Tourette's Syndrome

Case Study

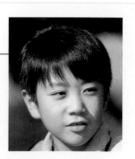

Steven's Tics

Over the past few weeks, Steven's parents have noticed that he often blinks his eyes in an exaggerated fashion. They have become very concerned. Steven denies that there is something bothering his eyes and reports no irritation or itch. Steven's parents have also noticed that when he is playing baseball, the eye blinking seems to be much more prominent. Steven's parents recall a period, about a year ago, when he was 7 years old, he had a weird tightening of his neck muscles in an odd sort of repetitive twitch. This had gone on for weeks and then disappeared as mysteriously as it had begun. He was otherwise healthy, with a good appetite, and seemed to be enjoying school and his various activities.

His doctor asked a lot of questions about the twitches and specifically asked if he had any unusually persistent and irritating vocal habits, such as, whistling, sniffing, or throat clearing. He performed a full examination, including an eye and neurological examination. He reassured Steven's parents that this was most likely a simple motor tic. He explained that this was common, especially in young boys, and tended to come and go but usually settled down with no treatment. It was not unusual to see it get a bit worse during times of stress, for example when he was up to bat for his Little League baseball team. Steven's doctor advised his parents to "play it down" and not draw attention to the tics, as Steven would not be able to control them even if he wanted to. He suggested that they see how things were going at Steven's next annual physical.

❶ What Are Tics and Tourette's Syndrome?

Tics

Tics are involuntary, rhythmic, repetitive events. They can be primarily movements (motor tics) or sounds (vocal tics).

Motor tics can be simple or complex. Eye blinking and mouth twitching are common simple motor tics. Complex motor tics involve more than one muscle group, like facial grimacing or arm flapping. Vocal tics include throat clearing, sniffing, and animal sounds, like barking. Uttering obscene words or phrases (coprolalia), repeating one's own words (palilalia), and repeating another's words (echolalia) are more unusual vocal tics.

Tics are common in children under the age of 10 — up to 10% of children will have a tic, which is usually transient. Motor tics are more common than vocal tics. Tics occur more often in boys than in girls. Most tics disappear within several months. In a minority of these children, tics will persist and become chronic. Some tics progress to Tourette's syndrome.

Did You Know?

Controlling Tics

Tics can be suppressed for variable lengths of time (minutes to hours). Some children manage to suppress tics during school, and then have multiple frequent episodes once they get home. Typically, however, they cannot be stopped just by willing them away.

When should we contact our doctor?

A tic is not an emergency but may require medical attention if the tic is persistent, interfering with function, or is bothering a child. In most children, symptoms improve substantially or disappear with time, usually after puberty.

▶ Tic Red Flags

Consult your child's doctor if your child has any of the following symptoms associated with a tic:

- Persistent complex motor tics — for example, facial grimacing or hand flapping
- Persistent vocal tics — for example, throat clearing, whistling, or barking
- Any other rhythmic/repetitive movement (tic) that is persistent and appears to bother your child (or you!)

Tourette's Syndrome

Tourette's syndrome is rare, affecting approximately 1 in 1,000 children. Tourette's is a tic disorder that starts in childhood or adolescence, lasts for more than 1 year, and is characterized by both motor and vocal tics. Motor and vocal tics do not necessarily occur at the same time, and their severity can vary significantly at different times. Tics may occur daily or intermittently, and they cause marked distress or interfere with social, occupational, or other important areas of functioning.

The tics are aggravated by physical factors, such as hunger, fatigue, and anxiety, as well as by certain medications, particularly stimulants that are sometimes used to treat attention deficit hyperactivity disorder (ADHD). See Attention Deficit Hyperactivity Disorder (page 58).

❷ What Causes Tics and Tourette's Syndrome?

The exact causes of tics and Tourette's syndrome are not known. It is believed that tics are caused by abnormalities in certain areas of the brain, and may be related to chemical imbalances in those areas. The neurotransmitter (chemical substance) that has most frequently been incriminated is called dopamine. Genetic factors also seem to play a role.

❸ How Are Tics and Tourette's Syndrome Treated?

Most tics in children are simple motor tics that are transient and require no specific treatment. In the meantime, you can try the following techniques:

- Try not to draw attention to the child's tics, and don't tell your child to stop — he cannot control the tics and you may make him anxious, which can increase the severity and frequency of the tics.
- When symptoms are disabling, behavior therapy, relaxation techniques, and medication may be helpful. A number of community associations have been established to provide education and support for affected children and their families.
- Children with chronic tics or Tourette's syndrome should undergo comprehensive medical evaluation. It is important to establish that the symptoms are not caused by other neurologic or psychiatric conditions, or by medications or illicit drugs. Coexisting disorders, such as ADHD, must be identified and treated.

Doc Talk Children with isolated tics do not usually have associated conditions. However, many children with Tourette's syndrome also have attention deficit hyperactivity disorder (see ADHD, page 58), learning disabilities (see page 263), and obsessive-compulsive disorder. Some children develop symptoms of depression, sleep problems, social difficulties, and self-injurious behaviors because they may be teased and become socially isolated.

Toothache

What Can I Do?

▶ Help your child develop good oral hygiene to prevent tooth decay and toothache.

▶ Take your child to see a dentist as early as 12 months of age or within 6 months of the first tooth eruption.

▶ In the case of injury to the teeth or toothache, see the list of indications for urgent assessment as well as tips for immediate management strategies.

❶ What Is a Toothache?

A toothache refers to pain that a child may feel in or around a tooth. Commonly, tooth pain is felt from a tooth that is temporarily sensitive.

❷ What Causes a Toothache?

Toothaches that endure are often a warning sign that your child may have decay or a cavity. Less commonly, toothache may result from injury to the tooth or gums. Occasionally, it can be pain coming from another location but sensed in the tooth (referred pain), such as from an ear infection or from inflammation of the temporomandibular joint (the joint that joins the upper and lower jaw).

RELATED CONDITIONS

- Bleeding gums
- Dental caries (decay)
- Dental trauma
- Teeth grinding

When should I see my child's dentist?

Call your child's dentist if:

- Toothache lasts more than 1 day.
- You are concerned that your child has dental caries or cavities that might lead to toothache.

▶▶ Toothache Red Flags

See your child's dentist immediately if there is:

- Severe tooth pain.
- Swelling of the face with tooth pain.
- Tooth pain with a fever.

❸ How Is a Toothache Treated?

- To help reduce pain, offer acetaminophen or ibuprofen.
- Apply a cold pack to the affected area for 15 minutes at a time. This can be soothing and reduce any swelling.
- If there is a history of injury, see your child's dentist.
- If the pain doesn't subside in 1 or 2 days, or it becomes severe, have your child assessed by a dentist to look for signs of caries or infection in the tooth.

❶ What Are Dental Caries?

Dental caries refers to the presence of one or more decayed lesions (with or without a cavity), missing teeth (due to decay), or filled tooth surfaces in any primary tooth. Although your child will eventually start losing his primary teeth and develop his permanent teeth, keeping his first set of teeth clean is very important. If there are signs that your baby's teeth have decay, they likely need treatment by a dentist.

Left untreated, decay can lead to worsening infection and pain. This can spread to the face or other parts of the body and make your child very unwell. Decay and infection can also spread to the jaw bone and damage the development of permanent teeth.

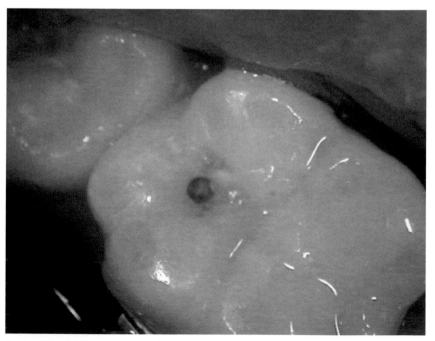

Tooth with mild decay

When should we first contact a dentist?

If your child shows any signs of dental caries, see a dentist. The first visit to the dentist should occur within 6 months of the first tooth eruption or when your child is 12 months old, whichever comes first. The dentist can determine if the cleaning you are doing at home is working. Going to the dentist at a young age will help make your child more comfortable with the routine and help to identify and fix any dental problems early.

❷ What Causes Dental Caries?

Caries are caused by bacteria, which break down the sugars we eat. This process, in turn, produces acid. The acid destroys the minerals that make up our teeth. The enamel of a baby's tooth is immature and susceptible to breaking down.

❸ How Are Dental Caries Treated?

Like many health conditions, prevention is the best treatment.

Prevention
- Do not put your baby or child to bed with milk, formula, juice, or sweetened water.
- If thirsty, give water rather than milk or something sweet to your child before bed.
- Clean your child's teeth after you breast- or bottle-feed him.
- Wean your child from the bottle by 12 to 18 months.
- Do not dip the pacifier in anything sweet.
- Do not let your child walk around with a bottle or cup of sugary fluids or milk.
- Parents and pregnant women should have their teeth cleaned to help prevent spread of the bacteria that cause caries to their infant or child.

How To: Clean Your Child's Teeth
Brushing
- A young child cannot clean his teeth properly and should get assistance from an adult. Teeth should be brushed at least twice daily. Brushing your child's teeth just before bed is very

Did You Know?

Fluoride Benefit and Risk

Fluoride makes the teeth stronger, making them more resistant to decay. If decay is already present, fluoride can prevent it from worsening and even reverse some of the decay that has already happened. Fluoride is added to most toothpastes and, in most communities, is added to the tap water. Too much flouride can cause fluorosis (staining of your child's teeth).

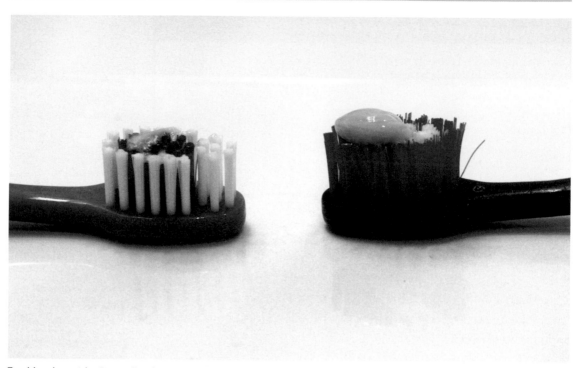

Toothbrushes with a "smear" and a pea-sized amount of toothpaste

important, to reduce the bacteria that sit on his teeth overnight, contributing to decay.

- From 3 months: Wipe gums with a soft washcloth after each feed.
- After first tooth eruption: Clean teeth with a soft brush, one appropriately sized for your child's mouth, at least twice daily. A tiny smear of toothpaste may be used on the bristles.
- While a toddler: Clean teeth with a soft brush. Use a pea-sized amount of toothpaste if the child is able to spit it out.

Flossing

It is important to clean the spaces between your child's teeth that cannot normally be accessed by a toothbrush. By the time your child is 3 years old, his teeth are usually close enough together that bacteria can get trapped between the teeth, and flossing should be started.

Snacking

Eating small, frequent snacks is a common way many children get their nutrition. However, continuous exposure to foods with sugar or starch can contribute to decay by prolonging the time the teeth are exposed to caries-producing bacteria. Avoid sticky treats (raisins, chewy candies), and after snacks, gently clean your child's teeth. If this is not possible, try giving your child some water to drink to help rinse the sugars from his mouth.

❶ What Is Dental Trauma?

It is very common for young children to injure their teeth. Injuries can range from a minor chip to a completely knocked out (avulsed) tooth. The most common teeth injured are the incisors at the front of the mouth. Any injury to the teeth should be assessed by a dentist.

Injuries to Primary (Baby) Teeth

Even though these teeth will eventually fall out, injury to the baby teeth has the potential for long-term dental problems. Even a small chip or loosened tooth should be assessed by a dentist because the injury can interfere with the development and alignment of the permanent tooth growing underneath.

Injuries to Permanent Teeth

Any permanent tooth that has been knocked out is considered a dental emergency!

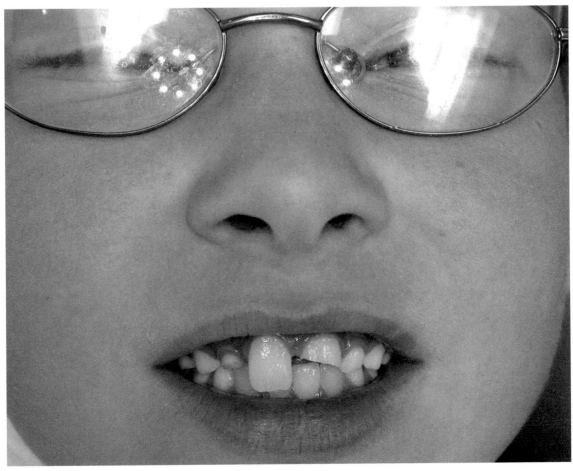

Chipped upper incisor

How To: Manage a Knocked-Out Tooth

- Find the tooth and pick it up by the top part of the tooth so as to avoid touching the root.
- Rinse the tooth off in water if dirty.
- Place the tooth back into the gum it came out of and hold it there.
- If unable to put it back into the gum, immerse it in a cup of milk and place it on ice.
- See a dentist as soon as possible (don't forget to bring the tooth!). The longer the elapsed time between tooth injury and seeing the dentist, the worse the chance of saving the tooth.

FAQs

Why does my child grind his teeth?

Up to half of all infants will grind their teeth at some point. This is most often noticed when the top and bottom two teeth have erupted. The reason infants grind their teeth is not entirely clear. Perhaps it is due to infants enjoying the sound and sensation of their teeth grinding — or perhaps it is to give parents yet another thing to worry about! Unlike tooth grinding in adults, grinding in infants is generally harmless. Fortunately, the vast majority of infants will outgrow this habit without any lasting damage to their teeth. No treatment is necessary — just ignore it.

My daughter's gums tend to bleed after brushing her teeth. Should I be worried?

Bleeding gums are most often a sign that your child has inflammation of the gums (gingivitis) from tooth decay and inadequate plaque removal. If your child regularly has bleeding gums, see your child's dentist for a cleaning and evaluation. Very rarely, bleeding gums can be a sign of a problem with the blood's ability to form a clot. These rare clotting problems are often associated with other signs, such as recurrent nosebleeds or easy bruising. See Bruising (page 98).

Doc Talk

Good oral hygiene is essential for preventing tooth decay and toothache. Brushing at least twice daily with fluoridated toothpaste and regular visits to the dentist for checkups and cleaning will help keep mouth bacteria and consequent cavities at bay. If you visit your dentist regularly, your child will become accustomed to preventive dental procedures and will be less likely to experience any fear or trepidation at the prospect of seeing the dentist.

Umbilical Cord Problems

What Can I Do?

▶ No special treatment is needed for the care of a newborn umbilical cord. Avoid applying alcohol, ointments, or other preparations to the cord or its surrounding skin.

▶ The cord will fall off on its own in about 1 to 3 weeks. Until then, fold down the top of the diaper to prevent irritation from the diaper rubbing on a fresh cord.

▶ If your baby has redness, swelling, or pussy discharge from the umbilical area, then seek medical advice urgently.

Case Study

Joshua's Belly Button

Joshua is a 3-week-old healthy baby boy whose umbilical cord fell off last week. His father was giving Joshua a bath and noticed that his navel had a little pink lump on it, with some watery discharge coming from the middle of it. He brought Joshua to the doctor the following day for a checkup and asked what was wrong with his son's belly button.

Joshua's doctor explained that when his cord fell off, a tiny connecting channel remained open where the cord used to deliver nutrients from Joshua's mother. As the tissue healed, the process was a little "overenthusiastic" and a fleshy lump, or granuloma, was created. Sometimes, infants can have a little bit of watery leakage from this sort of granuloma. It was not dangerous in any way, but it was a bit messy, so the doctor decided to cauterize it with some silver nitrate.

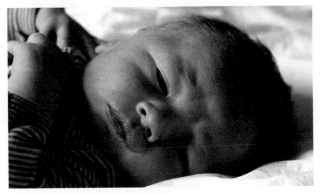

❶ What Are Umbilical Cord Problems?

Umbilical Cord Granuloma

The umbilical cord is the lifeline that provides nutrients to the fetus during pregnancy. At delivery, it is clamped and cut. Initially, the cord is thick, rubbery, and translucent, but after a few days, it dries out and shrivels up. The stump typically falls off between 1 and 3 weeks of age and the area becomes a belly button. A small amount of bleeding

RELATED CONDITIONS

- Hernia
- Omphalitis
- Umbilical cord granuloma

may occur just before or after the cord detaches. It usually stops almost immediately with gentle pressure alone and is not a cause for concern. In some cases, there may be a piece of small, pink, fleshy tissue called an umbilical cord granuloma. This does not hurt, but it can continue to create a small amount of discharge from where the cord was attached to the baby's belly. Often, your health-care provider will apply silver nitrate to remove the granuloma.

When should we contact our doctor?

Granulomas are not an emergency. Instead, you can ask your doctor at your child's next well-baby checkup if the granuloma warrants treatment.

⟫ Umbilical Cord Red Flags

Consult your child's doctor if your child has any of the following symptoms associated with the umbilical cord:

- There is redness, swelling, or pus around the umbilical cord
- Your baby is feverish, feeding poorly, or lethargic
- Your baby's cord stump has not fallen off after 4 weeks
- There is a lot of drainage from the umbilical stump

FAQ

How do I care for my newborn's umbilical cord?
Do nothing! The umbilical cord needs no special cleaning apart from normal hygiene. The cord falls off more quickly if left alone, and special cleaning with topical antiseptics has not proven to prevent infections, which are rare to begin with. Folding down the top of the diaper can prevent irritation.

Omphalitis

Rarely, the tissue around the cord becomes infected and inflamed and requires urgent treatment. This condition is called omphalitis.

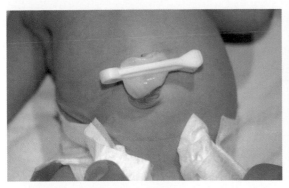

Normal cord at the time of clamping

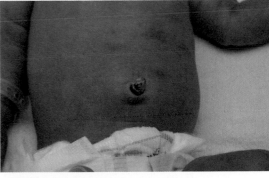

Dried and shriveled cord

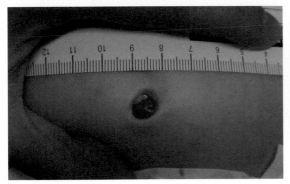

Umbilical cord granuloma

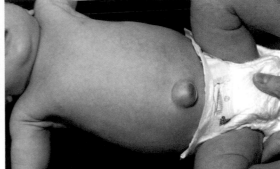

Umbilical hernia

Umbilical Hernia

Some parents will notice a lump protruding from their baby's belly button long after the cord falls off. The lump, which appears bigger with crying or straining, is an umbilical hernia. This hernia is usually caused by a temporary defect in the muscle of the abdominal wall under the belly button. The lump results from the abdominal contents protruding through the muscle, under the skin. It is painless and usually closes on its own in the first few years of life. It is much more common in Black infants and in premature babies. Although very large or persistent (beyond 3 years of age) hernias require surgery to repair, an umbilical hernia usually resolves without treatment.

Doc Talk Parents often ask whether they should give their baby a sponge bath so as not to wet the umbilical cord stump. There is no evidence that this is necessary; it is perfectly okay to bathe your baby with regular baby soap and pat the stump dry afterward.

Undescended Testicle

What Can I Do?

▶ If you notice asymmetry of your child's scrotum or cannot feel both testicles, bring this to your doctor's attention at the next well-child checkup.

▶ If your child has an undescended testicle at birth, do not be alarmed. Many will spontaneously descend into the scrotum in the first few months of life.

Case Study

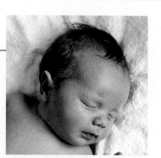

Tommy's Undescended Testicle

Tommy is a 7-day-old baby boy, born at term following an uncomplicated pregnancy. He was discharged from hospital the day after delivery and has been breastfeeding well and soiling diapers regularly. Tommy's mother brought him in to see the doctor to have Tommy's weight checked and to see if he was close to regaining his birth weight. Tommy's mom, having had two girls, felt a little nervous about having her first son. She had several questions for the doctor, one of which was: "Why is Tommy's scrotum really small on one side?" The doctor examined Tommy's scrotum and was able to feel the left testicle in the scrotum, whereas the right one was high up in the groin and could not be manipulated into the scrotal sac.

The doctor explained that Tommy's testicle had not fully descended into the scrotum. In time, it was possible that the testicle would complete its descent. If by several months of age, however, the testicle was not sitting in the scrotum, Tommy would be referred to a surgeon to have the testicle brought down into the scrotum and fixed there.

❶ What Is an Undescended Testicle?

An undescended testicle is a testis that has failed to move into the scrotum as a male fetus develops. About 3% of boys are born with one of their testicles undescended. By 6 months of life, only about 1% of boys have an undescended testicle. In boys born prematurely, up to 30% will have an undescended testicle at birth.

When should we contact our doctor?

Although it is not an emergency, make an appointment with your doctor as soon as you detect a problem with your child's scrotum or testicles.

❷ What Causes an Undescended Testicle?

During normal development in the womb, male fetuses experience a gradual descent of the testicles from the abdomen down into the scrotum. Typically, this process is complete by the time of birth. In many boys, the testicle has properly descended by birth, but it sometimes retracts into the body and cannot be felt in the scrotum. In other boys, the descent is incomplete at birth. Characteristics that distinguish an undescended testicle (cryptorchidism) from a retractile testicle are shown in the accompanying table.

Retractile Testicle	Undescended Testicle
• Very common • One or both testicles seem to "disappear" in cold temperatures or when the infant is excited; this is due to a retraction back up along the inguinal canal • Testicle can be felt in the scrotum in warmer temperatures • Always resolves on its own as the boy grows older	• Uncommon overall, yet very common among boys born preterm (premature) • More likely in babies who have low weight at birth • Scrotum may appear small and underdeveloped, or asymmetrical if only one testicle is undescended • Usually accompanied by an inguinal hernia on the affected side(s) • Typically requires surgical correction if still present after about 3 to 4 months of age

Diagnosis

Examination by a physician is necessary to make a proper diagnosis. Usually, if the physician does not locate both testicles in the scrotum of a healthy term infant in the first months of life, she will plan to re-examine the scrotum at 4 months of age.

❸ How Is an Undescended Testicle Treated in Infants?

The most common treatment is a surgical procedure in which the testicle is brought down and fixed to the base of the scrotum. This is usually performed by a pediatric urologist before 1 year of age, and has a low rate of complications.

> **Doc Talk** There are two main reasons for doing the surgery if a testicle remains undescended beyond the first several months of life. First, the future capacity to produce sperm is impaired if the testicle remains in the abdomen for too long. Second, surgery reduces the risk of undetected testicular cancer.

Urinary Tract Infection
(Bladder or Kidney Infection)

What Can I Do?

▶ To prevent urinary tract infections, help your child to avoid constipation.

▶ Strong-smelling urine often means that it is concentrated, for example when your child goes to the toilet after waking up. Drinking fluids should make it more dilute and less strong-smelling.

▶ If your baby has fever and vomiting or your child has pain from voiding (dysuria), increased frequency, urgency, or blood in her urine, have her checked for a urinary tract infection.

❶ What Is a Urinary Tract Infection?

Urinary tract infections are quite common, especially among girls and young women. Foul-smelling urine might be the first sign of a urinary tract infection in babies. The urine may also appear cloudy or hazy. Other symptoms may include fever, vomiting, frequent and painful urination, back pain, and sometimes blood in the urine.

Urinary Frequency

If your child is passing frequent but small amounts of urine compared to her normal voiding pattern, you should suspect a bladder infection. Note that beverages that contain caffeine, a diuretic, also cause increased urination.

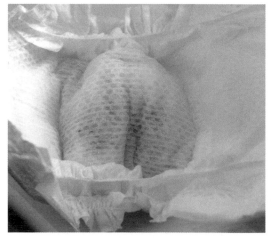

Urate crystals, signifying dehydration in a newborn baby

When should we contact our doctor?

If you suspect a urinary tract infection, then you need to seek medical attention. Symptoms may include:

• Fever, vomiting, back pain
• Frequent and/or painful urination
• Cloudy, hazy, or foul-smelling urine

➤➤ Urinary Tract Red Flags

In addition to the symptoms of infection mentioned, these other symptoms of concern require medical attention:

- If your child seems to be passing lots of urine (polyuria) and drinking more than usual (polydipsia), it may signify diabetes mellitus. Other symptoms of diabetes mellitus include weight loss and fatigue. Your doctor should take a urine sample and dip a testing stick in it to look for sugar. Under normal circumstances, sugar is not found in the urine.

- Any time blood in the urine is suspected, you should see your doctor right away. A urine sample should be tested for the presence of blood.

Burning or Painful Urination

Painful urination may be a sign of a urinary tract infection. In girls, it may also be due to nonspecific vulvovaginitis (see 409), which may be triggered by poor hygiene (common in young girls as they learn to use a toilet independently), irritants (for example, bubble bath), and tight, nonbreathable clothing.

Color of Urine

This table identifies some common color changes seen in urine and the possible underlying causes.

Color	Possible Causes
Pink/orange urine	Urate crystals are commonly seen in newborn babies as a pink/orange stain in the diaper. This is not blood; rather, it is due to the precipitation of urate crystals in the diaper. Apart from indicating dehydration, it is harmless. Make sure your baby is getting enough to drink.
Brown urine	Dark brown urine might be a sign of liver disease and can be due to bilirubin spilling into the urine. Normally, bilirubin is made in the liver and gets dumped into the gastrointestinal tract, giving the stool its usual brown color. Other accompanying signs to look for include yellow eyes (jaundice) and/or pale, clay-colored stools. See your doctor right away. See Jaundice (page 250).
Red/pink urine	The food your child eats (for example, beets) and certain medications can result in red/pink urine — not to be confused with blood in the urine. In other cases, blood may be present due to urinary tract infection, lower back trauma, or, rarely, a kidney stone. If you suspect blood in the urine, see your doctor.
Cola/tea-colored urine	This can also be due to blood, usually from inflammation in the kidneys, a condition known as glomerulonephritis. Your child may have had a sore throat or skin infection a couple of weeks earlier. She may also have a headache, pass smaller amounts of urine, and have a slightly puffy or swollen appearance, particularly around the eyes. See your doctor if your child has cola-colored urine.

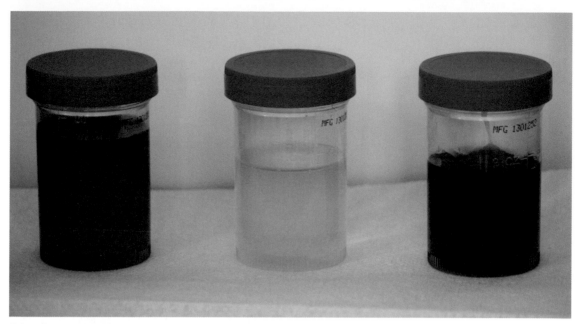

Color of urine: red/pink; normal; cola/tea-colored

Concentration

The kidneys have a natural ability to produce concentrated urine (dark urine) or dilute urine (light urine) depending on how much water your body needs. Certain foods and behaviors affect the concentration of the urine. Here is a list of factors:

- The amount of liquid your child drinks: if she drinks lots of water, her urine will be lighter.
- The outside temperature: her urine will be darker because of excessive sweating when it is very hot outside.
- Fever and illness: usually her urine will be darker due to less fluid intake and fluid loss from sweating.
- Time of day: her urine will be darker first thing in the morning after she hasn't had anything to drink all night long.

❷ How Are Urinary Tract Infections Treated?

Urinary tract infections are treated with a course of antibiotic therapy given by mouth. The type of antibiotic will usually depend on what bacterial germ grows in the culture of the urine sample provided by your child. Some of the common germs, for example E. coli, may be resistant to some of the commonly used antibiotics in children.

Did You Know?

Strong-Smelling
Occasionally, very concentrated urine is described as smelling "strong." Try giving your child a bit of extra fluids and see if the smell improves as the urine becomes less concentrated.

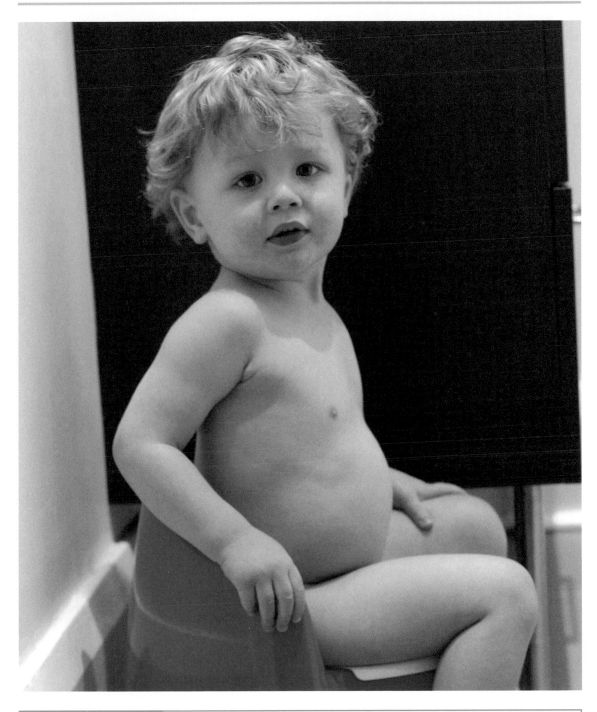

Doc Talk Constipation is one of the most common problems leading to urinary tract infections. The stool in the bowel prevents the bladder from emptying effectively, which means that some urine remains in the urinary system and is at increased risk of becoming infected. In children prone to urinary tract infections, it is really important to ensure that any constipation is effectively treated.

A B C D E F G H I J K L M N O P Q R S T U V W X Y Z

Vaginal Problems

What Can I Do?

▶ Don't let your child wear wet or damp bathing suits or underwear for prolonged periods of time.

▶ Teach your daughter simple hygiene measures (for example, wiping from front to back after using the toilet) that can help with both prevention and treatment of vulvovaginitis.

▶ If there is any vaginal bleeding in a prepubertal child, ensure that she is assessed promptly by your health-care provider.

Case Study

Catherine's Vulvovaginitis

Catherine is a 3-year-old who is healthy and active. She has been complaining for the last week that her "privates" are itchy, and her mom has noticed some redness in her vaginal area over the last couple of days. It is summertime and Catherine has been taking swimming lessons for the last 2 weeks. She also spends the afternoons in a bathing suit — running around the backyard with her brother, jumping through the sprinkler, and playing in the sandbox. Because it has been hot out and she is active, her mom has been giving her bubble baths every night before bed to keep her clean. When Catherine is seen by her doctor, he notices redness of the inner and outer labia of the vagina, with overlying small scratch marks. There is no discharge or foul odor. Catherine's doctor diagnosed her with vulvovaginitis and recommended that she limit time in her bathing suit by changing into loose cotton underwear immediately after swimming lessons. He also suggested eliminating bubble baths because they can be irritating and recommended Catherine have a barrier cream applied to her vaginal area several times daily until the area heals.

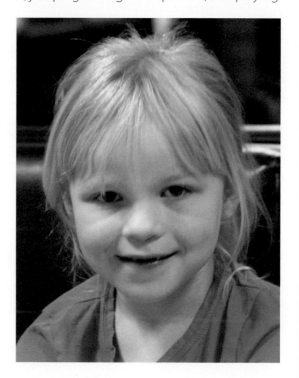

❶ What Is Vulvovaginitis?

Vulvovaginitis results from inflammation due to irritation or infection of the external genitalia. It is commonly seen in young girls prior to puberty. This occurs because girls at this age have low levels of estrogen. As a result, the lining of the vagina tends to be thin, relatively unprotected, and prone to irritation from feces and other irritants. This irritation can lead to burning, itching, redness, and pain when going to the washroom, and general discomfort in the genital area.

RELATED CONDITIONS

- Labial adhesions
- Vaginal bleeding
- Vulvovaginitis

When should we contact our doctor?

Consult your child's doctor if your child has burning, itching, redness, or general discomfort in the genital area that is not eliminated by the simple hygiene measures suggested on page 410.

⏩ Red Flags

Red flags that suggest this is something other than a simple irritant vulvovaginitis:

- Severe pain and/or redness are present, which suggests the presence of a bacterial infection that may require antibiotics. Your child's doctor may take swabs from the vaginal area to look for infection.
- Vaginal bleeding, which could have other possible causes. (See page 412.)
- Vaginal discharge, especially in prepubertal girls, which usually does not occur with simple irritant vulvovaginitis alone. Its presence often indicates inflammation of the vagina due to a bacterial infection or the presence of a foreign object.
- Vaginal itch with white "cottage cheese" discharge. Although yeast infections occur in very young infants, this infection is uncommon in older girls prior to puberty. Yeast generally attaches to genitalia exposed to more estrogen.
- Itchiness predominantly around the anus. This could suggest a parasitic infection, such as pinworms, which requires treatment with an oral anti-parasitic medication.

❷ What Causes Vulvovaginitis?

Anything that causes skin irritation can contribute to vulvovaginitis.

Suboptimal Hygiene

Most cases of vulvovaginitis are caused by suboptimal hygiene. Young girls who have only recently mastered going to the toilet independently are not the best of wipers, and bacteria from the anus or unwashed hands, or wearing dirty underwear, can cause irritation.

Chemical and Physical Irritation

Chemical irritation by scented or treated soaps and bubble baths can lead to vulvovaginitis. Physical irritation from clothing that rubs on this sensitive area and dampness can also contribute.

Bacteria

These are normally present in the child's throat, particularly streptococcus, and can be transferred to the vulva and produce inflammation or infection.

❸ How Is Vulvovaginitis Prevented and Treated?

Most vulvovaginitis cases resolve on their own with the implementation of simple good hygiene measures.

Do's and Don'ts

Do

- Encourage your child to wear loose-fitting cotton underwear. She may need to change her underwear a couple of times a day to stay clean.
- Apply a barrier cream (such as zinc oxide or petroleum jelly) several times daily until the area heals.
- Ensure your child is wiping from front to back when she goes to the washroom.
- Give your child a sitz bath for 10 minutes, 2 to 4 times daily, while area is inflamed.
- See your child's doctor if the itchiness is predominantly around the buttocks, rather than the vagina, or if there is foul-smelling discharge or bleeding.

Don't

- Let your child sit in soiled underwear for any period of time.
- Let her wear tight, synthetic underwear or tight-fitting pajama bottoms to bed.

- Let her wear a wet bathing suit after swimming. Remove wet clothing as soon as possible.
- Use soap or bubbles in baths, especially those with additives or scents. Assist your child in bathing daily, and thoroughly rinse genitalia in warm water.

How To: Prepare a Sitz Bath

- You can buy specialized sitz bathtubs that will fit over a toilet or chair.
- Your bathtub or a basin can act as a simple, cheap, and convenient place for a sitz bath.
- Use warm water and have your child sit in it for 10 to 15 minutes.
- The hips, buttocks, and vaginal area should be soaked in water.
- You can add ¼ cup (60 mL) of Epsom salts or 1 tsp (5 mL) of baking soda to the water. These can be soothing but are not essential.

❶ What Is Vaginal Bleeding?

Vaginal bleeding in an infant or child prior to the onset of puberty can certainly be alarming for a caregiver. The majority of cases are not serious, but most warrant prompt evaluation by a health-care provider. Your health-care provider will ask you questions to try to determine the cause of the bleeding and then examine your child. In some cases, you may learn that it isn't actually blood or that the bleeding is actually coming from elsewhere.

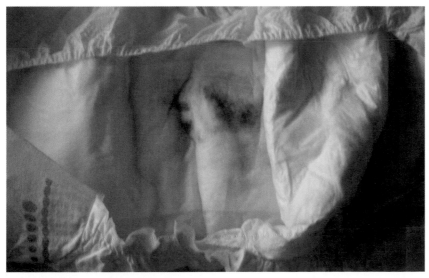

Diaper showing some vaginal bleeding

❷ What Causes Vaginal Bleeding and How Is It Treated?

Common Causes and Treatments of Vaginal Bleeding in Newborns
Neonatal Withdrawal Bleed

Newborn girls can have a "menstrual period" in the first week or two of life as a result of withdrawal of estrogen stimulation by their mothers. The bleeding may last a few days.

- **Suspect this condition if:** Your daughter is a newborn in the first week or two of life.
- **What to do:** No treatment needed.

Urate Crystals

Crystals from the urine can form in a diaper and look reddish, orange, or pink. These crystals are coming from the bladder, not the vagina, and can be confused with vaginal bleeding. They are often seen in the first few weeks of life, more commonly in infants who are dehydrated.

- **Suspect this condition if:** Your infant is within the first month of life.
- **What to do:** Urate crystals are not harmful. However, if your infant is breastfeeding and you suspect she may be dehydrated, have her evaluated by a health-care provider to ensure feeding is going well and that she is adequately hydrated. See Dehydration (page 150).

Common Causes and Treatments of Vaginal Bleeding in Children (Prepuberty)
Straddle Injury/Trauma

The genital area contains a lot of blood vessels, with little protection, and it can be easily injured, resulting in significant bleeding.

- **Suspect this condition if:** Your daughter has a history of a fall with injury to the vaginal area (for example, off a bicycle).
- **What to do:** All trauma to the genitals with bleeding should be evaluated promptly by a health-care practitioner to assess what treatment is needed.

Foreign Body

Young girls who have recently learned to use the toilet independently may accidentally leave small bits of toilet paper in their vagina. This can lead to irritation and bleeding. Some curious young children may insert toys or other objects into their vagina, leading to bleeding.

- **Suspect this condition if:** Your child has foul-smelling vaginal discharge. Your child has recently learned to use the toilet independently or has a tendency to hide or put objects where they don't belong!
- **What to do:** Your child should be assessed by a health-care practitioner so that any foreign body may be removed and the area cleaned.

Vulvovaginitis

The itching associated with vulvovaginitis can lead to small breaks in the skin, causing bleeding.

- **Suspect this condition if:** Your daughter has a red, itchy vaginal area.
- **What to do:** See the section on vulvovaginitis, on page 409.

Rectal Bleeding (Bleeding from the Bum)

Blood in the diaper or on the toilet paper may lead you to think that blood is coming from the vagina when it is actually coming from the rectum or anus. Most commonly, this is from an anal fissure. See Bloody Stools (page 90).

- **Suspect this condition if:** Your child has constipation and/or small cuts at the anal opening.
- **What to do:** Treat the underlying constipation. See Constipation (page 124). Apply petroleum jelly to the area for a few days so that the fissure can heal.

Urethral Prolapse

The urethra (the tube connecting the bladder to the outside of the body, where urine comes out) has an inner lining that may stick out at its opening. Exposure of this inner lining to clothing and soaps, for example, can cause irritation and bleeding.

- **Suspect this condition if:** Your daughter falls into one of these higher-risk groups: girls of Black and Hispanic ancestry between infancy and puberty, and girls with heavy coughing, constipation, or obesity (conditions that can increase pressure inside the belly).
- **What to do:** See your health-care provider, who will likely suggest giving sitz baths and may prescribe a hormonal estrogen cream to heal the urethra.

❶ What Are Labial Adhesions ?

Labial adhesions occur when the labia minora (the inner and thinner labia) become irritated and stick together. The inner labia can become stuck together in the midline. Sometimes, the adhesions are just at the front or back of the vaginal opening; other times, the adhesions can be virtually the entire length (front to back) of the vaginal opening. This can lead to difficulty having a normal, free-flowing stream of urine.

❷ What Causes Labial Adhesions?

Prior to puberty, a girl's external genitalia, or labia, are not exposed to very much estrogen. Because of this, they remain thin and more susceptible to irritation. As the irritation heals, the labia may fuse.

❸ How Are Labial Adhesions Treated?

Often, no specific treatment is needed beyond attention to hygiene, avoiding irritants, and regularly airing the area between diaper changes. If almost all of the labia minora are stuck together, if there are problems urinating, or if recurrent infections occur, your baby's doctor might prescribe a topical estrogen cream to be applied to the area of attachment. You will need to use a zinc barrier cream or petroleum jelly once separation occurs to prevent recurrences. The incidence of labial adhesions decreases at the onset of puberty, with the body's natural rise in estrogen levels.

Doc Talk Good hygiene measures are key for both prevention and treatment for most vaginal problems. As young girls strive for independence, especially when it comes to toileting and their personal hygiene, guiding and assisting your child with everyday hygiene remains important. Continue with this until she has fully mastered cleaning herself and understands the importance of these preventive measures.

Vomiting

What Can I Do?

▶ Rest assured that baby spit-up is normal as long as your child is gaining weight appropriately.

▶ Prevent dehydration. Offer small amounts of oral rehydration solution frequently.

▶ Seek emergency care if the vomit is dark green (bilious) or contains blood, or your child cannot keep anything down and you suspect dehydration.

❶ What Is Vomiting?

Vomiting is the forceful expulsion of the contents of the stomach. Vomiting should be distinguished from spitting up, or reflux, which is a normal, effortless regurgitation of stomach contents that occurs most often in infants in the first year of life, during and after feeding.

There are many reasons why your child might vomit. Some are not worrisome, while others require emergency medical attention.

Usually, vomiting occurs through the mouth, but sometimes it can come through the nose as well. Although this can alarm parents, it does not imply a more serious cause.

⯈⯈ Vomiting Red Flags

Seek immediate medical advice if your child shows any one of these red flag signs:

- Vomiting with blood (red or dark brown in color)
- Vomiting with bile (dark green in color)
- Projectile vomiting traveling up to 3 feet (1 m), particularly in the first 2 months of life
- Not keeping anything down for more than 6 hours
- Listless and not interested in feeding or interacting
- Dehydration with dry mouth, decreased urine output (not wetting diapers), or sunken eyes. See Dehydration (page 150).
- Severe headache, irritability, neck stiffness with the vomiting
- Severe headache with vomiting in the early morning
- Low back pain, urinary symptoms, or foul-smelling urine
- Severe abdominal pain

Color of Vomit

Health-care providers use the color of the vomit and associated features to help determine the cause of the problem and what steps need to be taken.

Color	Why Is It This Color?	What Does This Often Mean?
Curdled milk	Curdled milk suggests recently ingested milk, prior to digestion by the stomach juices. This is especially common in young infants.	• Reflux of stomach contents, known as gastroesophageal reflux
Yellow	Partially digested food that has been in the stomach for a while can take on a yellow, watery appearance as the stomach juices digest the food.	• Gastroenteritis (stomach flu) • Pyloric stenosis • Urinary tract infection
Green (bilious)	Presence of bile makes the vomit take on a dark green color. Bile is a digestive fluid that helps break down fats and is excreted into the intestines.	• With profuse or repeated vomiting from any cause, some bile can "reflux" into the stomach, causing green vomit. • Blockage of the bowels (intestinal obstruction) must also be considered. This can be seen, for example, when the bowel becomes twisted (volvulus) or when it telescopes into the adjacent segment (intussusception). See Abdominal Pain (Acute) (page 20).
Red, dark purple	If your child has just drunk red liquids, then it is more likely just the food color. Red vomit may also suggest the presence of fresh blood. Dark purple may suggest the presence of fresh blood that has clotted.	• The stomach lining may ooze tiny amounts of blood when inflamed or irritated from gastritis. • The esophagus may become inflamed from acid or trauma from gastroesophageal reflux with forceful vomiting.
Dark brown	Vomitus that resembles grounds of coffee suggests the presence of blood that has been in the stomach for a while.	• Breastfed babies can swallow blood while feeding if the mother's nipples are cracked or raw.

❷ What Causes Vomiting?

Overall, viral infections make up the most common cause of vomiting. Many infections tend to be associated with a fever, so its presence suggests some type of infection as the cause of the vomiting.

Viral Infections

Viruses involved in stomach flu can lead to vomiting. See Viral Gastroenteritis (page 209). Diarrhea, fever, abdominal pain, and cramping may result. Viral gastroenteritis is usually self-limited but contagious. Be sure your child stays well hydrated and washes frequently to reduce spread.

Other Causes to Consider

Gastroesophageal Reflux

In the first months of life, by far the most common cause of vomiting is gastroesophageal reflux (GER). This is a normal developmental process for many babies, caused by a somewhat inefficient valve between the esophagus and stomach. Babies' lax muscle tone and the tendency for most infants to lie flat after a feed also contribute to the problem. GER is the regurgitation of stomach contents and, provided that your baby continues to gain weight appropriately, appears comfortable, and has no fever, it would be appropriate to wait for this to gradually resolve. It usually does so by 9 to 12 months.

Pyloric Stenosis

If the vomit is projectile, traveling up to 3 feet (1 m), without bile, your baby may have an obstruction at the outlet of the stomach, a condition called pyloric stenosis. This condition classically occurs in first-born male infants from 2 weeks to 2 months of age. Vomiting tends to be progressive over a few days, gradually increasing to the point where every feed is vomited.

Bowel Obstruction

Any problem that results in obstruction of the bowel will usually produce vomiting. If the blockage occurs after the first part of the small intestine where bile empties into the gut, the vomit will be bile-stained, or bilious. For example, in rare occasions, the intestines can twist on themselves (volvulus) or telescope into the segment in front of it (intussuception), causing obstruction and bilious vomiting. See Abdominal Pain (Acute) (page 20).Intussusception causes an obstruction and affects the blood supply and nutrients to the piece of intestine being squeezed. This can result in a baby becoming pale and limp or cause bouts of severe abdominal spasms where she draws up her legs. Blood can sometimes be seen in the stool. Bowel obstructions are more common in children who have had bowel problems, especially those requiring surgery, which can result in scar tissue.

Did You Know?

Head Trauma
Commonly, children may vomit following a concussion from a head injury. Persistent or worsening vomiting following a blow to the head requires evaluation to rule out a bleed in the brain.

Causes of Vomiting

Possible Cause	Signs and Symptoms	Comments
Gastroenteritis (infection of the stomach and small and large intestines)	• Accompanied by low-grade fever • Poor appetite • May have diarrhea • Other family members and friends may have similar symptoms • Typically settles within 24–48 hours	• May lead to dehydration
Meningitis (infection of the lining of the brain)	• Accompanied by high fever • Headache, which in young infants may manifest as severe irritability • Neck stiffness • Extreme lethargy	• Any signs and symptoms of meningitis should prompt urgent medical attention, because, though rare, it can be life-threatening
Urinary tract infections (kidney or bladder)	• Frequent urination • Painful urination • Loss of bladder control • High fever • Foul-smelling urine	• May have a past history of kidney or bladder infections
Gastroesophageal reflux	• In the first year of life, especially first 6 months • Usually during or after a feed • Not forceful, more like regurgitation • Curdled milk	Seek attention if: • Not gaining weight or losing weight • Severe irritability and /or arching with feeds • Turning mouth away from feeds
Pyloric stenosis	• In the first few months of life • Projectile (i.e., the vomit travels at least a few feet forcefully) • Not bilious (dark green) in color • Progressively getting worse	• May lead to dehydration
Intussusception	• Bilious in color (dark green) • Severe abdominal spasms of pain with drawing up of legs • May be accompanied by blood/reddish color in the stool	• Requires urgent medical attention
Intracranial problem (for example, brain tumor)	• Severe headaches • Headaches in the morning • No associated fever or diarrhea	• Very rare • Other neurological problems are usually seen as well
Ear, throat, or chest infections (for example, whooping cough, pneumonia, and bronchiolitis)	• Vomiting from a forceful cough that tends to empty the stomach at the same time • Often mucus (phlegmy) • Tends to be in younger infants	Seek attention if: • Breathing difficulties (increased rate or effort of breathing)

Keeping Your Child Hydrated When Vomiting

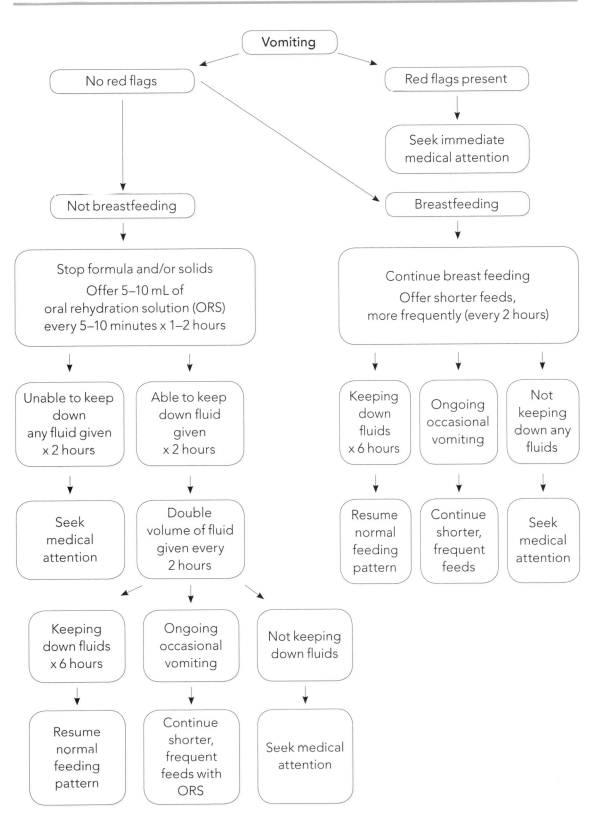

Neurological Causes

Children with conditions leading to a rise in the pressure inside the skull will often vomit. In fact, vomiting can be the first sign of such a problem. Vomiting, for example, can indicate the presence of a brain tumor. These, fortunately, are very uncommon and the child will usually also have severe headaches, particularly in the early morning.

❸ How Is Vomiting Treated?

Dehydration

Whatever the cause, persistent vomiting can lead to dehydration due to loss of fluids from the stomach. Dehydration will occur more rapidly in a child who has associated diarrhea and fever from excess water loss through the stool and skin. The younger the child, the more quickly he or she will become dehydrated.

Signs of Dehydration

- Decreased amount of urine in the diapers
- Dry tongue or mouth, without saliva
- Sunken eyes or soft spot (fontanelle)
- Decreased tears
- Listlessness or lack of interest in surroundings

Recurrence

If your child has only vomited once and appears well, continue normal care. Without any other symptoms (for example, fever and diarrhea), there is generally no cause for concern. If the vomiting recurs, you will need to determine the underlying cause and follow the guidelines outlined for treatment. Be alert to any red flags that may occur and require urgent treatment.

Doc Talk

For many years, doctors have not recommended any medicine for vomiting, because they were concerned that it could disguise the underlying problem and result in side effects, such as drowsiness. Parents have always been advised that they could give acetaminophen if necessary to treat the fever and/or the tummy cramps, providing your child can keep the medication down!

In recent years, there is increased evidence it may be beneficial to try a dose of anti-vomiting medication; for example, ondansetron (Zofran) for vomiting caused by viral gastroenteritis. This should only be done in consultation with your health-care provider.

Warts

What Can I Do?

▶ If your child has warts, discourage him from picking at them because this contributes to further spread.

▶ Try one of the wart treatments available from pharmacies without prescription and follow the instructions closely.

▶ Warts on the face or genitals, and those that are persistent or painful, should prompt a visit to your health-care provider.

❶ What Is a Wart?

Warts are flesh-colored, rough, bumpy growths of accumulated dead skin. They occur most commonly on the hands and feet. Warts are generally painless; however, when on the soles of the feet (plantar warts), they can be tender and uncomfortable.

❷ What Causes a Wart?

Warts are caused by viruses (human papillomavirus), which are not particularly contagious, though the virus often spreads from one location to another on the same child. Picking at warts and thumb-sucking contribute to this type of spread. Warts can also be spread by direct contact with various surfaces, such as towels and swimming pool decks, that have been contaminated by the virus.

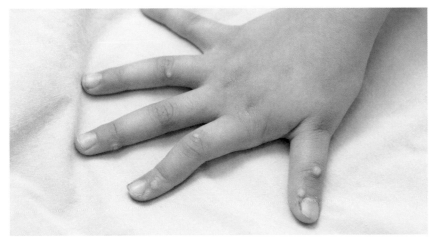

Multiple warts

When should we contact our doctor?

Most warts are painless and naturally disappear on their own over the course of several months to years. Several treatment options are available. In some cases, the wart is painful and will need medical attention.

▶▶ Wart Red Flags

Consult your child's doctor if your child has any of the following symptoms:

■ Warts that are persistent or painful

■ Warts that appear on the face or genitals

❸ How Is a Wart Treated?

Method	Comments
Wart-removing acids	Most preparations contain salicylic acid and are available without prescription. They can be purchased as a liquid, patch, or ointment. These should be applied once or twice daily and covered with adhesive tape to promote drying. The acid dries the wart tissue, which then turns white. You can use a razor blade or emery board to carefully shave down the dead wart tissue once or twice weekly.
Duct tape	Apply duct tape to the wart and change it once or twice weekly. This helps to dry and kill the wart tissue.
Liquid nitrogen	This is a painful option requiring multiple treatments and can only be done at a physician's office. It can be quite effective, but it is seldom used in younger children because of the associated discomfort.

Doc Talk   Genital warts are also caused by human papillomaviruses (HPV) and are contracted through sexual contact with an infected person. They are the most common sexually transmitted disease and certain strains can lead to cervical cancer in adulthood. While exceedingly rare in young children, vaccines against the HPV strains causing cervical cancer are recommended for young girls BEFORE they become sexually active.

Weakness

What Can I Do?

▶ Try to establish whether your child has true weakness, which requires investigation and treatment, versus general malaise, which often resolves spontaneously after an acute illness.

▶ Give your child acetaminophen or ibuprofen if you suspect the weakness is due to acute aches and pains. If it doesn't settle, then seek medical attention, especially if any red flags are present.

❶ What Is Weakness?

It is important to discriminate between generalized malaise (feeling "out of sorts") and true weakness. Feeling out of sorts is very common, especially when your child has a high fever from an illness, such as influenza. See Flu (page 207). With general malaise, your child may seem completely listless and spend lots of time sleeping. When the fever goes down, his activity level usually increases. This is not the same thing as true weakness.

When should we contact our doctor?

If you suspect your child has true weakness, he needs medical attention.

▶▶ Weakness Red Flags

Consult your child's doctor as soon as possible if your child has any of the following symptoms associated with weakness:

- Your child is unable to walk or climb stairs.
- He has other symptoms, such as numbness, tingling, seizures, or muscle pain.
- Your child has a depressed level of consciousness.
- He has an unsteady gait.
- He has delay in meeting his developmental milestones or regresses, with a loss of the ability to do things he was able to do before.
- His weakness is progressing from the legs and moving up toward the muscles of the upper body.

❷ What Are the Causes of Weakness?

True weakness is caused by a problem in the child's neurologic system somewhere along the pathway from the brain through the spinal cord and out the nerves that go to activate your muscles. This is relatively rare in children. When it does occur, it is more commonly due to viral infections that cause, for example, encephalitis (brain inflammation) or myositis (muscle inflammation). Strokes and brain tumors are exceedingly rare in children, but they, too, can present with weakness in the presence of other symptoms, such as seizures or progressively worsening headaches. There are also some genetic causes of muscle weakness, such as muscular dystrophy.

❸ How Is Weakness Treated?

The treatment for weakness is entirely dependent on the underlying cause. If you suspect your child has weakness or any red flags, consultation with your health-care provider is essential to initiate appropriate treatment.

> **Doc Talk**
>
> The majority of occurrences of feeling "weak" will actually be part of a general malaise associated with an intercurrent illness. This should get better quickly as the illness passes and may not be consistently present, improving with some acetaminophen or ibuprofen. If this is the case, then rest is likely the best treatment.

Wheezing

A
B
C
D
E
F
G
H
I
J
K
L
M
N
O
P
Q
R
S
T
U
V
W
X
Y
Z

What Can I Do?

▶ Seek medical attention for breathing that is rapid, if your child appears bluish around the lips, or if the muscles of the chest wall are being sucked in with each breath.

▶ If your child has recurrent wheezing, try to identify what the triggers are and avoid them.

▶ Do not expose your child to cigarette smoke.

Case Study

William's Wheeze

William is a 6-month-old infant who had been congested for a few days, but now his breathing sounds noisy. Since his older sister started daycare, it seems like everyone in the house constantly has a cold! William's parents have been coughing and have had sore throats over the last week, and his mother thought the baby had the same thing. But now she is worried because his breathing sounds different. She decided to make an appointment with their family doctor, who diagnosed William's symptoms as bronchiolitis with wheezing.

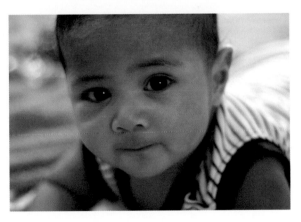

❶ What Is Wheezing?

Wheezing is a high-pitched whistling noise that is usually loudest when breathing out. It is caused by a narrowing of the breathing passages (bronchi and bronchioles) and increased mucus secretion in the lungs, causing obstruction of airflow. Think of the noise made by blowing out through a small or kinked straw. Wheezing is not the only cause of noisy breathing, and it can sometimes be difficult to differentiate wheezing from other causes of noisy breathing. Nasal congestion can cause very loud breathing, but the noise is lower-pitched and rumbling. Wheezing is best heard by listening over the chest rather than to noises that come from the nose and throat.

RELATED CONDITIONS

• Asthma
• Bronchiolitis

> ### When should we contact our doctor?
>
> If your child shows signs of breathing difficulty, you will need to seek medical attention. See the red flags below.

⯮ Wheezing Red Flags

Consult your child's doctor as soon as possible if your child has any of the following red flags associated with wheezing:

- Breathing appears to be fast.
- Chest muscles are sucked in with the increased effort to breathe.
- Your baby is not interested in feeding.
- Bluish color appears around the lips.

❷ What Causes Wheezing?

Common Causes
- Bronchiolitis/viral-induced wheezing
- Asthma

Less Common Causes
- Foreign body (food or object) stuck in an airway
- Fixed narrowing or compression of an airway
- Heart disease
- Gastroesophageal reflux
- Uncoordinated swallowing

Rare Causes
- Cystic fibrosis
- Inflammatory lung/immune problem

❸ How Is Wheezing Treated?

The mainstay of treatment is prevention of triggers that cause wheezing in your child. When wheezing is present, fast-acting, "reliever" medications such as salbutamol (Ventolin) can be administered to your child through inhalation, often with an aerochamber or a nebulizer. For children with recurrent wheezing, preventive medications such as daily inhaled steroids can help reduce the frequency of wheezing episodes. Occasionally, if wheezing is severe, oral or intravenous steroids may be administered to reduce inflammation in the lungs.

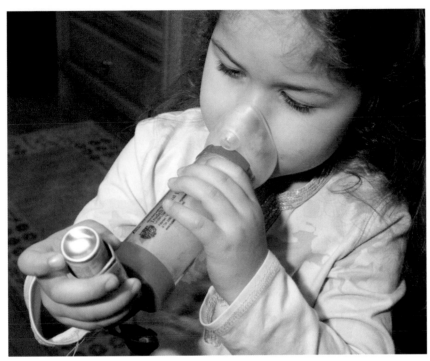

Child using an aerochamber with a metered-dose inhaler (puffer)

> **Did You Know?**
>
> **Aerochamber**
> There are a number of methods for delivering medications for wheezing. Which one your child uses will depend on her age and ability to use the device. All children using metered dose inhalers (traditional puffers) should do so with an aerochamber for optimal delivery of medication into their lungs.

❶ What Is Bronchiolitis?

Bronchiolitis

Bronchiolitis is one of the most common respiratory infections affecting young infants. It is caused by common viral infections that in adults or older children usually cause symptoms of a common cold but in young infants often affect their chest. A build-up of mucus and secretions develops in the small air passages in the lungs, leading to obstruction of airflow and wheezing. Most infants can manage at home while they recover on their own over a few days to a few weeks. Some will require hospitalization for monitoring and treatment. Although there is no medication that effectively treats the viruses that cause bronchiolitis, some infants with more severe symptoms may require oxygen treatment or the administration of fluids to prevent dehydration.

❶ What Is Asthma?

Asthma affects the small airways of the lungs and is diagnosed in as many as 1 in 10 children.

Symptoms and signs of asthma:

- Wheezing
- Coughing
- Chest tightness
- Shortness of breath

Children with asthma may cough for longer than expected after a common cold, have persistent coughing at night that interferes with sleep, or have a cough that develops with exercise. Some children will instinctively avoid exercise because they are aware that it might lead to asthma symptoms. The most common triggers of asthma in children are viral respiratory tract infections. Other triggers include allergies (such as to pets or environmental allergens) and exposure to smoke, cold air, and exercise.

❷ What Causes Asthma?

Inflammation causes swelling of the airways and an increased sensitivity of the airways causes them to constrict, or narrow, in response to triggers. Both these factors lead to narrow and hyperactive small air passages that make it difficult for air to move smoothly in and out of the lungs, as if you were trying to breathe through a straw. A combination of genetic factors (asthma tends to run in families) and triggers in the environment predispose a child to asthma. It is also more common in children with allergies (to foods or environmental triggers) and eczema.

❸ How Is Asthma Diagnosed?

In young children, repeated episodes of wheezing, persistent cough, or breathing difficulty in response to the common triggers suggest the possibility of underlying asthma. In between episodes, children usually appear completely normal. Sometimes, signs of chronic allergies (congestion and dark circles under the eyes) and eczema may be a clue that asthma is present. In severe cases of uncontrolled asthma, growth can be affected. In children who are older and coordinated enough to cooperate, lung function testing can be helpful in diagnosing asthma.

❹ How Is Asthma Treated?

Treatment of asthma involves both managing the symptoms and underlying inflammation and avoidance of any known triggers. Two types of medications are used: reliever medicines that act quickly to help when symptoms (wheeze, cough, shortness of breath) are present and anti-inflammatory medications that are used on a regular basis to prevent symptoms from occurring. Albuterol or salbutamol (Ventolin) are the common reliever medications and inhaled steroid medications are the most common and effective anti-inflammatory medication. It is important to avoid smoke and any known allergens. It is sometimes helpful for children to have allergy testing to learn about allergy triggers that might not be recognized. Some children tend to "outgrow" their asthma as they get older. For others, while asthma may be chronic, it can be effectively controlled with medication and education.

| **Doc Talk** | Wheezing is a common sign of asthma, but it does not necessarily indicate asthma. Bronchiolitis causes wheezing in infants in the first year of life, and infants who do develop bronchiolitis have a higher likelihood of recurrent but self-limited wheezing with cold viruses in the preschool years. Asthma is considered when repeated episodes of wheezing develop in response to cold viruses, allergens, exercise, or changes in the weather (that is, cold air or hot/humid and smoggy conditions). |

Resources

The amount of information available to parents is overwhelming and not always easy to evaluate. While the Internet has made access to health information easy, this access has come at the cost of parents needing to sift through loads of information to try to determine if the information comes from an authoritative source, or if it is even true. The fact remains: much of what is available on the Internet is based on very strongly held personal opinion and may not be based on good research or even make common sense. For a caregiver seeking advice about how to best care for a child when injury or illness strikes, having a reliable source of information from a professional organization or from official government sites is invaluable. While your child's health-care provider remains your best source of advice and counseling for your child, we hope that this book will be a good resource and starting point. For that purpose, we have provided a list of reliable and comprehensive international resources about child health.

Parenting Corner
America Academy of Pediatrics (AAP)
P.O. Box 927, Dept C
Elk Grove Village IL 60009-0927
Tel 847-434-4000
www.aap.org/parents.html
Authoritative information in an American context with links to other credible resources

Caring for Kids
Canadian Paediatric Society (CPS)
2305 St Laurent Boulevard
Ottawa, ON K1G 4J8
Tel 613-526-9387
www.caringforkids.cps.ca
Authoritative information in a Canadian context with links to other credible resources

National Institute of Child Health and Human Development
Bldg 31, Room 2A32
31 Center Drive
Bethesda, MD 20892-2425
www.nichd.nih.gov
Official site of the U.S. government office on children's health

Canadian Institute of Child Health
Suite 300, 384 Bank Street
Ottawa, ON K2P 1Y4
Tel 613-230-8838
www.cich.ca
An advocate for children's health in a Canadian context

About Kids Health
The Hospital for Sick Children
555 University Avenue
Toronto, ON M5G 1X8
www.aboutkidshealth.ca
Comprehensive source of practical guidelines for baby and child health

Motherisk
The Hospital for Sick Children
555 University Avenue
Toronto, ON M5G 1X8
Tel 416-813-6780 or 877-327-4636
www.motherisk.org
A reliable source of evidence-based information about exposure to drugs and chemicals during pregnancy and while breastfeeding

Child and Family Canada
www.cfc-efc.ca
A collective of more than 50 child health agencies

La Leche League International
1400 North Meacham Road
Schaumburg, IL 60173-4840
Tel 800-LA-LECHE
www.lalecheleague.org
Support for mothers who choose to breastfeed

National Advisory Committee on Immunizations (NACI), Public Health Agency of Canada
www.phac-aspc.gc.ca/naci-ccni
A source of information, official statements, and updates on vaccines used in Canada

United States Department of Agriculture
www.mypyramid.gov
The USDA's MyPyramid food guide

Food and Nutrition, Health Canada
www.hc-sc.gc.ca/fn-an/index-eng.php
A webpage called Food and Nutrition with links to Canada's Food Guide, information on labeling, and other resources.

Safe Kids Canada
http://www.safekidscanada.ca
A resource for current safety regulations and information.

American Academy of Sleep Medicine (AASM)
www.aasmnet.org
A source of accurate information on sleep and sleep disorders

American Dental Association
www.ada.org

Canadian Dental Association
www.cda-adc.ca

Acknowledgments

This book would not have been possible without the help of a number of individuals. We are sincerely thankful for the contributions, support, and advice of so many to make this a wonderful guidebook about child health for parents around the globe.

We would specifically like to thank:

Norm Saunders, who passed away too soon, before this book came to fruition. As a pediatrician, he continues to be the gold standard, a role model physician for all of us. This book would really not have been possible without the foundation he laid in his previous written work, his exemplary dedication to pediatrics and improving child health, and his enduring mentorship and guidance for how to approach any problem we face. As a great friend, colleague, and father, his integrity, courage, and wisdom continue to inspire us every day.

Our team of authors, Sherri Adams, Carolyn Beck, Stacey Bernstein, Zia Bismilla, Mark Feldman, Beth Gamulka, Sheila Jacobson, Irene Lara-Corrales, Elena Pope, Daniel Roth, and Michael Weinstein. Their expertise, dedication, and enthusiasm for writing and editing have been exceptional.

The terrific team at Robert Rose, Bob Hilderley, Bob Dees, Marian Jarkovich, and Kevin Cockburn at PageWave Graphics. They have been an amazing team to work with and have done an extraordinary job at making this book easy to read, attractive, and useful for every caregiver.

Our colleagues at SickKids, Denis Daneman, our pediatrician-in-chief, and Mary Jo Haddad, our CEO, for continually being supportive of our creative professional endeavors, for their leadership, and for their dedication to making the Hospital for Sick Children the most outstanding place to work. Thanks to Tiziana Altobelli for keeping us organized and enthusiastically going above and beyond the call of duty every day, and always with a smile.

Robert Teteruck and Diogenes Baena from Medical Photography at SickKids, who took many of the photographs in the book. Thanks, of course, to all of our models for so willingly allowing us to illustrate to our readers what we were trying to say in words.

And finally, thanks to our families, Lynn, Lyndsey, Bethany, and Megan, for their thoughts, insight, and helpful comments about the manuscript and for allowing this project to go forward. A special thanks to our spouses, Shelley and Justin, for their never-ending support and encouragement through the many, many hours of writing and assembling this book. And to all of our children, Sam, Danielle, Nathan, and Hailey, for making parenting an incredibly rewarding journey.

— *Dr. Jeremy Friedman*
— *Dr. Natasha Saunders*

Photo Credits

All photos by Robert Teteruck, Diogenes Baena and the Dermatology Clinic, © The Hospital for Sick Children, except: **page 2** © Gordon Soon; **5** © iStockphoto.com/Joe Potato Photo; **6** © iStockphoto.com/sjharmon; **36** © iStockphoto.com/Carlos Gawronski; **39** © Natasha Saunders; **42** (right) © iStockphoto.com/ArtAs; **46** © Natasha Saunders; **47** © Natasha Saunders; **52** © iStockphoto.com/ArtisticCaptures; **54** © iStockphoto.com/Richard Ellgen; **56** © Natasha Saunders; **61** © iStockphoto.com/cglade; **65** © iStockphoto.com/UrsaHoogle; **68** © iStockphoto.com/fatihhoca; **72** © iStockphoto.com/OJO_Images; **75** © iStockphoto.com/borchee; **78** © iStockphoto.com/biffspandex; **80** (middle) © Natasha Saunders; **85** © Natasha Saunders; **86** © iStockphoto.com/skynesher; **96** © Beverly Daniels Photography; **98** © iStockphoto.com/Soubrette, **102** © iStockphoto.com/Kalashnikov_O; **105** © iStockphoto.com/HKPNC; **107** © iStockphoto.com/slobo; **116** (top left) © shutterstock.com/andersphoto, (top right) © shutterstock.com/Glenn Price, (bottom right) shutterstock.com/R.Ashrafov, (bottom left) © shutterstock.com/eans; **122** © iStockphoto.com/rafalkrakow; **124** © Gordon Soon; **128** © shutterstock.com/Elena Blokhina; **136** © iStockphoto.com/Robert Mandel, **139** © shutterstock.com/Shahsuvar Asadov, **141** © iStockphoto.com/hidesy; **142** © iStockphoto.com/RuslanDashinsky; **146** © iStockphoto.com/JoannaZielinska; **147** (top left) © iStockphoto.com/perfectPhoto, (top right) © Natasha Saunders, (bottom right) © Natasha Saunders, (bottom left) © iStockphoto.com/michaeljung; **150** © Natasha Saunders; **154** © Natasha Saunders; **160** © iStockphoto.com/Gelpi; **163** © iStockphoto.com/RuslanDashinsky; **176** © Gordon Soon; **180** © iStockphoto.com/ArtAs; **186** © Alex McDonald; **196** © Natasha Saunders; **207** © iStockphoto.com/Renphoto; **212** © iStockphoto.com/Juanmonino; **214** © Natasha Saunders; **217** © Natasha Saunders; **221** © Gordon Soon; © iStockphoto.com/Maica; **230** © Gordon Soon; **234** © iStockphoto.com/princessdlaf; **235** © iStockphoto.com/debibishop; **238** (top) © Jeremy Friedman; **243** © iStockphoto.com/ArtisticCaptures; **246** © iStockphoto.com/eurobanks; **251** © Jeremy Friedman; **256** © iStockphoto.com/asiseeit; **264** © iStockphoto.com/MarsBars; **269** © iStockphoto.com/shutterbugger, **270** (top) © iStockphoto.com/KevinDyer, (middle) © iStockphoto.com/arlindo71, (bottom) © Jeremy Friedman; **276** © Natasha Saunders; **278** © iStockphoto.com/Blue_Cutler; **284** © Gordon Soon; **285** © iStockphoto.com/MelissaAnneGalleries; **288** © iStockphoto.com/princessdlaf; **297** © Natasha Saunders; © iStockphoto.com/Kevin Landwer-Johan; **306** © iStockphoto.com/digitalskillet; **310** (left) © Alex McDonald; **312** © iStockphoto.com/John Neff; **326** © iStockphoto.com/NI QIN; **332** © David Sheffe; **337** © iStockphoto.com/aabejon; **349** © iStockphoto.com/Shelly Perry; **352** © iStockphoto.com/ArtisticCaptures; **364** © iStockphoto.com/loooby; **366** © iStockphoto.com/AlexMotrenko; **370** © iStockphoto.com/Marina_Di; **371** © iStockphoto.com/Dejan Ristovski; **372** © Natasha Saunders; **374** © Natasha Saunders; **381** © iStockphoto.com/Renphoto; **382** © iStockphoto.com/blendcreations; **389** © Benjamin Kennedy; **390** © iStockphoto.com/Rich Legg; **394** © David Singer; **396** © Natasha Saunders; **397** © David Singer; **399** © Natasha Saunders; **401** © (top left) Alex McDonald, (top right) Alex McDonald; **402** © iStockphoto.com/Monique Heydenrych; **404** © Natasha Saunders; **406** © Natasha Saunders; **407** © Natasha Saunders; **408** © Natasha Saunders; **411** © Natasha Saunders; **425** © iStockphoto.com/susaro.

Every effort has been made to contact and obtain permission for the photographs in this book. If omissions and errors have occurred, we encourage you to contact the publisher.

Library and Archives Canada Cataloguing in Publication

Friedman, Jeremy, author
      The A to Z of children's health: a parent's guide from birth to 10 years / Dr. Jeremy Friedman, MB, ChB, FRCPC, FAAP;
Dr. Natasha Saunders, MD, MSc, FRCPC; with Dr. Norman Saunders, MD, FRCPC.

Includes index.
ISBN 978-0-7788-0460-4 (pbk.)

1. Pediatrics—Popular works.
I. Saunders, Norman, author II. Saunders, Natasha, 1979-, author III. Title.

RJ61.F747 2013   618.92   C2013-903353-X

Index

G

H